Finding the Fountain of Youth

Finding the Fountain of Youth

THE SCIENCE AND CONTROVERSY BEHIND EXTENDING LIFE AND CHEATING DEATH

Aharon W. Zorea

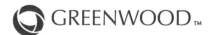

GREENWOOD™

An Imprint of ABC-CLIO, LLC

Santa Barbara, California • Denver, Colorado

Library of Congress Cataloging-in-Publication Data

Names: Zorea, Aharon W., author.
Title: Finding the fountain of youth : the science and controversy behind
    extending life and cheating death / Aharon W. Zorea.
Description: Santa Barbara, California : Greenwood, an imprint of ABC-CLIO,
    LLC, [2017] | Includes bibliographical references and index.
Identifiers: LCCN 2016051907 | ISBN 9781440837982 (hardcopy : alk. paper) |
    ISBN 9781440837999 (eBook)
Subjects: | MESH: Longevity | Life Expectancy | Aging—psychology |
    Aging—physiology | Health Knowledge, Attitudes, Practice
Classification: LCC QP85 | NLM WT 116 | DDC 612.6/8—dc23
LC record available at https://lccn.loc.gov/2016051907

ISBN: 978-1-4408-3798-2
EISBN: 978-1-4408-3799-9

21 20 19 18 17   1 2 3 4 5

This book is also available as an eBook.

Greenwood
An Imprint of ABC-CLIO, LLC

ABC-CLIO, LLC
130 Cremona Drive, P.O. Box 1911
Santa Barbara, California 93116-1911
www.abc-clio.com

This book is printed on acid-free paper ∞

Manufactured in the United States of America

To Emily, my own personal fountain of youth

Contents

Acknowledgments

The idea for this book was initially inspired by two people—one directly and one indirectly. The first was my wife of 17 years, Debbi Anne. She was diagnosed with breast cancer at the age of 38, and after a courageous battle and an untold number of treatments, she eventually left this world at the tender age of 45. Within days of her passing, Deb's grandmother Bernice Sander died at the age of 101. My wife was always in good physical condition and healthy, and yet she succumbed to cancer at a young age. She came from a family of long-lived individuals—several dying at age 100 or later. Yet, her father, Gilbert Sander, also died of cancer at the age of 54. His mother, Bernice, died at 101.

The seeming randomness of the ages of mortality was striking, and I knew I had to write something about the science and philosophy related to the end of life. I spoke with my editor, Maxine Taylor, and she suggested a discussion of the anti-aging movement. It was perfect and exactly what I had been looking for, and this book is the result. I would like to thank Maxine and the memories of my wife, Deb, and Grandma Sander for leading me on this path.

The prospect of antiaging and the modern quest for a scientific fountain of youth popped in and out of the narrative during my research for *Steroids* in 2014, but I was never directly involved with the movement. To jumpstart my research, I began with a series of public forums and open requests for "thoughts on aging and getting old" on social media. My goal was to gain a broad overview of the types of issues that most people thought about related to aging and dying. The response was overwhelming. I heard from family, friends, and complete strangers from all over the world. I expected to hear from older adults, but what I found was that most respondents were relatively young. It seems a large percentage of younger adults are clearly thinking about getting older and the prospects of moving beyond their youth. The idea of discovering a fountain of youth and somehow evading old age and death knows no age barriers.

These opening forums were extremely helpful, and it is impossible to thank everyone who participated in them. There were some individuals who were especially helpful, and I would like to thank Nikki Wentworth Allbaugh, Dawn Rafferty Bloechl, Eric Cairns, Amy Davis Clark, Kathleeen Corey-Pittman, Chris Drea, Angela Flemming, Karen Fowell, Patrick Hagen, Mary Hanrahan, Bethany Helmich, Barbi Hillesheim, Mara Ibra, Jane Sizer Jacobs, Jennifer Ann Johnsrud, Bushra Khan, DeAnna Kratochwill-Nitka, Candace McGrath, Shane Mitchell, Kim Mindham, Beth Ann Morgan-Aiken, Henk Newenhouse, Sharon Peralta, Thomas

Peralta, Karin Elizabeth Pettinger, Ashley Polcyn, Robert Rynes, Lora Schultz, Andrew Sharp, Evgeny Sklyarsky, Shell Smith, Paula de Vegh, Yvonne Venturelli, Linda Wahl, Lisa Lowrie Wanless, Clifton Wickstrom, Joy Gail Williams, Laurent Wouters, Brian Yam, Sharon F. Zales, and Rivka Zorea.

In addition, many of my professional colleagues provided helpful insights, including Dennis Carpenter (psychology), Tim Dunn (philosophy), Brandon Fetterly (chemistry), Jennifer Gavinsky (biology), Colleen Halverson (English), and Jessica Laeseke (UW Extension). Other invaluable staff members include the dedicated library staff at UW-Richland, who helped me process more than 900 sources, especially Director Todd Roll, his assistant Le Suong Cina, and Krisann Holthaus, Karin Tepley, Eric Hoffman, Allen Fortney, Jennifer Tagliapietra, and Kayla Schultz.

I would also like to thank all my contributors: Nicholas Agar, Bishop Robert Morlino, Dale Murray, S. Jay Olshansky, Jill Rinzel, and Zoltan Istvan, especially those with whom I had longer conversations with, including Rabbi Tuvia Bolton, Amer Haleem, Gregory Johnson, Louis Kinsley, Jeff Kleiman, João Pedro de Magalhães, as well as Nate Simmons (on behalf of Bishop Morlino). In addition, there were numerous experts in the field who did not contribute, and yet who still provided helpful encouragement, especially Nick Bostrum (University of Oxford), Bruce Carnes (University of Oklahoma), Eric Claeys (George Mason University), Donald Critchlow (Arizona State University), Muriel Gillick (Harvard Medical School), Leon Kass (American Enterprise Institute), Dawn Kiefer (editor of the *Richland Observer*), Adam Lee (Daylight Atheism), and Frederica Mathewes-Green.

Numerous local physicians provided insight during various stages of the research process, including Andrew Wright (Richland Medical Center), James Dickman III (Richland Medical Center), and James Dickman II (Krohn Clinic, Black River Falls). I would also like to thank Michael Kloess (Our Lady of Hope Clinic in Madison) and Jodeen Hosmanek, and Moshe Zorea for reviewing the final manuscript and to give a very special thanks to Dorothy Thompson, who provided helpful insight at every stage of the research and writing process.

My family and friends have been wonderful and encouraging throughout this project. I would like to say special thanks to my colleagues and neighbors Faye Peng and Stephanie Kernik for their patience and a special thank you to my friend Madison Vande Hey for keeping me on task and on schedule. My wife and boys (Jacob and Jonah) have been both generous and tolerant of the many hours spent researching and writing. They provide the only real temptation for my ever wanting to remain young.

Introduction

Who wants to live forever? It might seem that we all want to live forever—at least, we all want to look forever young, be attractive, act vibrantly, and live with the strength, excitement, and sexual virility of youth, provided we also have the resources to support such a lifestyle. Finding the fountain of youth is a little like winning the lottery: it seems to promise solutions for long-standing problems in our lives. If there were only enough money, if we could only cure this disease or that illness, and if we could somehow stop the course of aging, then the problems of human life would perhaps vanish.

Yet, we also know that such promises are probably not true. We may dream of winning the lottery, but there are too many stories of lottery winners blowing through their money in only a few years and falling more in debt than they were before winning. We also know stories of wealthy heirs who seem to live lives of self-destruction, continually addicted to something because their wealth provides little incentive for learning how to struggle, persevere, and live a meaningful life. In the same way that we know money cannot buy happiness, we also suspect that the fountain of youth would not guarantee happiness either, and may, in fact, only come at a price that we may be unwilling to pay.

We may know all these things, but we still buy the lottery ticket and we still search for scientific solutions to hide or evade our age. The American antiaging market, which includes cosmetics and supplements, was more than $40 billion in 2016, and related health and exercise markets were the same. These figures do not include the billions spent by advertising firms and entertainment media outlets that use images of youth and beauty to sell products, storylines, and ideas to an eager public. The modern antiaging movement thrives in the 21st century because many consumers yearn to defy their age, to retain their youth, and to permanently postpone the pains of disease and death.

This book is about the journeys in science, technology, and moral values that have made the possibility of finding immortality on this earth believable. In premodern times, the quest for eternal youth was limited to myths, magic, and superstition. Yet, around 500 years ago, the scientific revolution opened new pathways by which these dreams might someday become reality. For many centuries, science, faith, and philosophy easily intermixed into a growing antiaging movement that believed longer lives were possible and that God supported the prospect. After the shift in secular philosophy during the 19th century, that same antiaging movement believed that extended life spans were inevitable, but it also suddenly concluded that God's view of it was irrelevant. By the 20th century, science and faith had grown into philosophical competitors, and faith in human ingenuity seemed at odds with the older faith in divine order. As modern culture became more secular, the antiaging movement grew stronger and had a more intense sense of urgency to discover any solution for age-related conditions and diseases and to generally extend the human life span. In the 21st century, there is a very sincere belief in some quarters that youth can be maintained and preserved and that death can be delayed or even evaded altogether.

Finding the fountain of youth is not about a physical journey; it is an intellectual and emotional journey of faith. The dream of human immortality remains as it was in ancient times, but our hope in mankind's ability to solve almost any problem has increased exponentially. The idea of living extremely long lives without disease is no longer limited to fantasy and mythology. A sizable portion of our modern culture believes we have found the fountain of youth through scientific ingenuity. Just as our cell phones, computer chips, social media, and audiovisual technologies seem to be improving so rapidly that we may soon reach a point of total immersion, so too we believe that biochemical researchers are making revolutionary strides in medicine and health. The promise of a scientific fountain of youth seems nearly within our grasp.

THE MANY FACES OF ANTIAGING AND THE FOUNTAIN OF YOUTH

Who leads this modern search for the fountain of youth? In the 21st century, the antiaging movement is a cultural phenomenon that transcends any single set of principles or guidelines. No single voice or personality can claim unique access to the fountain of youth; instead, a variety of interests have independently aligned to gradually and consistently move the priorities of antiaging forward with increasing speed. Each group is motivated by its own agenda, but common desires bring them together to create a cultural consensus. The diverse motivations mean that individual interests are often not consistent and are occasionally at cross purposes with each other. Nevertheless, the antiaging movement reflects a dominant priority in modern culture.

Some of the earliest vanguards of the antiaging movement were leading researchers in biochemistry, evolutionary biologists, and geneticists. Gerontologists study the process of aging and are especially drawn to potential solutions for age-related conditions and diseases. Not all gerontologists support the antiaging movement, but most of the clinical research conducted on the subject has been led by scientists who study aging. Some are biologists who study the life spans of various organisms to find comparative characteristics in humans. Some are geneticists who are trying to identify the chemical sequences in a variety of different genomes so as to isolate the genes related to aging, repair, and regeneration. Academic researchers were the first to give legitimacy to the idea of scientifically delaying, halting, or even reversing the aging process. Prior to the advent of modern biochemistry, the pursuit of the fountain of youth was more philosophical than practical—few serious observers paid it much attention. Now, in the modern era, antiaging researchers receive ample recognition, legitimacy, and respectability from the wider public.

Legitimacy and public support mean more public and private funding. Scientists continue to lead the way in antiaging research, and it is from their work that the antiaging movement grows and develops.

In addition to academic researchers in white lab coats, there is a broad movement among amateur enthusiasts who write about, talk about, and generally support and pay for the ideals of the antiaging movement in social media on the Internet and through magazines and periodicals. The popular antiaging movement may include some academics, but it is usually led by people with strong communication skills who convey an excited vision of future potential. They form chat groups to pass along the latest news on supplements, diet and exercise routines, and exciting new technologies that may counteract the effects of aging. This group of enthusiasts support antiaging research, but they do not always require hard data or clinical evidence to guide their excitement. Often described as "futurists," it is the very prospect of humanity's potential for overcoming long-standing obstacles that most drives their enthusiasm.

Beginning in the 1970s and really blooming in the 1990s, the amateur antiaging movement attracted the attention of popular mainstream media. As the public demands, so too the market provides. Some of the most powerful driving forces in the antiaging community are the businesses and retailers who advertise and sell products that promise to maintain youthful beauty, athletic vitality, and sexual attractiveness. These may include large cosmetics and drug manufacturers, but just as often, they involve smaller companies that market supplements, diet and exercise plans, and specialized technologies to maximize health and longevity. These manufacturers are often only indirectly related to the academic researchers, but they are directly tied to the amateur enthusiasts who are their largest consumer base. For this reason, there is considerable tension between the scientists who study the precise biochemical process of aging, the marketing firms who make sensational claims of miraculous results, and the enthusiasts who target both sides as critical allies.

Meanwhile, as the scientists face off against the businessmen and the enthusiasts attempt to cling to both sides, there is a larger and more socially potent side of the antiaging movement that slowly pushes everything forward. The cultural icons of the entertainment and media industry all promote ideals of youth and beauty and sex, which constantly stimulate research, the marketplace, and popular enthusiasm. Hollywood sets the standards of fashion and "coolness" that the rest of the culture aspires to. In the early 21st century, these standards are heavily drawn from the examples set down by the Baby Boomer generation, but they are continually augmented by each successive generation (Gen X and Millennials), who are working to achieve the power and prestige of their predecessors. As the older generations age, they become the most ardent advocates and role models for practical antiaging solutions: diet, exercise, facelifts, reconstructive surgery, Botox injections, steroids, and human growth hormone. Each of these is used heavily by those who must always look beautiful on screen or on a magazine cover. The gossip columns all talk about it, and the public knows about it. As a result, the artificial pursuit of antiaging has become an accepted part of modern culture. The public is drawn to the culturally established standards, and the antiaging movement provides potential solutions for achieving them.

Finally, the antiaging movement in the 21st century ultimately owes its support and growth to the common lay consumer who often knows nothing of its existence. The man or woman on the street who buys the latest antiaging skin cream or herbal supplement does not know the history of the movement or even of the idea of prolonging life. They buy the product because it is part of their local cultural priorities: they want to look handsome or pretty, and they want to fit in with the expectations of their friends. Names like Ray Kurzweil and Aubrey de Grey mean nothing to them, and the historic ideas of progress, vitalism, and transhumanism mean even less. Yet, these consumers support the marketplace, which reinforces the trends of cultural icons, which magnifies the enthusiasm of movement insiders, which ultimately empowers the scientists to pursue further research. The antiaging movement is felt in almost every aspect of modern society because fundamental priorities have largely been accepted and embraced by the general public.

THE SKEPTICS

Images of youth, beauty, and sex appear almost everywhere. If modern culture is mesmerized by the antiaging movement, who could oppose it? The historic truth is that the antiaging movement has always had its share of staunch opponents that are not always the same groups and not always for the same reasons. Up until the 21st century, it would be safe to say that the critics of the movement largely outweighed its supporters. It is only recently that popular culture fell under the influence of an antiaging ideology, and only because its primary opposition suffered a corresponding decline in cultural influence.

From its start in the 15th century, the Western antiaging movement and its goals of extending the human life span had little to do with cosmetic appeal and the sexiness of youthful beauty. The goal of living extremely long and active lives was tied more strongly to vocation and the fulfillment of God's will on earth. Most of the very early antiaging researchers were clergy, and the Church was generally supportive of scientific innovations that improved the conditions of health and well-being. Yet, to be fair, the primary goal of this early stage of the movement was less about radically extending the human life span and more about making the most out of the gifts that God had already bestowed on the world. For hundreds of years, the primary critics of the growing antiaging movement simply believed that it could not be successful and was doomed to failure. These were not necessarily leaders of the Church; they were more often competing intellectuals who disagreed on one or more scientific points.

The general disbelief in mankind's ability to overcome the natural limits imposed by nature most often came from scientists themselves. This remains true even in the 21st century. Though the bulk of antiaging research is conducted by gerontologists in biochemistry, evolutionary biology, and genetics, it is not true that the majority of gerontologists support the antiaging movement. A very large consensus, especially among practicing physicians who specialize in geriatrics, simply do not believe that the human life span is changeable. If cures were found for all the current age-related diseases, they would expect a new wave of hitherto unrecognized diseases to rise up and take their place. Most gerontologists believe that the conditions of old age can be improved, but they do not believe that the gradual decline and loss of vitality that follows aging will ever be slowed or reversed. This sort of opposition is not based as much on faith as it is on the experience of practical application. Those who work with the elderly, the infirm, and the dying do not readily believe that these conditions will be cured.

Another sort of opposition is quite confident in the scientific potential to resolve aging and to continually extend the human life span. It is not the futility but the success of the antiaging movement that leads to their concern. The environmental movement often voices fears about how increasing life spans might add to overpopulation problems and potentially offset the ecological balance. Political voices from both sides of the aisle often raise the specter of an ever-increasing aging population to justify their plans for taxation, social services, and health care. Economists debate the eventual impact of higher retirement ages on the dynamic pressures of job growth, job training, and new job creation. In all these cases, though, the concern is less about the guiding principles of the antiaging movement and more about particular implications that may arise as a result of its success. These sorts of opposition rise and fall with the development of particular technical solutions.

There is, however, another category of opposition that is more fundamental in nature and based primarily on differences of faith. In the early periods, as long as the antiaging movement presumed God's ultimate sovereignty over life and the overall course of human events, there was no inherent opposition from religious believers. During the 19th century, however, the antiaging movement assumed a new direction that stripped science and biology from any connection to God and divine purpose. Charles Darwin and Thomas Huxley were extremely influential in pushing a view of science that was detached not only from the need for divine agency but also from any moral or religious explanation or justification. By the start of the 20th century, the antiaging movement had developed into a new belief that humans were ultimately responsible for the direction of evolution. As such, all the traditional presumptions about death and disease as natural conditions of life were questioned and, in many cases, cast aside by new theories that believed anything was possible through careful scientific planning. If death was merely a by-product of evolution and mankind could exert control over the course of evolution, then new scientific research might overcome death itself. In terms of philosophy, the antiaging movement toppled the sovereign position of God over creation and substituted humanity in his stead.

Beginning in the mid-19th century, but especially during the 20th century, the strongest source of opposition to the antiaging movement came from religious believers. Not only do they believe that scientific research goals are futile (because God, and not man, is ultimately responsible for the sufficiency of life), but they also believe that the priorities of eternal youth and radical life extension are in themselves contrary to faith and morals. The pursuit of a practical fountain of youth—regardless of whether it is ever successful—can become immoral when it places too much emphasis on material standards of beauty as a basis of happiness and success and too little emphasis on immaterial standards of virtue and character. Perhaps more explicitly, the dream of living eternally on earth runs counter to the dream of living eternally in heaven. This subtle opposition of faith served as the greatest obstacle to the ascendency of the antiaging movement. As modern society became more secular and began to lose its traditional presumptions of faith, the antiaging movement assumed a more dominant cultural position.

Though religious opposition remains the strongest source of criticism of the values and priorities of the antiaging movement, they are not alone. Other nonreligious philosophical positions also question the value of continually pursuing ideals of youth and beauty that are difficult to achieve and impossible to maintain. Mostly, the nonreligious opposition to antiaging comes in the form of general anti-industrialism or from countercultural opposition. Those who oppose capitalism and its emphasis on a consumer society are usually equally opposed to the artificial standards of youth and beauty that are arbitrarily set in place by marketing and advertising campaigns. Similarly, there is a growing antiageism political movement within the community of retired persons who resent the marginalization of those older adults who no longer fit the popular stereotypes of healthy, active, strong, and relevant or socially meaningful lives. In both instances, opposition to the antiaging movement stems from the related cultural pressures that seem to exclude all those other definitions of happiness and success that are not related to age and physical appearance.

For most of the history of Western civilization, opponents of the antiaging movement held the day. Even in ancient times, the various legends of magical fountains of youth were always told as morality tales, warning listeners about the dangers of envy and of the futile brooding for lives free from pain and struggle. Though old age and death were rarely heralded as positive qualities in life, they were nonetheless recognized as unavoidable realities. Wishing their end would not make it so, and such desires might lead one to forget and ignore the gifts that are ever present. It is from the modern world of science and technology that the inevitability of death and disease found their challengers. Yet, the very long tradition of skepticism remained strong. It is only in the 21st century that such skepticism began to waiver.

THE LAYOUT OF THE BOOK

This book is divided into three major sections. The first section is arranged chronologically and tells the story of when, where, and how the idea of a magical fountain of youth entered into the mythology of human civilization. The universal desire to somehow evade death is seen in widely diverse cultures around the world, yet only a few places came to believe such desires were practically obtainable. Chapters 1 and 2 trace the origins and spread of the myths, while chapters 3, 4, and 5 explain how those ideas found their way into Europe and eventually evolved into a modern antiaging movement. The history of the pursuit of eternal youth and immortality tells a great deal about the moral and ideological struggles that continue to confront the movement today.

The second section shifts from scientific history to scientific practice. Moving from a chronological to a topical narrative, the chapters are organized according to key questions that help define the various approaches to antiaging. Each chapter may be read independently, which means that they may be read in any order without fear of losing general continuity. Chapters 6 and 7 discuss preliminary definitions of life and death, while chapters 8 and 9 provide an overview of current methods for looking and feeling youthful—regardless of whether they result in an extended life span. The last three chapters (10, 11, and 12) discuss the most current approaches to treating age-related conditions and diseases and to avoiding both. The most popular products and recommendations of the antiaging movement for healthier and longer life spans are discussed with current research. The overall effectiveness of any particular suggestion is open for debate.

The third and final section provides an anthology of essays on the antiaging movement by experts in a wide variety of fields. These experts were chosen not so much because they are leading voices in the movement (though some of them are) but because they are experts in their particular fields. Each essay answers a question related to how the world might change if the antiaging movement is successful. The first question begins with an expert in genetics and comparative biology who answers the basic question of whether or not aging can ever be "cured." This same question is tackled by a sociologist who is an expert in biodemography. After this, the humanists and social scientists weigh in. A psychologist and a visual artist consider the cultural implications of a culture where extended youthfulness is more common than old age. A historian considers the sociopolitical implications of extended life spans based on literary discussions of the past. Two philosophers examine the potential impact of extremely long life spans on ethical reasoning and individual decision making. Finally, the last question brings the collective viewpoints of six different religious leaders on how the antiaging movement would affect faith. These experts include a Catholic bishop, a Protestant minister from the Church of Scotland, a Chasidic Rabbi from a yeshiva in Israel, an Islamic scholar, an agnostic academic, and an atheist, transhumanist presidential candidate.

The antiaging movement is interdisciplinary by nature because it is felt in almost every aspect of modern society. From these origins, *Finding the Fountain of Youth* reflects the broad spectrum of views. Much of the story is told from the perspective of those struggling to promote the idea of technological and biomedical progress. At the same time, the voices of those who resist or resent that sort of progress are ever present. Many of the leading figures in the modern antiaging movement are still alive, and their recommendations are easily found in their published books and articles—so too are their critics. This book does not intend to promote or oppose any particular recommendation, plan, visionary outlook for the future. It simply tells a story of a long, growing movement that has become dominant in contemporary culture.

SECTION ONE

The History of Antiaging from Myth to Modern Science: A Chronological History of an Idea

The fountain of youth is more than a mythical legend; it is an idea of hope that can be traced throughout most of human history from all parts of the globe. Originating more than 5,000 years ago, this idea evolved into a popular fable used to teach important lessons about the necessity of disease, aging, and death. Later versions evolved into a scientific possibility, inspiring hope that immortality might be possible given enough hard work and human intelligence. The modern antiaging movement owes its origin to ideas that began millennia ago.

This section tells the story of how the idea of a fountain of youth moved from mythology to science. The myth of a magical source of life spread around the world into regions mostly untouched by direct contact with the Middle East and Europe. After 2,000 years, they found their way into the Far East, where they were no longer treated as myths alone. During classical China, the prospect of attaining immortality on earth became a practical and pragmatic goal. While Europe and the West continued to view the fountain of youth as nothing more than a fable, Taoist alchemists pursued radical life extension in China as a scientific priority for almost a thousand years. It was not until the expansion of Arab traders into the Middle East that the pragmatism of Chinese alchemy found its way into Europe—albeit in a different form. By the start of the modern era, Europe had begun viewing the fountain of youth differently. It remained a myth in literature, but it became a practical goal in terms of science. Beginning around the 15th and 16th centuries, Western intellectuals seriously explored the possibility of extending the natural human life span through the new scientific method.

The next five chapters are generally arranged chronologically, with some broad regional emphasis. The first two chapters tell the story of how myths were transformed into scientific goals. Chapter 1 discusses the origins of the fountain of youth as it is found in mythology around the world, dating from around 2500 BCE in ancient Mesopotamia to the early 1500s CE among the North American Indians. Chapter 2 tells of the journey of religious-scientific practices in China that passed through the Middle East and finally became seeds of modern scientific research in Europe. Stories of practical immortality cross both time and distance, and in the process, a new pseudoscience of alchemy entered the West and prepared the way for modern chemistry.

The next two chapters tell of the birth of the modern secular antiaging movement in the West. Chapter 3 discusses how the ideal of a prolonged life span emerged during the scientific revolution to become the basis for the modern antiaging movement. It begins with the religious goal of maximizing God's gifts on earth and ends with the secular goal of maximizing life on earth without God. Chapter 4 follows the same story into the 20th century. Evolution and the revolution of secular science propelled the modern antiaging movement as a practical idea worthy of serious study. The last chapter tells how baby boomers took ownership of the antiaging movement, legitimized its research, and eventually dedicated both private and public research funds. In the 21st century, the fountain of youth is no longer a myth. It has become a multibillion-dollar business.

The ideal of obtaining immortality on earth carries significant moral and religious implications, whether it is found through a magical fountain of youth or through its modern equivalent of scientific research. In both cases, immortality on earth means evading immortality in the heavens. As a cultural priority, the antiaging movement is strongly tied to fluctuations in popular views of faith and spirituality. As Western society has become more secular, the desire to find a practical and real fountain of youth has become increasingly more urgent. The massive 21st-century antiaging marketplace reflects modern cultural priorities that place greater emphasis on life in the moment and less emphasis on life hereafter.

Chapter 1

Myth, Magic, and Folklore: Immortality in the Eras before Science

The history of the antiaging movement begins with stories that inspired people to see the dream of eternal youth as a realistic possibility. Stories of the fountain of youth were born out of traditions of religion and myth and served as morality tales that taught the necessity of death and the importance of living a just life. Ordinary people sought the secrets of immortality, but in these stories, their quests almost always fail in the process. Though the heroes may not have been able to escape the pains of death, they usually found some sort of immortality in the positive memories of future generations. Stories of the fountain of youth inspired listeners to live lives worth telling stories about.

The fascinating aspect of the fountain of youth mythology is that we can see traces of it in the folklore of cultures around the globe. These stories do not belong to a single civilization, nor are they limited to a single historic era. The dream of some kind of magical spring or device that heals the sick and brings life to the dying seems to pervade all advanced civilizations. Yet, there is an important connection between a civilization's level of technological development and its hope in finding the secrets of eternal youth. Like a seed that only waits for the proper nourishment to rise up and pierce the surface, so too objectives of the modern antiaging movement lay dormant in the fountain of youth myths that were shared by dozens of cultures until such time as technology promised some hope of fulfillment. As the advent of science changed the definition of what was and was not impossible, we see a gradual transformation of age-old myths into practical scientific objectives creating a new antiaging movement. In this chapter, we explore just how deeply the fountain of youth symbolism pervades the imaginations of civilizations in both the East and West during the eras before the scientific revolution.

THE STORY OF THE STORY OF THE FOUNTAIN OF YOUTH

The magical fountain of youth that restores youth and vigor and protects against sickness and aging has inspired explorers and scientists since the birth of the modern age. Some version or another of the fable had circulated among European lore masters since the 12th century, but it was not until the early 16th century, when

Juan Ponce de León set out in search of the magical spring during the early days of the Spanish explorers, that it became most famous. The story of his quest is itself quite romantic, and many versions have been retold. In one iteration, Ponce de León is a naive idealist chasing native legends; in another, he is an old man desperately seeking the secrets for keeping the affection of his young bride. It is a subject of both classical literature and modern films. If the fable of the fountain is fantastic, then the story of the Spanish explorer has seemingly mirrored its subject.

Unfortunately, the historical reality is sometimes a bit less romantic. As a historical figure, Ponce de León left little evidence, and some basic facts, such as the exact year of his birth, remain uncertain. Older accounts usually claim he was born in 1460, but modern sources now argue he was born much later, in 1474. No birth records exist, but there is a court case from 1514 in which de León testifies that he was 40 years old at the time of the hearing. It only matters because a more accurate birthdate would help correct the image of him as either a young idealist or an old man. Similarly, older accounts claim he was an officer under Christopher Columbus during his second voyage to and from the New World in 1493. Yet, if he had been born in 1474, he would have only been 19 and would have only been a mere sailor, if he had made the journey at all. There is fairly strong evidence that Ponce de León sailed out in 1502 with Nicolás de Ovando, the new governor of Hispaniola (modern-day Haiti and Dominican Republic). It seems, however, that de León was not an ordinary sailor because, after only a few years, he sought after and received permission from the Spanish Crown to settle and explore the neighboring island that Columbus had named San Juan Bautista (after Saint John the Baptist). The de León family was respected in Spain, and it is likely that their favored son, Ponce, whether at 28 or 42 years of age, was somehow connected to the royal court.

Within a few years, Ponce de León had established the first settlement on the island of San Juan Bautista, become its first governor, and chosen to name his town Puerto Rico (or "the rich port city"). Documents from the Spanish courts indicate his administration only lasted two years before it was interrupted by Diego Columbus, who sued to assert his father's claim of governorship of all the islands that he had discovered. Under feudal law, the right of discovery was passed down to the heirs, which meant the son of Christopher Columbus could claim the governorship of the island of San Juan Bautista, even if Ponce de León had established its first settlement. The case went back to the courts in Spain, and even with the support of the king, Ponce de León was forced to defend his claims. It is from these court papers that we find most of the historical evidence of Ponce de León's life.

While the courts debated who held the right to governorship, Ponce de León was forced to look elsewhere to find a stable position. He heard rumors from the natives of a rich island named "Bimini," supposedly located in the Bahamas, which includes nearly a thousand islands north of Cuba. With 65 men and three ships outfitted at his own expense, Ponce de León sailed northward from Puerto Rico and traveled from island to island. After a month, he spotted the shores of a vast new land that seemed to have no obvious ends. He made the discovery on Easter morning, which was known as the "Feast of Flowers" (or *Pascua de Flores*) in the Spanish calendar, and as there were lush flowers growing all along the coastline, Ponce de León named the new land *La Florida* (the place of flowers). Historical evidence suggests his only goal in discovery was simply to claim new lands for the Spanish Empire and to secure a new governorship for himself.

Ponce de León assumed Florida's coastline was just one more island, like the hundreds that dot the ocean in that region. His initial discovery occurred further up the eastern coast, just north of modern St. Augustine. He decided to travel southward to trace the boundaries of the "island" until he came into the Keys down at its southern end. He rounded the mainland and ventured northward up the western side of the Florida coast. The land seemed vast, and throughout his journey, he and his ships came across stiff resistance from local natives. Seeing the "island" was much larger than he expected, Ponce de León was forced to end his expedition short. He sailed back to Spain and met with King Ferdinand to report on the new discovery. The king gave him a knighthood and granted him the right to explore, settle, and govern the new lands of Florida.

It was seven years before Ponce de León made it back to the New World. Nevertheless, he eventually organized and equipped two ships with 200 men to settle and colonize the territory and claim his new governorship. He settled on the western coast and was only there a few months before he was attacked by the same natives he and his men had encountered during their first trip. The onslaught was significant, and the settlers were overwhelmed. Ponce de León lost many of his men and barely escaped with his life. He was shot in the thigh, and the entire operation was moved back to Cuba. After a slow decline, possibly from poison in the arrow, Ponce de León died in Cuba in 1521. He was later buried in Puerto Rico.

The historical records made during his lifetime show that Ponce de León was actively exploring the Florida and Caribbean islands, and there is ample evidence of his quest for gold and his struggles to guarantee his right to govern Puerto Rico and Florida. There are, however, no references to the fountain of youth. The story of his quest to find the elusive island of Bimini and its fountain of invigorating springs was published some 15 years after his death. The first mention of the story appeared in 1535, in Gonzalo Fernández de Oviedo's *General History of the West Indies*. The author described Bimini as a land believed by the natives to contain a spring that would "renovate or respout and refresh the age and forces of he who drank or bathed themselves in the fountain." This story was repeated nearly 20 years later in another historical account written by Francisco López de Gómara (*The History of the Indies*, 1553), which described the fountain as one "which transformed the aged to youths." Yet another 20 years passed, and the next version, recounted in the *Memoirs* of Hernando de Escalante Fontaneda (1575), described Ponce de León as an old man searching for the Garden of Eden and a new Jordan River to "become young from bathing in such a stream." From that point forward, the historical events had occurred long past the memories of living men, and the story of Ponce de León and his quest for the fountain of youth took on a life of its own. By the 19th century, the story was a popular subject of painters, who often portrayed an aged Ponce de León in a long, flowing white beard.

Origins of a Legend

There is other evidence that the story of a fountain of youth somewhere in the New World had been circulated around the Spanish royal court as early as 1514, which was a year after Ponce de León discovered Florida. An Italian scholar named Peter Martyr d'Anghiera was living in Spain during the time of Columbus's exploration, and he was given the charge of educating the young nobles of the court. In a letter to his friend Pope Leo X, he reported that there were numerous stories coming in from the New World of a spring with rejuvenating waters. He said these stories were "most seriously told to all the court" and were not easily dismissed. Initially, Peter Martyr d'Anghiera seemed willing to explain them away as a simple healing process that came from God's natural providence. Later, however, more reports came in, and some were from three high-ranking officials who had returned from the Caribbean islands and reported firsthand testimony of miraculous healings as a result of the magic springs—the father of one of the men's servants had been rejuvenated. The stories so dominated the gossip at court that Peter Martyr d'Anghiera had to explain to the Pope that if such waters existed, it was simply a gift from God. Just as God allows snakes to rejuvenate themselves by shedding their skins, why would He not also provide such treatments for man? Pope Leo X did not comment, and the church never took an official position on the fountain of youth. But there is ample evidence to suggest that the Spanish court had been heavily drawn into these tales. Yet, there is no mention of Ponce de León in any of them.

Did the natives tell such tales of "healing waters"? Since the 1500s, Europeans had had access to many myths and legends told by the Native Americans of North America. But very few had been recorded directly from the Caribbean, nor were many written down during the 16th century. Professional attempts to collect and record the oral traditions of Native Americans did not occur until the 1800s. In that time, there was an Iroquois myth that spoke of "healing waters" saving an Indian village from certain death by plague. In the story, a young Indian named Nekumonta was living in a small village that was struck by a plague. After watching each member of his family slowly succumb to the disease, he discovered his wife was showing symptoms of the illness and would quickly follow suit. In desperation, the brave Nekumonta set out to find healing herbs. He was led by various creatures, such as rabbits, bears, deer, and other spirits, to find a secret spring "which carried life and happiness wherever they went." He brought the water back, saved his wife, and revived the rest of the village. From that point on, he was known as "Chief of the Healing Waters."

It is not impossible that the story of a magical fountain of youth reached the Spanish court by way of the New World. The Iroquois were a group of nations that settled from what is now upstate New York down to Virginia, which is a fair distance from Florida. Many of the Native American myths seem to share some common themes and often spread considerable distances among related nations. At the same time, however, the internal elements of the story suggest it is not as old as initially thought. Indian villages did not suffer widespread "plagues" until after their immune systems came in contact from diseases carried over from the

Old World. Just as the Black Plague swept through southern Europe shortly after the rise of direct trade connections between the Mediterranean and the Far East, so too a similar sort of disease swept through the New World shortly after the arrival of the European explorers. That would date the creation of the Nekumonta myth to sometime after the 1500s.

Ponce de León and his men were the first Europeans to set foot on North American soil, and the spread of diseases likely took some decades before devastating the eastern coastline. The timing of the fervor among Spanish officials coming as it did upon the discovery of the New World and the Florida mainland suggests some connection, but it may not have come from the North American natives. Other historians trace the mythology of "healing waters" that restore youth and vigor back to Hindu legends from the 700s BCE. Since that time, numerous versions of the "fountain of youth" can be found among ancient writings in the Far East, and some of the specific legends may have reached Spain by way of the Arab traders during the 14th and 15th centuries. There is also a strong folklore of healing springs in the Gaelic and Celtic mythology, located very near to Spain. There is good reason to think that the legend of the fountain of youth did not come from the Native Americans to the Spanish but instead came from the Spanish to the Native Americans, who later incorporated the motif into one of their own myths.

The fact remains that the fable of the fountain of youth managed to wind its way into the highest houses of Spain. For that, the evidence is very clear. The fountain motif was likely already present in the local folklore, but it was brought to the forefront of urban legends through the excitement of the discoveries of the New World. During the late 1400s and early 1500s, the Spanish court must have been an exciting place, with new tales and new stories routinely coming in from all quarters. It is no wonder that the fountain of youth became associated with the tragic life story of Ponce de León, whose death made it impossible for him to refute. He was yet one more legend from the New World, and it was a perfect opportunity to include another legend that was popularly remembered but perhaps not particularly identified.

For our purposes, the most compelling part of the story of the fountain of youth legend is how it was possible that the serious men and women in one of the world's most powerful nations at that time, Spain, could have been persuaded for even a short time to believe that there existed some stream in a distant land that gave healing and eternal youth. Some historians have argued that the fountain legend was attributed to Ponce de León by his enemies, who wanted to portray the late explorer as an impetuous and reckless adventurer who died in a futile quest for a mythical treasure. That does not explain, however, why people such as Peter Martyr d'Anghiera took the story so seriously. Peter Martyr was a Renaissance scholar and a historian of the exploration age, and he was very well respected in the Spanish court. It seems clear that whether or not Ponce de León ever thought about the fountain of youth, or was motivated by its discovery, the people back home surely did.

The 1500s were the beginning of the scientific revolution, and the Spanish court was heavily influenced by the new science coming out of the Italian Renaissance. Men such as Lorenzo de' Medici, Leonardo da Vinci, Niccolò Machiavelli, and

Nicolaus Copernicus emerged during this era and helped launch the new Christian humanism of the scientific revolution. These new artists and scholars took pride in being above such superstitions as myths, magic, and folklore and initially coined the label the "Dark Ages" to describe the medieval period out of which they had sprung. How could such a fantastic story as the fountain of youth have received such serious attention?

The answer is a bit deeper than what we might be tempted to think. A survey of the myths and legends from the ancient world, through the Middle Ages, and up to the modern era reveals a consistent trend in stories that deal with immortality and antiaging remedies. The oldest accounts in precivilized societies, the ones most dominated by magic and superstitions, make very few references to miraculous life extension. Among the native cultures of North America, there are hardly any references at all. Tales of men who seek to evade death began to emerge along with the first civilizations in the East and the West, but they are mostly morality plays that warn the listeners not to strive for something that they can never obtain. The first systematic attempt to evade the consequences of old age arose in China during the first century, roughly 2,000 years into their civilization. It was very influential for a period of almost a thousand years but always faced opposition from other cultural forces that argued the prolongation of life was futile or even immoral. In the West, the pursuit of human immortality on earth was never seriously pursued and was also relegated to the fringes of mythical superstitions. It was not until the emergence of the Renaissance that ideas from the Far East merged with practices of the West through the cultural diffusion of trade and conflict. The pseudoscientific quest for extraordinarily long life emerged from the study of alchemy, and it is out of this tradition that our modern scientific revolution arose. Ironically, it is only through science that the quest for eternal life began to be seriously considered.

Rather than reacting to the absurdity of the fountain of youth, the Spanish court at the cusp of the modern age more easily believed such tales because the promises of modern science gave life and vitality to the dream of finally discovering some solution to aging and death. The fabled fountain of youth in the New World was only a shortcut to another goal that was becoming more seriously considered among the new modern men. Now that science was beginning to understand the ways of nature, it was possible to conceive of finding a cure for anything—even old age and death.

DEATH DEFIANCE IN ANCIENT RELIGIOUS MYTHOLOGY

Epic of Gilgamesh

The fountain of youth story has roots that extend deep into the mythological traditions of cultures throughout the Eurasian world. The basic elements of the story include a stream of water, often near a tree, on a remote island that gives life and youthful vigor to all who drink or bathe in it. Beginning in the Near East, we can find many of these elements in the *Epic of Gilgamesh*, which is considered the oldest surviving work of literature in the world, dated sometime between 2500 and 1800 BCE. We also see similar elements in the funerary texts carved into the walls of the pyramids of Saqqara, which date from the Fifth and Sixth Dynasties of ancient Egypt (roughly 2350 to 2200 BCE). It is possible to see some of these elements in the tree of life in the biblical retelling of the Garden of Eden. The dates when these stories were first written cannot accurately reflect the times when they were first told around a fireside, perhaps hundreds of years earlier, maybe even a thousand. The point is that Western civilization is peppered with stories from both religious and literary traditions that tell of an unapproachable mystical land where life may be preserved indefinitely.

The *Epic of Gilgamesh* is a story about an ancient king of Uruk, which was a real city that is recognized by historians as the birthplace of civilization—the very first city in the world. This story, though, is set at a time after its founding. Gilgamesh is a king with supernatural strength, wisdom, and physical prowess. He is described as one-third man and two-thirds god. He was cruel and ruthless, and he built up his mighty kingdom by oppressing his people with forced labor and harsh punishments.

The gods heard the cries of his people, so they sent a savage man named Enkidu, who was as powerful and mighty as Gilgamesh, with the intent of providing the king with an opponent whose strength matched his own. The two wrestled against each other in a long-fought struggle, until Gilgamesh eventually emerged as the victor. Yet, the struggle caused both men to understand each other, and they became fast friends who agreed to set out to find their adventures together. After mighty deeds of daring and valor, the two men eventually offend the gods so much that the council of the gods decree that one of the two men must die. Enkidu falls ill and suffers greatly before dying. Gilgamesh is heartbroken at the loss of his friend, but he is even more distraught at the realization that if Enkidu could die, so too could he. Despite his wealth, power, and strength, he was still mortal and would eventually suffer a fate similar to that of his friend.

In desperation, Gilgamesh seeks out Utnapishtim, who is sometimes described as the "Mesopotamian Noah." He was the man who the gods warned about the upcoming flood that would destroy mankind and who built a massive ark to hold all the seeds and animals of the world. As a reward for his service to the world, Utnapishtim had been granted eternal life by the gods. Gilgamesh sought to find Utnapishtim to discover the secret of immortality. After journeying past the far reaches of the world and coming up against many supernatural obstacles, Gilgamesh finally finds and meets Utnapishtim on a far-off island across the seas. There he learns the story behind the flood. The gods wanted to destroy mankind, but one of them, Ea, the god of wisdom, deliberately warned Utnapishtim to save mankind through the great ark. After the floodwaters receded, the gods decided they would never again try to destroy mankind, but they concluded that each individual man would have to die. In the Sumerian king lists, all the kings before the flood are listed as having ruled many hundreds of years. But after the flood, the reigns were significantly reduced. Gilgamesh was only the second king of Uruk after the great flood. His father reigned 100 years, and Gilgamesh's son is listed as reigning only 30 years. The lives of all men after the flood remain relatively short.

Gilgamesh was told, however, that there was a fountain of healing waters on another island, and beside it grew a magical plant of immortality. Another journey takes Gilgamesh to the long-sought-after island, where he discovers the fountain and the plant. He takes the plant with him so that he can share it with his kin at home, but along the way, while he stoops down to drink from a stream, a snake darts in and steals the plant. The snake becomes young again by shedding its skin. Gilgamesh returns to Uruk with nothing, but the story concludes with his beginning to understand the wisdom of the gods. Gilgamesh must die, as all men will, but his works and his people will live on.

Throughout the tale, Gilgamesh is warned against trying to achieve immortality by various wise characters, yet he presses on undaunted. It is not until he loses the last opportunity for escaping death that he begins to reflect on the meaning of individual human life and the permanence of human civilization.

Egyptian Pyramid Texts

Around the same time that the various stories of the *Epic of Gilgamesh* were being composed, a very similar story of death and rebirth was being told by the priests and scribes of ancient Egypt as they constructed the pyramids of Saqqara. By the end of the Fifth Dynasty of the Old Kingdom, the pyramid shape of the pharaohs' tombs had been perfected by Egyptian engineers. Within each pyramid are at least two main chambers where the sarcophagus with the mummified remains of the pharaoh reside. On almost every square inch of the chambers' walls and ceilings, hymns, spells, and other incantations have been painted that tell the story of the soul's journey after death. The Pyramid Texts were copied and replicated in several of the tombs erected during this era. These texts were intended only for the pharaoh, and few people besides the scribes who wrote them would have ever seen them. As such, they are not considered literature but are instead described as "sacred texts." Priests wrote them on the walls as a sort of permanent utterance of prayers to the gods to ensure safe passage of the pharaoh's soul to the netherworld, where it would receive eternal life.

The Pyramid Texts are written as a series of spells to help guide the pharaoh's body to heavens, where it will become reanimated with life. The spells speak of the journey as if the utterances both describe and cause the events to happen, including such details as how the soul climbs ladders, flies up to heaven, and is ferried across waters on reed rafts and other mighty boats using a variety of ferrymen. As the soul confronts each obstacle, the priest's incantations provide the secret solution for overcoming it, after which the soul is purified and continues to travel again. In one section, after a sequence of purifications and many stages of travel, a series of utterances tell of the pharaoh boarding a ferry to "the great island in the midst of the Marsh of Offerings" on which is found "the tree of life" that sustains the gods. With the help of the food and drink on that island, the pharaoh is given the sustenance needed to live among the gods. The gods then welcome the soul and set the pharaoh up "as a prince among the spirits, the imperishable stars of the north sky."

The original Pyramid Texts were written without decoration and were intended to be kept in utmost secrecy because they were spells reserved for the pharaoh alone. Later, after the collapse of the Old Kingdom, Egyptian cosmology changed, and the spells were adapted and enhanced for more general use and were written on the insides of the coffins during the First Intermediate Period and the Middle Kingdom (2150–1650 BCE). These "coffin texts" were later compiled during the New Kingdom (1550–1170 BCE) and made available as a separate text painted on papyrus, which became known as the *Book of the Dead*. These were often richly decorated scrolls that were placed in the coffin or tomb as a sort of mystical protective formula to ensure safe travel for any soul who wanted to reach the afterlife.

Both the *Epic of Gilgamesh* and the Pyramid Texts arose from oral traditions that must have predated their initial codification by many hundreds of years. Most

Who Was First, Egypt or Mesopotamia?

The Gilgamesh poem was transcribed in many languages by successive civilizations over the course of many centuries (Akkadian, Hurrian, Elamite, Assyrian, Persian) in the Mesopotamian region. It is difficult to know whether the earliest surviving cuneiform tablets are from the original era or were simply transcribed copies of even older tablets that are no longer in existence. The story is usually written over 11 tablets, but no single copy exists with all the tablets intact. Fragments of tablets from eras spanning 1,500 years have been assembled together to recreate a single narrative, but only about 85 percent of the story is accounted for. Additionally, it is likely that the poem is based on an oral tradition, which means that the story may have existed as a tale told by priests long before it was written down. Modern historians do not agree on its origin, and estimates for the birth of the Gilgamesh story range anywhere from 2700 to 1400 BCE.

Guesses about the date are only important because some elements of the Gilgamesh story can also be found in the Pyramid Texts in Egypt. These funerary hieroglyphics were carved in the walls of Fifth and Sixth Dynasty pyramids that were built toward the end of the Old Kingdom in Sakkara, Egypt. The oldest of these texts are estimated to be from around 2350 BCE, so historians are undecided whether the *Epic of Gilgamesh* influenced the Egyptian Pyramid Texts or the texts influenced the epic. Some scholars suggest that the imagery of the tree of life in the Garden of Eden is itself an echo of these same elements as well as the other associations with human mortality and the great flood. Tradition holds that the stories of Genesis were written down by Moses sometime during the 1400s BCE, though recent historians sometimes place the date of the codification of Genesis between 1000 and 500 BCE. Genesis was most likely written down after the first two texts, but scholars are undecided as to whether the Pyramid Texts and the *Epic of Gilgamesh* were written first.

historians place the date of conception for certain elements at around 3,000 BCE or before. At that time, physical contact between Mesopotamia and Egypt would have been extremely limited, if there was any contact at all. Yet, the storylines from these two texts share some similarities. They both reference a mystical island where there is a tree of life and special foods or drink that restore health and life to those that consume them. In the Egyptian texts, the pharaoh is assumed to have already died, so he can only reach this mystical island through metaphysical means. In the Mesopotamian story, the island is physically present on this earth, but the means of reaching it is still magical and far beyond the capabilities of normal mortal men. It is only because Gilgamesh is two-thirds a god that he is able to reach it. The significance is that, in both instances, the fountain of youth or tree of life is held to be far off and inaccessible to common folk.

The promise of everlasting life for the soul, if not necessarily for the body, was commonly held throughout Western civilization. What we see in these very early stories is the use of water as a literary device for ensuring immortality (the cleansing of mortal wounds) and the distant island as the literary device for keeping this source of immortality out of the reach of ordinary people.

Greek and Roman Reflections

Greek civilization emerged about a thousand years after Mesopotamia and Egypt, and though there are no explicit references to a fountain of youth in their collective mythology, there are related stories that describe distant mystical lands where the rules of sickness and death seem to have been suspended. Greek civilization arose among the islands and coasts of the Aegean peninsula, and their myths often include journeys to fantastic islands and to other secret abodes. There are numerous stories of quests for magical items, such as the golden apples of Hesperides in the Hercules myth, but these items are usually used as simple distractions and do not carry any powers of rejuvenation.

There is a reference to rejuvenation toward the end of Jason and the Argonauts and their quest for the Golden Fleece. According to the legend, Jason is sent on the quest to prove his worthiness to claim the throne from his uncle, King Pelias. He sails to the land of Colchis, where he must satisfy the near-impossible demands of King Aietes to procure the Golden Fleece. Along the way, he falls in love and marries Medea, the daughter of King Aietes, who is largely responsible for Jason's eventual success. There is no indication that the fleece has special powers except that it came from a magical flying sheep that is used by the gods to protect the heroes of another story. In Jason's tale, the only reference to rejuvenation comes after the voyage is completed and Medea promises to make King Pelias young again. The promise, of course, is only a trick to win the king's trust so that Medea can kill him—which she does. The Golden Fleece itself does little except to entice men to take on grand adventures, and no one associated with it gains health or any prolonged life. Both King Pelias and Jason end up dying tragic deaths, directly or indirectly, at the hands of Medea, who originally helped Jason to procure the object.

The motif of the Golden Fleece evolved over the course of the Roman era and during the Middle Ages. Later commentators speculated as to the real meaning of the myth, and because Romans were less inclined to believe in magic or gods as active agents in real history, they usually interpreted the myth in more practical terms. During the time of the first Roman emperor, Augustus, the Greek historian Strabo argued that the Golden Fleece was a symbol used to describe the start of Greek trade contacts with the Colchis region, which was known for its gold, silver, and iron. The locals used sheep fleeces to line their mining troughs, and Strabo explained that the myth arose from the fact that these fleeces tended to take on a golden hue as a consequence of the mining process. This practical view was echoed by the Roman historian Pliny the Elder more than 100 years later.

From these reinterpretations, others evolved that were less obviously connected to the story of the myth itself. Between the 7th and 10th centuries, several references link the Golden Fleece to alchemy, which is the science of trying to turn base metals into gold. In this interpretation, the Golden Fleece is actually a book in which the secrets of alchemy are collected. Parchment was made of sheepskin (called vellum), and therefore a fleece was a thinly veiled reference to a book, rather than a literal sheepskin. In the 12th century, Eustathius of Thessalonica cited an ancient source that asserts the Golden Fleece is actually a method of writing in gold on parchment. The story of Jason, then, recounts the efforts of the Greeks to discover that artistic technique. These theories were repeated frequently by historians of the 19th century, with many variations. By the 21st century, the story of Perseus was retold for modern audiences by Rick Riordan, an author who attributes rejuvenating powers to the Golden Fleece in his books. No such references exist among the ancient sources, but the image of the Golden Fleece seems to lend itself to reinterpretation.

The Greek myths did speak of a distant land called Hyperborea, which is "beyond the north wind" and home to a magical people who live for a thousand years. Beyond the cold regions dominated by perpetual winter, Hyperborea is a land of perpetual spring. The people who live there never get sick, never suffer from old age or disease, and never become embroiled in wars. Instead, they spend their lives singing and dancing and worshipping their patron god, Apollo. When the Hyperboreans choose to end their lives, they leap into a magical lake, where they transform into white swans.

The Greeks accepted the existence of Hyperborea as if it were a real location that mortals might try to reach if they had the power to do so, but they also believed it was mostly inaccessible. In the myths, the land is protected by high mountains and a fierce, cold wind, and the lands beyond the mountains are inhabited by cruel warriors who are constantly at war with each other. The final approaches are guarded by magical beasts that are half eagle and half lion (griffins), which makes ordinary access all but impossible, except for those heroes with some divine assistance. Once arrived, however, Hyperborea is friendly and peaceful. The mortal (though half god) hero Perseus travels to the land in search of the secrets of Medusa, and he is welcomed by the inhabitants. Another mortal (though, again, half god), Hercules, also travels to Hyperborea on two separate trips with no repercussions.

The Greek historian Herodotus included Hyperborea in his history of the island of Delos, which includes a shrine to the god Apollo. He recounts how the people in Delos believed that they were receiving annual tributes from the land of Hyperborea through indirect channels. According to legend, the Hyperboreans send escorts to bring the offering to the shrine in person, but these escorts are inevitably waylaid and never return to their homeland. As a protective measure, the Hyperboreans then send their tributes to their closest neighbors, who pass them along indirectly from nation to nation. The tributes are always hidden within wheat-straw, of a kind foreign to the Greek islands, which therefore seems to affirm the distant source of the tributes. Later historians usually included Herodotus presumptions in their descriptions of world geography and placed Hyperborea as an island of temperate weather in the far northern reaches, beyond the snowy regions.

By the first century, Pliny had described Hyperborea with great scientific detail, though mostly following the pattern set down by Herodotus. The difference was that Pliny also included myths from India, which must have reached him through the communication of the Silk Road. The Indian Vedas describes a land to the north, located near the Himalayas, called Uttarakurus. This land resides beyond the cold reaches and is inhabited by people who live to be many thousands of years old. In the Vedic traditions, these men are far from peaceful and are described as invincible: very tall men with a high tolerance for pain and incapable of being harmed. Later historians theorized that the Indian Aryans found the tribes in their northern frontiers to be too difficult to defeat; therefore, they attributed supernatural powers to the entire race in their sacred histories. At the time of later Rome, though, these Vedic traditions were accepted as a misunderstanding of basic geography. Both Pliny and, later, Ptolemy included references to a land similar to Hyperborea in their descriptions of Indian geography and concluded that the Indians were confusing their land (Uttarakurus, or "Attacori," as identified by Pliny) with the one known to the Greeks as Hyperborea. In both places, the weather is always very temperate, and the inhabitants never suffer from disease, old age, or death, except at their own desire.

There is no magic spring of eternal youth in Greek mythology, but the quest for immortality and long life appear periodically within the stories. Almost always, though, the means for evading death are prohibited to humans. Even when granted through special edict, the immortality is viewed as a curse or as a gift beyond the capacity of mortal men to deal with. In the myth of Tithonus, a mortal with whom Eos is condemned to fall in love, Zeus appears to grant his wish for immortality. He makes Tithonus immortal but deliberately withholds the corresponding gift of eternal youth. Over time, Tithonus becomes more and more decrepit and senile, until he is incapable of either movement or coherent thought. This gift proves to be a curse for both Tithonus and Eos, who is forced to love someone who has no viable life. From these Greco-Roman traditions, Western civilization maintained the promise of escaping death, which is the primary characteristic of the fountain of youth, but nevertheless reaffirmed the impossibility of ever successfully obtaining it.

THE FOUNTAIN IN SECULAR MYTHOLOGY

Chinese and Japanese Islands of the Blest

The idea of a mystical island containing a tree of life and the food of immortality was clearly present in the collective knowledge of the first great societies since very early times. The West was not unique This same motif can be found in places thousands of miles and thousands of years removed from Mesopotamia, Egypt, and Greece. During the Warring States period (475–221 BCE) of ancient China, more than 1,500 years after the *Epic of Gilgamesh* and the Pyramid Texts were first written, a shamanistic practice called *fangshi* emerged among emperors who sought to find the key to immortality (called *xian*). Sima Qian (145–86 BCE), the first Chinese historian, wrote about beliefs that had become dominant about 200 years before his time and which persisted another 500 years after his death, when they gradually merged into Taoism (which is discussed in more detail in chapter 2. The goal of *fangshi* was to develop physical techniques that prolonged the human life span to the point that the practitioner became an immortal. Sima Qian assumed the practices were genuine and that most of those who had successfully achieved immortality were currently living among the three "Islands of the Blest."

The Islands of the Blest (Penglai, Yingzhou, and Fangzhang) were formed from mountains that rose out from the sea, but they are almost impossible to find because the winds always turn against the sailing ships. Even more disturbing is that the islands are perpetually hidden behind luminous clouds. If a ship from the outside world comes too close, the islands sink into the waters and reemerge later. Those practitioners of *fangshi* who achieve immortality can transcend their earthly bodies and magically transmigrate to these islands, where their bodies reform upon reaching the land. Other mortals who manage to find a way to sail to the islands the old-fashioned way and conquer the mystical defenses are rewarded with palaces of gold and silver and the secret to eternal life. On the islands is a fountain of life, which pours forth from a jade rock. Beside the life-giving stream grows the herb of life, which is a fungus-like substance that enables men to cheat death and live for at least a thousand years.

The precise number of these islands ranges from three to five, sometimes as many as ten (two groups of five), depending on the writer. They all share very similar characteristics in that they are almost impossible to reach by ordinary means; they contain fountains of youthful vigor and herbs of long life; and they are usually filled with jewels and other precious things. Though obviously legendary, several Chinese emperors thought them real enough to send out expeditions in search of their whereabouts.

Sima Qian relayed the story of Xu Fu, who was sent out by China's first emperor, Qin Shi Huang (221–210 BC), to discover the sacred fungus and bring it back to the court. Xu Fu later claimed he was intercepted along the way by a sea god who asked what form of payment the explorer was willing to give for the secret of immortality. Xu Fu showed the offerings that were sent with him by the emperor, but the god rejected them as insufficient. Xu Fu was allowed to reach the island of Penglai to see that the herb of life actually existed, but the god insisted that he would need many young girls and other youths before permitting any of the herbs to be taken off the island. Xu Fu sailed back and reported the story to the emperor, who was convinced enough to send another fleet with over 3,000 children along with various craftsmen to appease the god and buy access to the plants. Xu Fu sailed off, but he was never heard from again. Undaunted, Qin Shi Huang devoted the rest of his life to finding the magical elixir of immortality and eventually died from ingesting mercury, which he (and other Taoist practitioners) believed would extend his natural life span.

Some modern historians, however, believe that Xu Fu actually arrived on the island of Okinawa, Japan, and settled there with the children and craftsmen and founded a distant colony of his own. In part, this theory is supported by the many Japanese legends that also tell of Xu Fu and his quest for the magical island of Penglai. There are even shrines dedicated to Xu Fu (whom the locals call Jofuku), and the locals believed he found the magical herb and is still living hidden away somewhere in the Japanese mountains. According to these Japanese traditions, the Chinese Islands of Blest are known as the Horaizan, and like their Chinese counterparts, they also feature three high mountains. The tallest mountain is called Harai, and that is where the tree of life grows, with roots of silver, branches of gold, and fruit of precious jewels. Growing in the shade of this tree of life is a magical moss (sometimes described as a grass) that contains the same properties as the herb of life in Chinese mythology.

One of the Japanese myths tells the story of Sentaro, who traveled around Japan to visit the shrines of Jofuku and pray that he might also discover the secret of immortality. After a week of prayer and fasting at one such shrine, Jofuku appears to him in a translucent cloud and explains that only hermits are allowed to learn the secret of eternal life. Before leaving, though, he promises to send Sentaro off to one of the islands of perpetual life. Fashioning a tiny crane out of paper, Jofuku instructs Sentaro to sit on its back. Magically, the crane grows to an enormous size, and Sentaro is sent off on a journey of more than a thousand miles to Mount Harai. Upon arrival, the paper crane shrinks back to a tiny size and flies into his sleeve.

Sentaro discovers a very beautiful country, but he is surprised to find the people to be generally miserable and unhappy. They all yearn for sickness and death in the same way that Jofuku had previously yearned for health and long life. They spend their fortunes seeking deadly poisons that never work, and instead of wishing each other good health and long life, they wish each other sickness and death. The story ends with Sentaro praying that Jofuku will release him from this immortality. Suddenly, the paper crane flies out of his sleeve again and grows large enough to carry Sentaro back to Japan. Along the way, Sentaro begins to despair and to have second thoughts about living out his remaining years at home. Almost immediately, his crane falters, and Sentaro is cast into the sea, where he is almost swallowed up by a shark. Moments before his death, Sentaro prays again for life and wishes he had never entertained thoughts of death.

The story ends with Sentaro waking up in front of the shrine of Jokufu. He initially believes the entire experience was a dream, but an angel appears before him and reminds Sentaru about what had happened. The angel warns, "You now understand that neither the desire for perpetual life nor the wish to die are things to be granted to a human being. Life such as you lead on earth is the best possible thing desirable." Very much like the epiphany given to Gilgamesh, the hero Sentaro is told that humans are supposed to make the best of their time on earth and that a good life will endure in history far longer than the individual who lived it.

There are other Japanese myths with very similar plotlines that feature various versions of mystical islands with the fountains of youth and herbs of life. There is a fantastic story of a Japanese explorer named Wasobioye who has adventures that are remarkably similar to those of Jonathan Swift in *Gulliver's Travels*. In one episode, Wasobioye is in a disabled ship that is cast adrift through a sea of mud for days, until he finally comes across a beautiful island with three high mountains. There is a well of sparkling water on the island, which refreshes him immediately. Wasobioye then meets up with Jokufo, who is living on that island, and Jokufo introduces Wasobioye to a city of immortals. From there, the story follows the same line as the legend of Sentaro, with the inhabitants being bored of their long lives and daily seeking ways to kill themselves. Though, in this story, Wasobioye manages to escape and continue on his way to discover other fantastic lands. Basil Chamberlain first translated this folktale in 1879, but it is not certain whether it has any particularly ancient origins. There are no local monuments to Wasobioye, as there are for Sentaro and Jofuku. As with many myths, it is possible that the story of Wasobioye was influenced by later Western contact, perhaps even including Jonathan Swift's story of Gulliver.

Gaelic Traditions of Bran

Meanwhile, back in the West during the 5th century, St. Patrick was kidnapped by Irish raiders off the coast of Britain and brought to Ireland. After escaping back to Britain, he sought ordination and later returned to Ireland to spread Christianity throughout the island. Over the course of the next hundred years, Christian monasticism spread over the waters from the Gallic coast of France to the southwestern coast of Ireland, and Ireland became a center of monastic traditions in the West for more than a thousand years. Irish monastics wrote mostly in Latin, and many of the oldest legends and folktales from the pre-Christian Celtic traditions were written down during the 6th century, when the people remembered both the ancient ways and the new ways. Though most of these original manuscripts were burned or destroyed during the Viking raids of the 9th and 10th centuries, the contents of these stories were often recopied during the peace that followed the Norse assimilation. Several collections of ancient Irish myths can be found in manuscripts that date from the 11th through the 14th centuries.

A common theme among Irish legends involves adventures and sailing, especially in those set in the relatively recent eras after the rise of city-states and Bronze and Iron Age technologies, but before Christianity. The sailing myths provided ample opportunities for fantastic journeys to far-off lands. At least two Irish myths include stories about springs or lakes that rejuvenate and give eternal youth to those who drink or bathe in them. One of the oldest tales is the *Voyage of Bran*, which tells the story of an Irish prince who lives at a time before Christian influences. One day Bran is bothered by mysterious music sung by women, which he can hear but cannot see the source of. The music causes Bran to fall into a trance, during which he meets a strange woman who sings a song about a magical island where the most beautiful women in the world live. The weather on this island is always sunny, and there is never a shortage of food, nor any sickness, disease, or death. The woman ends her song by inviting Bran to come and visit the island. After Bran awakens, he organizes a group of 27 men in three boats to go out and find the mysterious island.

Shortly after setting sail, Bran and his men meet the Irish god of the sea, who is riding a chariot driven by a golden horse over the waters as if it were flat land. The god also sings to Bran and afterward provides directions for how to find the mysterious island. After some minor adventures, the crew finds their way to an island, where a queenly woman stands waiting on the shore. Though initially hesitant, Bran and his men are drawn in and come to live on the island, and Bran and the queen live as man and wife. The women on the island are beautiful, and there is never a shortage of food. Time passes as if there is no time at all. After what seems like only a few years to the men in Bran's company, they decide to sail back to Ireland. The queen warns the company that they will regret it if they leave and further cautions that they not set foot on dry land. The company sails back to Ireland anyway.

Upon arriving, and while still in their boats, the company comes across a man on shore. Bran introduces himself, but the man has never heard of Bran except as a tale in ancient legends. One of Bran's men leaps out of the boat and runs to shore, but as soon as he touches the dry land, his body turns to ashes, as if it had suddenly aged hundreds of years in a single instant. Bran realizes that they can never return to Ireland, so he tells the man on shore of all their adventures and asks that the man write it down and record it. Bran and his crew then sail away, never to be heard from again. The *Voyage of Bran* includes some references to a special tree made of silver with golden apples, but the primary source of the eternal life appears to have been the island itself. It is a variation of the typical fountain of youth theme.

There is another Irish story called the *Voyage of Maíle Dúin* that contains more explicit elements of rejuvenating waters. It may not be as ancient a myth because the main characters are all Christian, but it was probably written down around the same time; both stories are included in the same 11th-century manuscript collection. It is likely that the story is an adaptation of an older theme. The *Voyage of Maíle Dúin* includes many more adventures than the *Voyage of Bran*, and though elements are quite similar, the variations are unique enough to consider them separate legends.

Maíle Dúin is a chieftain's son who grows up in his aunt and uncle's castle. His biological father is murdered by raiders, so his mother gives him over to her sister so that she can live the rest of her life as a nun. Maíle Dúin is raised as a prince with three stepbrothers, though he never knows his true origins until he becomes an adult. Once he discovers that the nun who had watched over him is actually his mother and that his father had been murdered by pirates, Maíle Dúin sets out to avenge his father's death. He receives special instructions from a local druid and then sets out with 20 companions, including his three stepbrothers, who swore they would swim alongside the boat if they were left behind. After a day's travel, Maíle Dúin comes across an island and finds his father's murderers. But before they can set ashore, the weather suddenly turns, and storms cast the ships back out to sea. Maíle Dúin and his crew then spend many years traveling from island to island in search of the first one they had encountered, and along the way, they face fantastic and harrowing adventures.

Similar in style to both Homer's *Odyssey* and Jonathan Swift's *Gulliver's Travels* from 17th-century Ireland, each island encountered by Maíle Dúin and his crew presents the party with a sort of temptation. Sometimes the crew members are able to resist these temptations, and at other times, they fail, usually resulting in loss or suffering. At one point, the crew comes across an island of beautiful women. But unlike the story of Bran, the voyagers are held against their will, and Maíle Dúin has to cut off the hand of one of his companions to escape. There are no references to time or enduring youthfulness in this tale.

Shortly thereafter, though, the voyagers come across an island inhabited by a hermit who explains that he had originally arrived with a group of 15 pilgrims, but after many years, he is the only one still alive. The voyagers are welcomed and given supplies, but as they are getting ready to depart, they see a group of very large birds acting peculiarly. The younger birds are stripping the feathers off a single aged bird. After the feathers are all gone, the old bird swims in a nearby lake. When it emerges from the water, it is young again. Maíle Dúin's crew see that the lake is bewitched and fear it will turn young men into old men. Nevertheless, one of the members jumps into the lake and suddenly becomes young and healthy. Unlike most of the fountain of youth myths, the youthfulness and health last for the natural duration of the man's life, but he does eventually die. There is no indication of immortality. The story of the voyage ends with the crew arriving back at the original island, and Maíle Dúin forgives, rather than kills, his father's murderer. They all return to Ireland in joy and gladness.

The voyages of Bran and of Maíle Dúin were both largely incorporated into the hagiography of a later figure with a similar name, Saint Brendan. Brendan was an actual person who was born in Ireland toward the end of the fifth century. He helped to build a number of monastic cells around the Irish coastal lands before traveling to the English islands and founding numerous churches and monasteries on both shores. He is most famous for a seven-year voyage in which he traveled to the "Land of Promise." The oldest manuscript that recounts the story of Saint Brendan also contains the stories of Bran and Maíle Dúin, though they are all treated as separate tales. References to the story can be found in earlier manuscripts, which suggests the biography of the saint was probably composed during the seventh century, not very long after his death in 577.

According to legend, Saint Brendan receives a vision of the Promised Land while in his monastic cell perched atop a very high mountain in southwest Ireland. In the vision, he is instructed to set forth and search for the land, so Saint Brendan takes many monks with him—different versions of the story put the number at anywhere between 18 and 150 monks. They travel to a series of islands in much the same way that Maíle Dúin does, with the difference being that almost all the stories and obstacles are deeply imbued with religious meaning. For example, Saint Brendan encounters the soul of Judas Iscariot chained to a rock in the middle of the ocean because God permits him a brief retreat from the tortures of hell every Sunday. They also visit an island inhabited by talking birds that are actually the souls of young children who have died but whom God has permitted to live happy lives on earth. Saint Brendan's crew also skirts by the very edge of hell, where demons and other spirits assail them, but their ships pass through safely under the protection of God's grace. The voyage is marked by much prayer and fasting and a continual reliance on God's guidance and will.

When they finally arrive at the Land of Promise, it is clear to the voyagers that the land is as much protected by the forces of the immaterial realm as it is present in the material realm. When Saint Brendan and his monks arrive on the island, they find two streams issuing out of the side of a hill and pouring into the bay. One looks foul, while the other looks still. The monks are terribly thirsty, but Saint Brendan warns them not to drink or to take anything from the island without the permission of the inhabitants. Immediately following, a very old man appears and introduces himself as the abbot of a religious community that was founded on the island. Saint Brendan and his men are invited to join in vespers and afterward to share a meal of white bread and pure water with the two dozen monks who live there.

They had all taken vows of silence, but the abbot is permitted to explain their story. He and the other monks had been living on the island for 80 years, since the arrival of St. Patrick. Every morning, a fresh loaf of bread is provided to feed each monk, and the water is taken from one of the two streams on the island. The water and the bread both provide life-giving nourishment so that the monks neither age nor ever grow sick. Saint Brendan asks whether he can stay on the island, but the abbot responds that he and his men are not meant to do so. They have to return to Ireland and continue God's work there.

The interesting part of Saint Brendan's voyage is that the "Land of Promise" was included on most ancient maps from around the 10th century until as late as the 15th century. Legend held that Christopher Columbus first journeyed out to Ireland to research the records of Saint Brendan before he set out on his own voyage. There is little evidence to prove that Columbus made this research trip, but it is known that the map he used for his maiden voyage in 1492 contained a large island in the middle of the ocean labeled "Saint Brendan's Island." The story of Saint Brendan's voyage was retold many times throughout the Middle Ages, with versions in Dutch, Norse, Anglo-Norman, Occitan (an archaic romance language from southern France from the 10th century), and Catalan (another old romance language from Spain) and numerous versions in Old English. Though the story of Saint Brendan attributes the power of rejuvenation more to God's will than to the life-nourishing spring, it is clear that the story of a fountain of youth was held within the folktale tradition of the English, French, and Spanish people long before Ponce de León set out on his famous expeditions.

Bran of the British Isles

The folktales and mythology of the Celtic people spread easily from Ireland to Britain, Scotland, and Wales. Historically, the Welsh are those people who lived in the south and west of England when the Romans invaded the islands during the 1st and 2nd centuries and who resisted the later invasions of the German Saxons during the 5th and 6th centuries. The Welsh folktales, therefore, reflect the closest connection to the mythology that existed prior to the Roman and European influx. Some of the most famous tales, including King Arthur, and other ancient Celtic myths and poems were written down in a number of manuscripts, beginning with Geoffrey of Monmouth in the early 12th century, the *Black Book of Carmarthen* from the mid-13th century, and the *White Book of Rhydderch* and the *Red Book of Hergest*, both from the 14th century. References to these books suggest that the original copyists were transcribing tales that had been in circulation for many centuries before their inclusion in these books. In some cases, the myths may date back to before the Roman occupation. These books all contain copies of old Welsh poetry from around the same time as many of the other legends of ancient Welsh gods and heroes.

The name Bran appears in various forms throughout the Welsh tales, as it does in the Irish versions across the water. Sometimes it is Bran, Brân, Bren, or Bron, and sometimes it is elongated as Brennos, Brennius, or Brannos. It is not clear whether the variations were intended to describe the particular exploits of the same individual or whether the same name was used to describe a multitude of people sharing similar characteristics. Regardless of how the name is spelled or the time period in which the story is framed, the name Bran is usually associated with rejuvenation.

The earliest references to Brennus appear in Roman histories as one of the Celtic barbarians storming the northern gates of Italy. Several versions describe Brennus as a victorious general who becomes king of Britain and establishes law. In the ancient Welsh language, the name Brennos can be translated as "raven king," and the raven is invariably used as the symbol for all the versions of Bran. In these early stories, there is no identification with rejuvenation; they mostly describe supernatural courage and strength before Roman occupation forces. In later tales, dating probably from the 6th century during the conflict that followed the withdrawal of Roman forces, the figure of Bran emerges more as a Celtic god than as a fighting soldier. One such tale mimics the Irish version of the *Voyage of Bran* and tells of a journey to an island full of beautiful women, except that in the Welsh version, the principal character is a semideity named Bran Fendigaid, who is a Celtic god of regeneration and identified as the son of the sea god Llyr and the grandson of the Sun god Belenos. There is no archeological evidence for Fendigaid except that the castle associated with his legend is named *Castell Dinas Bran*, which is derived from the word *raven*.

The 14th-century manuscripts of Rhydderch and Hergest tell stories of "Bran the Blessed," an ancient Welsh king who is a giant with magical powers. In an effort to ensure peace between Ireland and Britain, Bran agrees to the marriage of his sister Branwen to the Irish King Matholwch. Unfortunately, Bran's brother is unhappy about the union, and he mutilates the horses of the Irish king during the prewedding visit of the two families, greatly embarrassing Bran. To pay for the offense, Bran offers a magic cauldron to the Irish king. This cauldron can be made smaller or larger at will, and it will heal and even resurrect from death the body of anyone who is thrown into it. After a year, King Bran discovers that his sister is being abused by the Irish king, and he launches a war in response.

As a giant, Bran is able to wade across the Irish Sea carrying his armies on his back. Once in Ireland, he pursues King Matholwch, and numerous, very bloody battles ensue. The magic cauldron is then used to heal and revitalize the Irish forces, which makes the battles much bloodier and longer than they would have been otherwise. During the war, Bran's brother sees how the Irish are reviving their dead, so he lies among the corpses and pretends to be dead. When they throw his body into the cauldron, he sacrifices himself by extending the cauldron so large that it bursts asunder.

In the end, the Irish are victorious, and like Ponce de León in a story a millennium later, Bran is wounded in the thigh with a poisoned dart and dies in Ireland. Immediately following his death, the crops and lands back in Britain fall into drought and blight for seven years. While he lies dying, Bran instructs the seven survivors of the campaign to cut off his head and take it back to Britain to be placed on the White Mount (where the Tower of London now sits) to serve as a magical defense against sea-born invaders. His men carry out his instructions, but they are delayed along the way because Bran's head continues to talk and regale them with joyful tales and constant feasting. This delay lasts for 80 years without any of the crew growing older, until one day when they finally come to their senses and choose to finish the task they had begun. Bran's head eventually arrives in London and is placed in its protective position. Legends say that the head remained in place until King Arthur removed it, claiming that he would protect Britain on his own. Until very recently, ravens were housed in the Tower of London as a symbol of Bran's protection.

The key elements of rejuvenation later became interwoven into the legends of King Arthur from Robert de Boron's story of the Fisher King and the Holy Grail. This story dates from the late 12th century and tells of Joseph of Arimathea, who uses the cup from the Last Supper to catch the blood flowing from the side of Christ before laying his body in the tomb. As the vessel that held the source of eternal life, the chalice (or Holy Grail) becomes permanently imbued with the power of healing and rejuvenation. The connection to the Celtic traditions comes in with

Joseph's brother-in-law, named Bron. He and several followers take the Grail to England, where they found a monastery to look after their charge. Bron is called the "Rich Fisher" because he is charged by Jesus in a dream to provide a fish to lay beside the Grail on the table where it is kept. There are 12 chairs around the table, and only the most worthy are allowed to sit there. Anyone who attempts to sit there but is unworthy faces the punishment of Judas Iscariot and is cast into hell. Those who are worthy may feast at the table and enjoy immortality while they are there. Onlookers cannot not see anything on the table except the Grail, while those who are among the worthy see the entire feast. Though the Grail guarantees eternal life, those who stand as caretakers only hold the position for a limited time—none of the stewards attempt to retain their lives indefinitely.

Over the course of two centuries, Robert de Boron's story was retold by a dozen other writers, and the story became deeply connected with the Fisher King, King Arthur, worthiness, and the right to rule over Britain. Numerous elements link the later stories with the stories of Bran the Blessed, but the Grail is always connected with rejuvenation, even though the main thrust of the stories rarely focus on that aspect alone. As a literary device, the Grail is used as a sort of litmus test to judge the worthiness of the knight seeking it. The fountain of youth clearly evolved as a literary motif from the healing waters in the *Voyage of Bran* to the Holy Grail in the King Arthur legends. Yet, the idea of a sacred, nonearthly object providing healing and rejuvenation for those very select few who could obtain it is constant. The Arthurian tales spread all throughout Europe and were a dominant theme in medieval mythology.

MYTHOLOGY IN PRECIVILIZED SOCIETIES

The dream of the fountain of youth is not necessarily universal to human nature. The ideal of living a long life without sickness or disease is a luxury of civilized societies. In precivilized societies, where there was limited technological development, the daily routine was focused on getting enough food to eat and surviving the winter months. The traditional definition of a "civilized" society is one that can create a city without outside help. Specifically, it is a society with a concentrated population, a specialized division of labor, and a complex government that is able to redistribute resources to sustain the specialization. In plain terms, it means that there are enough people cooperating together to create a surplus of resources that allows part of their population to concentrate on planning, inventing, and thinking. Cities paved the way for advanced technologies such as writing, metallurgy, irrigation, and the wheel, which in turn made it possible to accumulate greater surpluses to sustain ever larger populations. In precivilized societies, there was always a lack of resources, which meant that daily life was dominated by a constant struggle for adequate food supplies and sufficient shelter. In a culture where hunger, disease, and deprivation was ever present, the dream of eternal youth was much less common, and the dream of any sort of fountain of youth is difficult to find.

Pacific Islanders

Not all precivilized societies lived under a constant scarcity of resources. In some cases, populations remained small because there were few avenues for external migration. For example, the cultures that migrated from Southeast Asia throughout the Pacific Islands were somewhat limited in the concentration of their population. They may have been without advanced technologies such as metallurgy and writing, but their political hierarchies were often quite complex. Recent archaeological evidence combined with linguistic and DNA analysis suggests that the first migration to Australia and New Guinea was over a land bridge just before the last ice age, around 40,000 years ago, and a second migration occurred over water around 4,000 years ago. The archipelago of islands off the coast of New Guinea were slowly populated by an early Lapita culture beginning between 2000 and 1500 BCE, but the majority of the Polynesian islands were populated between 500 BCE and 300 CE, which is a little more than 1,500 years before the first Europeans landed on Hawaii and its surrounding islands.

During the last wave of migrations, Polynesians developed a double-hulled canoe that held 40–60 people and allowed them to transport pigs, dogs, chickens, and a variety of starter plants for their farms. As they came from relatively advanced precivilized societies that were well acquainted with agriculture, the pioneering settlements were able to exploit both the sea and the land for their food resources. Island populations generally grew quickly, and the complex social hierarchies of the island villages provided ample opportunities for Polynesians to see their chieftains living luxurious lives with ease and prosperity. Long life in such conditions could be very pleasurable.

It should not be surprising, then, to find references to something like a fountain of youth among the myths and legends of the Polynesian society. The native cultures throughout the South Pacific islands, from Fiji to Hawaii, shared many common songs, ritual practices, and mythology. There was no writing, but the oral history remained strong. There are many clues to the extent of intercommunication that must have occurred between islands at some more distant period. The stories of the first voyages out to the islands still retain the names of their leaders and even descriptions of their cargo. Throughout the Polynesian culture, there are common deities that mostly differ only in name. The same trademark characteristics and related stories can be found on numerous islands, even though they may be separated by a thousand miles or more. On most of these islands, including New Zealand, Tonga, Samoa, Tahiti, and Hawaii, there is a common story of the "water of life" (*wai-ola-loa*), which heals those who are sick, brings beauty to those who are deformed or ugly, and brings the dead back to life.

Ka-ne, the lord of water, is one of the four main gods in the Polynesian pantheon, which is extremely important in an island culture that is always surrounded by water. According to Polynesian legends, Ka-ne protects the living water in a lake on some island far beyond the horizon and somewhere in the heavens. The mystical island is usually spoken of as an abode of the gods, but there are also legends of its being a very real island that is accessible to mortals in the material realm. In 1823, a British missionary named William Ellis recorded an early account of the interisland navigation between Hawaii and Tahiti, and the water of life figures prominently in the stories. According to their oral history, a priest known as Kamapiikai, or "a child running over the sea," went sailing off with 40 men in four double canoes in search of this special island. He receives a vision from one the gods, who commands Kamapiikai to sail from Hawaii to Tahiti. The priest and his crew are gone for 15 years, but they eventually return and speak of an island named Haupokane, which loosely translates as "lap of Ka-ne." It has sandy beaches, rich fruits, and ample shellfish. Kamapiikai says the local natives are all beautiful and wealthy because they bathe regularly in the lake of living water, which heals those who are sick and brings beauty to those who are ugly or deformed. These stories captivate his listeners, and he makes two more trips to the same island, taking many of his followers with him on each voyage. After the fourth trip, though, he never returns.

The oral traditions speak of Kamapiikai as a historic figure, rather than a legendary myth. The missionary William Ellis immediately connected the story with Ponce de León and his quest for the fountain of youth. Given the relatively late date in which these legends were recorded, it is difficult to know whether the stories are authentically Polynesian or reflect some later influence of European explorers who shared their own mythical tales.

There are, however, dozens of Polynesian myths that speak of Ka-ne's living water of life. Most of them do not speak of actual historical events but instead involve fantastic tales that include mystical encounters between men and gods. One such myth is set in the distant past. A king suddenly falls sick and is close to death. His sons seek help to heal their father, and they are told to seek out the water of Ka-ne, though they are also warned that it is difficult and dangerous to find. The eldest son swears to procure the water to become his father's favorite and thereby inherit the kingdom. He asks his father's permission to go. The father initially refuses because the path is too perilous. But he eventually relents, and the prince goes on his way. After traveling for some time, the prince comes across a dwarf in the middle of a forest path who stops him and asks why he is in such a hurry. The prince rudely replies that it is none of the dwarf's business and continues on. The offended dwarf responds by making the path tangled, narrow, and increasingly difficult. Eventually, the prince falls to the ground and is swallowed up by the vines controlled by fairies and gnomes.

When the eldest son fails to come back, the second son says that he too will go out and find the water of life and thereby gain his father's favor. Like his elder brother, the second son is mostly concerned with trying to win the kingdom as a reward. He follows the same path as the eldest son and eventually comes across the same dwarf who asks the same question as before, "Why are you in such a hurry?" The prince replies just as rudely as his brother and pushes the dwarf out of the way. Soon, he too is caught up in the winding road that narrows into a magically tangled web of vines. And like his brother, he eventually falls down and is swallowed up among the brush.

Finally, when the second son fails to return, the third and youngest son sets off to find the water of life. However, he is mostly motivated by the desire to find and rescue his brothers as well as to save his father. He is not thinking of the kingdom. Along the way, he comes across the same mysterious dwarf who asks him where he is going. The youngest prince politely replies that he is seeking the water of life of Ka-ne, and he asks the dwarf to help him with this quest. The dwarf replies that because the prince answered gently, he will give him a special staff that will reveal the true path and lead him to the castle of a king who holds the fountain of the water of Ka-ne. The dwarf also gives explicit instructions for how to foil the two dragons that protect the castle and how to escape from the sorcerer king. The young prince follows the instructions and returns with a bag full of the magic water. He meets the dwarf again and asks if he might use the water to bring his brothers back to life. The dwarf warns him that the brothers had evil hearts, but he agrees to let the young prince do as he desires. Following the dwarf to where his brothers lie buried in the vines, the young prince uses a few drops of the water and revives them both.

On the way home, the two brothers become jealous that the youngest had succeeded where they had failed, and they immediately seek ways to kill him. The youngest prince, oblivious of these schemes, leads the way back home and helps various kings along the way. After failing in repeated attempts to kill the youngest prince, the two brothers finally manage to switch out the living water of Ka-ne with saltwater. When they arrive home, the young prince gives the saltwater to his father, who nearly dies from drinking it. The other brothers then produce the water of Ka-ne and thereby revive their dying father. The father is very angry with the young prince, and he sends him out of the kingdom while the two wicked brothers stay.

Eventually, the kings who had been helped by the young prince come to give tribute for his aid and explain everything to the king. A magical princess also appears and reveals the truth of the young prince's honesty, which convinces the father of the error. The brothers are banished, and the prince grows up to inherit the kingdom and marry the magical princess. In the larger picture, we see that, like Gilgamesh, the young prince learns that it is a virtuous life that guarantees immortality (in memory) rather than the water of Ka-ne.

It is difficult to trace which myths grew out of the native traditions of the Polynesians and which may have been influenced by later European explorers. One unique characteristic, though, of that more ancient category of Ka-ne myths is that the living water is never seen as a tool for gaining permanent immortality. The stories involve magical journeys to find and retrieve the living water of Ka-ne to bring life to those who have died, but those who manage to make use of the waters all eventually die, as do the people who are temporarily revived by them. Unlike the more traditional stories of the fountain of youth, the living water of Ka-ne is almost always a temporary solution. For both the gods and humans, death remained inevitable and inescapable in Polynesian culture.

North American Indians

The same research that provides a timeline for the migration of the Polynesian culture throughout the Pacific Islands, also suggests that the North American Indians may have arrived in a second wave of migration that followed closely after the closing of the Beringia land bridge around 4000 BCE. There is some debate on this sequence, and though there are very similar traits between the Aleutian natives and the Polynesian islanders, there is a great deal of disparity between the ethnic and linguist ties within the other regions of North America. While the South Pacific populations generally enjoyed a relatively stable standard of living based on agricultural surpluses, the seminomadic natives of North America were not as fortunate. Hunting and the constant pursuit of food dominates Native American mythology in those regions north of Central America and the Aztec and Mayan civilization base.

As mentioned at the start of the chapter, there is a myth of "healing waters" found among the Iroquois that lived in the country spanning from modern upstate New York down to Virginia. The fountain of youth image is found in the story of Nekumonta and his quest to save his dying wife through the magic of healing waters that are revealed to him by various spirits who appear to him in the form of woodland animals. There are also elements of the legend that suggest it may have developed after European contact, particularly the fact that the village is suffering from a plague. The vast majority of tales among the North American Indians include very few hints of immortality from any source, or even unusually long lives. They usually focus on hunting and overcoming the scarcity of food. Both the humans and gods are subject to death, and hunting remains the primary occupation of both the material and immaterial realms.

Animism dominates Native American mythology—the belief that spirits inhabit all objects and places. More than just an abode, the objects are themselves "alive" with the spirits, and so they can think and speak and feel emotions. The trees, the wind, the rivers, the rocks, and certainly all animals share a distinct presence of life that cannot be muted. The stories of gods and demigods include these entities as separate characters that interact and engage with humans on a routine basis. The earth is the source of all living things from the ground and the sky, and it is looked on as the ever-vigilant father watching over all creation. Legends of ancient heroes often pass from one animal form into another as they journey on. Almost every story involves hunting, which is the primary occupation of the humans and the gods. As daily life was dominated by a constant pursuit of food, it was natural for every story to include some element of that routine, whether the story is set in this world or in the next.

An animistic worldview does not easily distinguish between the material and the immaterial realms. Just as there are unseen spirits that enliven the rocks and trees, so too there is an unseen world that is ever present in other aspects of our material lives. This is a critical distinction between ancient and modern perspectives, and it is not unique to the North American Indians. The same fluid exchange between the material and immaterial realms dominated ancient Egypt. The pyramids of Saqqara were built as an eternal representation of a mortal life. The pharaohs were given food and household objects made of stone because they were permanent and eternal, and the priestly incantations were carved into the walls and surfaces of the pyramids as perpetual prayers that would permanently sustain the unseen life of the soul.

Unlike the ancient Egyptians, though, the North American Indians did not have advanced civilizations with perpetual surpluses of resources that could guarantee a luxurious standard of living for some segments of society. For the Egyptians, eternal life for the pharaohs meant a life of continual opulence, much like how they lived in the material world. For the North American natives, no one escaped the need to hunt or the search for food and sustenance in the material world, so the dream of some magic stream or object that guaranteed eternal youth without sickness or disease offered little attraction.

Perhaps equally important is the fact that the animistic worldview also does not believe in death as a final end. There may be no promise of eternal youth in this material realm, but there is also no concept of death as an end of life. In both African and Native American mythology, the veil between the earthly and spiritual realms is so fluid that death is viewed simply as a doorway into another world that is as alive and real as the present world. Gods and men always die, but they continue to live in the spirit world in much the same way that they had inhabited the physical world. There is no concept of nothingness or a final conclusion to life. Death is a passageway, perhaps even an escape, but it is not a cessation of life.

This concept of ever-present life both in the material and immaterial realms is extremely important in understanding the origin and vitality of the antiaging movement. Even as an ideal, the quest for immortality must assume that the present world is more real than the existence after death. The North American Indians did not invent a fountain of youth legend because there was little advantage to living long lives that defied the inevitability of death. To a lesser extent, the same is true for the Pacific Islanders as well. Though their precivilized societies enjoyed greater access to ample resources, death remained inescapable for both gods and men, and the distinction between the material and immaterial realms was difficult to define precisely. Their stories of the fountain of youth did not guarantee eternal life; it only provided a mechanism for overturning an accident that could have been avoided.

CONCLUSION

The fountain of youth is a mythical story that seems to be as old as our oldest civilizations, though no older. The dream of finding some magical spring that heals all sickness and defies death can be found in almost every advanced civilization throughout the world, and the mythology of each region reflects that ideal. Yet, the dream is almost always elusive. From the *Epic of Gilgamesh* to the Chinese "Islands of the Blest" and the *Voyage of Bran*, the myth of a magical stream of rejuvenation always remains just out of reach for the common man. The heroes of these stories may find the mystical islands and bathe in the mystical streams, but with few exceptions, they are never able to achieve true immortality on earth. Even for those semidivine creatures who live near the fountains, life is not really eternal. The Hyperboreans inevitably jump into the lake and are transformed into swans, and the inhabitants of the Chinese and Japanese Islands of the Blest are forever seeking ways of ending their lives.

In this way, the fountain of youth serves the function of a morality tale for those cultures that speak of it. This is the kind of story you tell your children when they ask why there is sickness in the world or why some good people must die. In these stories, people seek out eternal youth, but they invariably fail because either the gods will not allow it or because the heroes are incapable of accomplishing the tasks necessary to achieve such a prize. The fountain, then, becomes a literary device that represents an earthly desire that cannot, and perhaps should not, be attained. Gilgamesh is an extreme example of a seemingly perfect life—he knows no poverty, he has no restraints on his actions, and he can enjoy every pleasure the world has to offer—and yet even he becomes sad and miserable. He realizes that death is inevitable and has to understand it as a necessary part of life to escape his sadness. Gilgamesh changes his life and lives in a way that serves as a monument for later generations, and that is how he plans to live beyond his allotted time. These stories pose hypothetical questions to our children: if you could do anything, without punishment, what would you do? And would you be happy? The answers are intended to inspire youth to adopt a life of some moral restraint to experience the satisfaction of a life well lived. Happiness does not come from worldly pleasures alone, but from the discipline of moral character. In this way, the fountain of youth stories share an almost universally human characteristic.

As long as the possibility of ever obtaining eternal youth remained an impossibility, the fountain of youth always remained just the stuff of legends and simply a myth. The antiaging movement did not begin with the first myth. The earliest stories really taught the listeners to accept death, and not to avoid it. At the same time, though, the constant presence of these myths ensured the ideal of eternal life on earth, even if only as an impossible dream. It is this foundation that the antiaging movement relies upon.

As the technology developed over time, and as civilizations became more adept at manipulating the natural world to overcome the struggles of daily life, that ideal fountain of youth became less of a myth and more of a practical objective. When Christopher Columbus seemingly defied the boundaries of the known world by traveling west to go east, the possibility of discovering other secrets became all the more real. The royal court in Spain came to seriously believe in the possibility of finding the fountain of youth because the discovery of an entirely new world meant that nothing was impossible—even the stuff of legends might become possible. The story of Ponce de León was rewritten to reflect a genuine hope of such new discoveries. The later scientific revolution inspired confidence in mankind's ability to overcome any obstacle, and it is from that confidence that the antiaging movement was born.

In this chapter, we examined the origin of the dream of immortality on earth. In the next chapter, we examine how the changes in religious faith helped to slowly move that dream from the realm of myth to the realm of possibility. In the second chapter, we follow the path of alchemy from the religious traditions of the Far East to the pseudoscientific mysticism of the West. Out of that pathway, chemistry and the scientific revolution will be born, and the antiaging movement will begin in earnest.

Chapter 2

Changes in Religious Faith and the Rise of Antiaging Science

Myths reflect the priorities of each culture, and religious belief plays a critical role in defining those priorities. As long as men and women believe that the unseen world of deities and spirits has more power over the course of human events than humans, the pursuit of long life and eternal youth is seen as futile. In this chapter, we examine the religious presumptions of Europe and the West, of China and the Far East, and of those civilizations in between, such as India, Persia, and the Middle East. For most cultures of the premodern era, religious impulses tended to discourage widespread antiaging movements. The one exception is in China, where the Taoist religion during the 1st and 2nd centuries BCE was almost entirely defined by the pursuit of eternal youth. Yet, even in China, Taoism was eventually overwhelmed by the contrasting religious values of Buddhism. By the turn of the 11th century, Taoism had changed from a religion to a philosophy, and its antiaging practices had evolved into a mysticism no longer tied to eternal life on earth.

At the same time, Western societies were also changing their priorities. Increased trade contacts between the Middle East and the Far East during the 11th and 12th centuries brought Taoist practices in the form of alchemy and other pseudoscientific theories from China into the West. Though Islam was not conducive to antiaging movements, the Arab traders were always interested in gathering new ideas and practices. They replicated Chinese theories of alchemy, mostly with the hope of changing base metals into precious metals, and alchemy traveled to Europe through Arabic manuscripts following the Crusades and the Christian expansion into Muslim Spain. Neither Judaism nor Christianity deemed eternal youth on earth as a realistic or desirable pursuit, but they were not inherently opposed to prolonging the duration of the natural life span provided it was within God's will. New ideas from the Middle East merged with European Scholasticism and combined with other events, resulting in the Italian Renaissance and the rise of Christian humanism toward the end of the 14th century. Over the course of the next 200 years, the Renaissance helped usher an end to the Middle Ages in Europe, and the ideology of antiaging took on a decidedly scientific tone.

Though still strongly religiously based, the new humanism provided the perfect environment for increasing confidence in mankind's ability to change the natural world. When the theories of alchemy spread among the intellectuals of Europe around the 16th century, the optimism of Western humanism transformed alchemy into the first science-based antiaging movement in Europe and the West.

POLYTHEISM AND THE EASTERN RELIGIONS

Animism, Monotheism, and Science

Precivilized societies depended on daily hunting or gathering to survive and often adopted animistic religious practices as a natural response to their immersion in a hostile world. Animistic societies, such as the North American Indians, believed that spirits inhabit all the elements around them—the rocks, the rivers, the animals, and even the sky and earth. The visible and invisible worlds were closely intertwined, and the fortunes or fates of mankind were almost entirely at the mercy of unseen forces. In the Far East, an animistic worldview persisted even after the rise of Hinduism, Buddhism, and Taoism. In the West, animism faded as the three monotheistic traditions of Judaism, Christianity, and Islam became dominant. Though some minority religious views were present along the frontiers, by the 10th and 11th centuries, the vast majority of people in Western culture adhered to one of these three faiths. Animistic beliefs were pushed to the periphery of society and were usually opposed and suppressed as pagan practices or as expressions of witchcraft or the occult.

During the late Renaissance period in Europe (1400s and 1500s), the study of alchemy, or any other mystical pathway for prolonging the natural duration of life, was viewed with some skepticism. European monotheism did not approve of mystical solutions for evading death. This was not the case for the Far East, whose animistic cultures presumed life existed in all things, animate or inanimate, and the earthly life of humankind was just one manifestation of a life force that might be found in any being or object. Between the 3rd and 7th centuries, Taoist alchemists in China were very popular and endorsed by most civic leaders. In part, the difference between the Far East and the medieval West lay not in their belief of life, but rather in their understanding of death.

Animistic cultures blurred the line between life and death because they believed earthly life expresses itself in any number of variations, both in this material world and in the next immaterial world. When animistic cultures also introduced ideas of reincarnation, such as what occurred in India and in China, the understanding of death becomes even more fluid. In China, prolonging earthly life involved the manipulation of unseen forces that transcended the material and immaterial realms. As such, these Chinese antiaging practices were never science based. Instead, Taoist alchemy depended on the mystical manipulation of unseen variables and was more mystical than scientific.

Monotheistic cultures under Christianity and Islam were also skeptical of purely scientific solutions to matters of life and death. For more than a thousand years, the Judeo-Christian and Islamic religions all thrived without developing any exclusively secular or scientific worldview. Yet, monotheism presupposed a predictable order to the natural world, and in this way, it was Europe's monotheistic culture that helped to eventually transform alchemy from a mystical superstition into one of the cornerstones of modern science. This evolution occurred over the course of about 400 years and rested on two religious principles. The first was the monotheistic belief that the material world is a deliberate creation of a single God: one God, one law of nature, and thus one scientific process. The second, was the Judeo-Christian belief that all men are endowed by God with free will.

By the 16th century, the West had developed a scientific revolution, but the Middle and Far Eastern civilizations had not. This is important in understanding the differing forms that the antiaging movements took in the East as opposed to the West. When the first large-scale public movement to defy death emerged in China during the 1st and 2nd centuries BCE, there were few scientific principles involved. Instead, the animism of China rendered the antiaging practices of Taoism into a sort of systematic spiritualism that presupposed certain rules of the immaterial realm. Yet, when the same practices found their way to Europe around the 15th and 16th centuries, they developed into prescientific disciplines based on rules of material nature. In this way, the emerging antiaging movement in the modern West relied more heavily on popular science than it did on religion. It was no longer a product of animistic beliefs, but a by-product of monotheism.

Origins of Confucianism and Taoism

There were no native monotheistic traditions in the Far East, and the remnants of animism remained strong until late in the modern era. Even in the 21st century, we can find animist practices and devotions among the more rural areas of India, China, Japan, and Southeast Asia. For most of its early history, Chinese religion was dominated by animism and related practices of shamans and state priests.

The earliest Chinese civilizations emerged along Yellow and Yangtze river valleys sometime around 2000 BCE, with the first historic dynasty, the Shang, emerging around the mid-18th century BCE. Chinese politics was mostly isolated, and their philosophies developed with little outside influence. Their most formative period was during the Zhou Dynasty, which is often divided into two periods: Western Zhou in 1122 BCE and the Eastern Zhou in 771 BCE. The loose government systems fell apart around the 500s, when China fell into a 180-year Warring States period. The disorder ended with a period of harsh unification that resulted in the consolidation of China's first empire during the Xin Dynasty, around 221 BCE (followed immediately by the Han Dynasty in 210 BCE). It was during the formative period toward the end of the Eastern Zhou Dynasty that China developed two new philosophical traditions: Confucianism and Taoism. These were both native to China and compatible with animism, and they both remained critical components of Chinese culture in the modern era.

According to Chinese tradition, Confucius was an administrator for a minor king during the Warring States period and was responsible for advising the practical government of the realm. He may have only served in office for a short time, but after his retirement, Confucius attracted a great many disciples who looked to

Chinese Timeline

2000 BCE	First Chinese cities
1750 BCE	First Chinese Dynasty (Shang)
1122 BCE	Start of Western Zhou Dynasty
771 BCE	Start of Eastern Zhou Dynasty
475 BCE	Breakdown of Zhou into Warring States Period
	Era of Laozi
	Era of Confucius
221 BCE	Unification of Xin Dynasty
210 BCE	Start of Han Dynasty
	Success of Confucian philosophy
	Success of Taoism philosophy
	Migration of Buddhism from India
220 CE	Breakdown of Han Dynasty
	Success of Taoism as a religion
618 CE	Start of Tang Dynasty
	Decline of Taoism begins
	Popularity of Buddhism begins

him as an authority for the answers to modern social problems. The sayings and teachings of Confucius were written down in a book called *Analects* and are mostly political and philosophical in nature. There is little religious commentary, though most of what there is might be as compatible with animism as with any of the other state religious practices.

At a time just slightly earlier than Confucius, another public servant named Laozi is said to have been the archivist of a king during the Zhou Dynasty. He was also consulted frequently for his wisdom and advice. After the Zhou Dynasty fell into the fragmentation of the Warring State period, Laozi disappeared from politics and headed to regions outside of China in the north. According to Chinese tradition, as Laozi was crossing the northern border, the official in charge recognized who he was and asked him to write down all of his teachings before leaving the country. The resulting book is titled *Tao Te Ching*, or *The Way and Its Power*. Unlike Confucius, the teachings of Laozi are mostly mystical and less related to politics and society. They are more closely tied to the animistic understanding of a harmonic relationship between the visible and invisible realms.

Initially, Taoist teachings spread in much the same way as Confucianism—it was seen as a philosophy for understanding the natural world. Like Confucius, Laozi was portrayed as a wise teacher, and his writings were viewed as an authority on politics and social order. By the second century, though, another parallel tradition emerged that viewed the writings of Laozi as divinely inspired. His book was reassembled under a new title called *The Way of the Celestial Master* and assumed the status of scripture for Taoism, which became a new religion. Laozi moved from

A Compilation or an Actual Man?

Several stories of Laozi meeting with Confucius claim that Laozi was the senior administrator of the two. Yet, the biographical information for Laozi was written about 400 years after his time, so there is some historical debate as to whether Laozi was an actual person or just a name attached to a compilation of several teachers who wrote on similar ideas around the same time. One reason for this debate is because the literal translation of Laozi is "Old Master," which could be applied to almost anyone.

wise teacher to divine founder. Unlike Moses or Jesus or Muhammed, Laozi did not reveal a unique faith based on a single monotheistic order. Taoism was polytheistic and assumed animistic beliefs, so Laozi taught individual believers to achieve sustained happiness by harnessing the unseen powers of the immaterial world. As a religion, Taoism mostly focused on the pursuit of achieving eternal youth and living immortal lives on earth.

Taoism quickly became popular in China. From the 3rd to the 7th centuries, it was the dominant religion and coexisted alongside local animistic devotions. The success was relatively short-lived, however, and after the rise of the Tang Dynasty (618–907 CE), Taoism was slowly replaced by Buddhism. Though originally imported from India, Chinese Buddhism was almost as old as Taoism and was adapted to fit Chinese culture. It gained ascendency toward the end of the first millennium, and by the 13th century, Buddhism had become the dominant religion in China. Taoist priests, monasteries, and other institutional markers all disappeared. Taoist teachings remained alive among intellectuals, but they largely reverted to their original incarnation as a mystical philosophical tradition.

Taoists, Alchemy, and the Elixir of Life

Hundreds of books were written on Taoism during its height from the third to the seventh centuries, and at least a third of these dealt with specific practices that could extend the human life span. When *Tao Te Ching* was first written, the primary focus was to introduce the concept of *Tao*, or "the way." Laozi devoted 33 chapters to explaining what the *Tao* is and how it is responsible for all that moves and lives in the universe. In Western culture, we might understand the concept of *Tao* as a mix between natural law and vitalism. In modern terms, it might almost be equated with "the Force" in the *Star Wars* films. In China, however, the meaning was even more powerful because the animistic worldview presumed that all things, animate and inanimate, were imbued with spirits that maintained their very existence.

By the second century BCE, the *Tao* was interpreted as the means for obtaining almost magical powers. If one could tap into the very life force that moved through all things, then one could accomplish anything. The promise of great power was overwhelming, and the philosophy was embraced at the highest levels. Traditional accounts suggest that China's first emperor, Qin Shi Huang, was so taken by Taoist philosophy that during his final years he devoted untold resources toward the discovery of the elixir of life, which included the Xu Fu expedition sent off to find the mystical Islands of the Immortals. In the end, reports suggest that Shi Huang met his death from ingesting alchemistic potions that were intended to make him immortal (though, in fact, they were likely made of mercury, which poisons the body by damaging the nerves, liver, and kidneys). Despite the emperor's obvious failure at achieving immortality, the theories upon which his treatments were based remained very strong in China.

Perhaps the earliest Chinese alchemist was Wei Po-yang (sometimes called "the Father of Alchemy") who wrote a manuscript on the subject in 142 CE. He refers to previous antiaging texts, and it was those practitioners who likely poisoned (accidently) Emperor Qin Shi Huang. In the third century, a Chinese philosopher named Ge Hong attempted to reconcile Taoism, which focuses on interior peace, with Confucianism, which focuses on exterior relationships. He wrote two books explaining how Taoism could be reconciled with Confucianism and lead to immortality. The first, *The Inner Chapters of the Master Who Embraces Simplicity*, was written to prove that immortality is possible and accessible to anyone who can discipline themselves enough to fully tap into the power of the *Tao*. His basic theory is that the length of life is not determined by the gods or by spirits; their role in the world is simply to keep track of each person's sins and virtues. Life comes from an energizing spirit that lives within the body, and long life is achievable by practicing techniques to keep that spirit inside the body and to prevent any of it from escaping.

Ge Hong describes the spirit of life as *Qi*, or "breath," and at times he meant the word in both literal and figurative terms. He wrote, "people reside with *Qi* and *Qi* resides within people. From heaven and earth down to ten thousand things, each one requires *Qi* to live. As for those who excel at circulating their *Qi*, internally they are able to nourish their body; externally, they are able to repel illnesses." According to this theory, if a person wants to avoid sickness, aging, and death, all he or she has to do is recirculate his or her *Qi* and prevent it from ever escaping.

Unfortunately, most mortals lose their *Qi* during the ordinary course of life, through breathing, eating, and sexual behavior. But Ge Hong argues these habits can be changed, and he lists five basic techniques of discipline for achieving immortality: (1) breathing, (2) calisthenics, (3) sexual practice, (4) dietary restrictions, and (5) alchemy. Breathing is the first and most critical stage. Practitioners were taught to "circulate" their breathing so that no breath could escape the body. This involved intense rituals of inhaling, holding the breath, and then partially exhaling only to "catch" the breath again in the throat and swallow it back down into the stomach. Once in the stomach, the breath was believed to move throughout all parts of the body to provide the necessary nourishment for life. This is where calisthenics became most important. Practitioners were encouraged to move their bodies in various positions to force the breath into all corners. This is the source of modern yoga practices.

Discipline in sexual practice was based on the same principles. As sexual desire is quite natural, practitioners were encouraged to engage in sexual activity frequently—but they were not supposed to reach orgasm because ejaculation would lose the precious Qi. Instead, they were supposed to bring their partner to orgasm and then draw in their partner's Qi. Ideally, the practitioner would involve multiple partners—as many as 10 in a single night. Understandably, the Taoist sexual practices were somewhat socially disruptive and were later targeted by Buddhists who pointed to these habits as examples of immoral and licentious living. For the Taoists, it was not immoral at all, but a necessary tactic for obtaining longer life.

Proper antiaging techniques required intense discipline. Those practicing breathing exercises would begin by fasting from all food or drink for many hours or until all the excrement had left the body. After a careful washing ritual accompanied by various prayers, the practitioner would enter a whitewashed room, sit in the middle of the floor on a simple mat, and meditate on the principles of Taoism. They would grind their teeth frequently to intimidate the evil spirits and then proceed to carry out very long expirations. At first, they would hold their breath for a period of 3 normal breaths and then do so for 5, 7, 9, and finally 12 breaths. Holding your breath for a period a 12 breaths was called a "small series." Believers were encouraged to practice until they could hold their breath for 10 small series, which was called a "large series." Ultimately, it was not until the practitioner could hold his or her breath for two large series that any positive antiaging effects would be realized.

Ultimately, proper breathing was believed to provide enough nourishment so that practitioners would not have to eat at all. Of course, if they had not yet achieved the discipline of perfect circular breathing (or nonexhaling), they were encouraged to limit their food intake to those items that were least likely to decay and to those colors that seemed brightest. Cereals were not allowed (rice, wheat, millet, oats, or beans), but red fruits and other items that do not seem to tarnish were. Color was as important as texture, so foods that were bright and shiny in color (red, orange, or yellow) were more powerful than those that were brown, white, or black. These rules stemmed from the "you are what you eat" theory, so anything that was prone to decay would create a body that was prone to aging. Anything that seemed long-lasting and full of life would create a long-lasting body.

Taoism and Transmutation

The dietary regulation eventually led to alchemy's more famous endeavor: transmuting lead into gold. According to the Chinese, gold was the only metal that would never corrode, and because you are what you eat, gold was viewed as the perfect food. Taoist practitioners who consumed gold in its most pure form could escape all need for breathing or eating and would live forever—it was the elixir of life. Unfortunately, eating raw gold was not sufficient. Successful practitioners had to discover perfect formulas for rendering the metals into the form most effective and then consume it.

Ge Hong and others were particularly drawn to mercury as the necessary ingredient for the elixir of life. When found in its natural, unrefined state, mercury is bonded with sulfur in a compound called cinnabar. It looks like a red rock and may occasionally form into very pretty bright red crystals. When crushed and heated, cinnabar is transformed into mercury in its liquid state, which is bright and shiny and seems to flow effortlessly as a liquid metal, even at room temperature. Taoists loved the color red, and they loved gold. Mercury seemed to have both qualities. Ge Hong believed that the two elements of gold and mercury were the only imperishable things on earth and that together they would provide the elixir of life. He wrote, "As for forging of gold and cinnabar, the longer one burns them, the more marvelous their transformations. When gold enters flames, even after one hundred firings, it will not disappear. If you bury it forever, it will never decay. If one ingests these two substances, they will refine that person's body, and make it so that he or she will neither age nor die."

No matter how adept someone might become at breathing, eating, and having sex, true immortality required the proper elixir of life. As Ge Hong explained, "Even if one performs breathing exercises and calisthenics, as well as ingests herbal medicines, this can only extend the years of your life span, but it will not save you from death. Ingesting divine cinnabar will make your life span inexhaustible. You will last as long as heaven and earth, be able to travel on clouds and ride dragons, and ascend at will to the Heaven of Highest Clarity." (Just to be clear, modern science now understands that mercury is extremely toxic and should never be ingested or even touched.)

In actual practice, the Taoist disciplines were heavily based on animistic beliefs. Not only was all life tied together by the *Tao*, but each part of life was inhabited by a spirit. There were more than 36,000 spirits in the human body,

Yin and Yang and Immortality

Ge Hong's second book, *The Outer Chapters of the Master Who Embraces Simplicity*, explained how those who have mastered Taoist immortality were also best at ruling kingdoms. He never did gain a ruling position in any government, but his teaching was very popular. It was his duality of "inner" and "outer" chapters that formed the basis of what modern students describe as "yin and yang," where complete unity involves combining opposites together. Ironically, it was this combination of opposites that helped to pave the way for Buddhism to become more compatible with Confucianism and eventually replace Taoism as the dominant religion.

Ge Hong wrote several other books detailing the lives of Taoist practitioners who (according to tradition) actually achieved immortality. He was highly respected as a Master of Learning and awarded numerous honors during his lifetime. At the age of 50, Ge Hong quit the public life altogether and went to live on a mountaintop, where he practiced his antiaging strategies for 10 years. He died, nonetheless, at the age of 60.

with multiple deities inhabiting and animating each organ. At its core, alchemy in Taoism was all about transmutation at all levels: transmutation of the body and transmutation of the spirits. Immortality was possible when the spirits that were responsible for corruption, decay, disease, and old age were exchanged with those that were responsible for permanence and constant youth. The spirits of gold and mercury would merge inside the human body and replace all the existing corruptible spirits that dominated the breath of life with new, incorruptible ones. The basic antiaging theory of Taoism was to arrange the proper alignment of spirits or deities that would stave off all the evil spirits, encourage all the good spirits, and recirculate the life force (the Qi) to perpetually feed those good spirits.

As most people had very limited access to gold, or mercury, which was needed to create the perfect elixirs, Taoist practitioners were forced to find ways of transforming easily accessible base metals such as lead or iron into precious metals. Ge Hong readily admitted that it was difficult to obtain the necessary resources to create the perfect elixir, and his efforts to transform lead into gold never succeeded. Yet, his Taoist theories remained undaunted.

ALCHEMY: THE STRANGE JOURNEY WEST

Chemistry and Alchemy

For historians, the spread of alchemy from China to Europe is difficult to follow. Taoism did not move westward. It was mostly a Chinese invention, and it spread eastward into regions that the Chinese Empire gradually influenced through conquest or trade, such as Korea, Japan, and Southeast Asia. As a religion, Taoism required the animistic environment of China and the Far East to thrive. Nevertheless, many alchemic practices made their way westward through India to be discovered by Arabic scholars. Islam is monotheistic and not at all conducive to Taoism as a religion; it does not support antiaging mysticism. But Arabic scholars were deeply interested in alchemy as a means for transmuting base metals into precious ones—turning lead into gold.

The ancient West already had a limited history of transmutation unrelated to Chinese Taoism, but when historians speak of ancient Greek or Egyptian alchemists, they are usually referring to those very early experimenters who investigated chemical reactions. The term *alchemy* is a later Arabic invention and is not used by either the Greeks or the Chinese. The Greek word *cheō* means "to melt or to fuse" and was usually used in conjunction with metallurgy. It was a thousand years after the Greek Golden Age, during the height of Arabic scholarship, that the term *al-khymeia* was coined, and it was only used generally to mean any transformation of one substance into another. It was not until relatively late in the 17th century that the term *alchemy* was only used in reference to the transmutation of lead into gold.

The first reference to Egyptian alchemists in ancient sources (that still exist) comes from a decree issued in 300 CE by Emperor Diocletian ordering all Egyptian writings related to *khemeioa* be burned. Scholars often interpret *khemeioa* as the root for the Arabic *al-khymeia* (alchemy). Yet, the decree had nothing to do with Diocletian's fear of mysticism or magical arts. During the 3rd century, the declining Roman Empire suffered a period of constant civil war that exhausted the treasuries. To pay their soldiers, many emperors inserted lead cores into their gold coins. At the same time, they used silver-plating techniques rather than genuine silver for their smaller specie. These practices made the gold and silver reserves last longer, but the result was rampant inflation that seriously undermined the Roman economy. It was to this regard that Diocletian issued his famous decree: he passed a series of laws that were intended to stabilize the money supply. In the process, he ordered the destruction of all instructions that could be used to disguise lead (or other base metals) into something that might pass as gold or silver. In essence, Diocletian was destroying documents that might lead to counterfeiting.

There are very few scraps of writing that still exist of other ancient alchemists, and they all seem to indicate that the craft was mostly focused on techniques for making cheap metals look like they were gold or silver. Unlike China, there does not seem to be a long history of transmutation prior to the Arabic ascendance in the Middle East. There is one famous authority, Zosimos, from the third century of Egypt, who is said to have written 28 books on alchemy, but only a few fragments remain today. It is not clear whether he genuinely believed he could change the physical composition of lead into gold or whether he knew he could only transform its outer appearance. He wrote of "tingeing" and "dyeing" metals, as if to change their colors. It is possible that he was precisely the kind of scientist that Diocletian was most concerned about, because his techniques might be used to plate or otherwise disguise base metals. There are too few of Zosimos's writings to be absolutely certain about what he meant, and the later Arabic scholars who refer to Zosimos as the ultimate authority usually do so to substantiate their own credibility and are not always to be relied upon.

The Arabic Alchemists

Islam emerged as a distinct religion in the early 600s CE in the wilderness of Mecca in modern Saudi Arabia. At the time, the Arabian coast was a trading crossroads between Mesopotamian states in the north, North African states to the southwest, and the Byzantine Empire in the west and northwest. The land was mostly desert and had only been permanently inhabited for less than a thousand years prior to the rise of Islam. The lands had no unified political state; the Arab peoples were mostly ruled by their tribal customs.

Beginning in 610, the Prophet Muhammad received recitations from the Angel Gabriel, which lasted for more than 20 years. These recitations were initially memorized by Muhammad's followers, but they were eventually written down shortly after the Prophet's death. The basic message of Islam is to lead believers into a complete submission to God. In practical terms, that meant that tribal laws were subject to God's law, and one of Muhammad's first actions was to serve as judge to reconcile differences between conflicting tribes. Before his death, Muhammad had developed a significant following, which turned into a powerful army of believers. Within a decade, Islamic forces had expanded in all directions, sweeping across Saudi Arabia and into North Africa. By 661, they had taken most of Persia, Syria, and Egypt. By 750, multiple Muslim empires spanned from Spain to the Indus River.

Most of the Muslim possessions had previously been under Byzantine rule, which means that the majority of those living in their realms remained Christian or Jewish (paganism was quickly fading). The Egyptian city of Alexandria had previously been under Byzantine rule and was the center of learning in ancient times. When the Muslims arrived, they came in direct contact with thousands of Greek and Latin manuscripts on every conceivable topic. The new rulers embraced the corporate knowledge of those that preceded them and even hired Christian administrators, architects, and other scholars to help govern their new political empire. At the same time, they also deliberately sought training for their own people to become as versed in the Greco-Roman knowledge base as the Byzantines had been. This triggered a "translation movement," which lasted for almost 200 years, where books from the leading Greek and Roman thinkers were translated into Arabic and held in the Islamic capitals—first in Damascus and later in Baghdad.

Alchemy was among the subjects that were explicitly targeted for translation. In his history of alchemy, Lawrence Principe recounted a story from the 10th century about a meeting between an Arabic ambassador to the caliph al-Mansūr and the Byzantine emperor Constantine V. An incident supposedly occurred in the late 700s, when the Byzantine emperor was showing off all the wonders of Constantinople to the visiting ambassador. One storehouse held many bags filled with white and red powders. According to the account, the emperor ordered a pound of lead

Monotheist Religions and Their Sacred Texts

Monotheistic believers hold that a single God revealed truths about faith and morality to mankind through a series of prophets. In Judaism, those revelations were eventually written down in an anthology of books that we now identify as the Old Testament, with collected commentaries that were eventually written down in the Talmud (two versions: one from Jerusalem and one from Babylon). In Christianity, believers claim that those same revelations were enhanced through the incarnation of God himself in the form of Jesus, and those revelations were gathered together in what we now identify as the New Testament, with commentaries written down through the writings of early church fathers and other ordained members of the teaching arm of the church. In Islam, believers claim that further revelations were made through the Prophet Muhammad and compiled in what we now identify as the Koran, with collected commentaries of the Hadith (or traditions of the faith) written down through several compilations.

to be melted down, and in front of the ambassador, the emperor threw a small amount of the white powder into the mixture, transforming the metal into silver. The emperor then ordered a pound of copper to be melted down and threw in a pinch of the red powder; it all turned into gold. The ambassador reported what he saw, and his caliph immediately ordered the translation of all Greek texts related to alchemy into Arabic.

Obviously, the incident never actually happened—at least, not in the way it was told. Modern science knows that no such powder exists or could exist. Nevertheless, the anecdote was sincerely reported in the 10th century, and it illustrates the kind of alchemy pursued by Arab scholars of that time. Unlike its Greek and Egyptian predecessors, Arabic alchemy was not limited to chemical reactions only but clearly sought to transmute base metals into precious ones. Historians still have a difficult time determining how, or when, ancient alchemy shifted from a science of all chemical reactions to a discipline that included the mystical transformation of one metal into another. While there are no direct links between Chinese Taoism and Arabic alchemy, there are other strong connections between China and the Middle East that make the correlation seem highly likely.

The Silk Road and the Monotheistic Filter

By the early 800s, Baghdad was the newest center of Islamic learning as well as a crossroads for intercultural communication. It lay in a critical juncture along the Silk Road, between the Far East through India and the farther West through the Byzantine Empire. Chinese manuscripts may not have passed along that route, but Chinese trade goods and other ideas frequently did. As early as the second century BCE, Roman markets in Italy were selling silks from China.

In ancient times, individual traders did not journey the entire path, but hundreds of intermediary traders made smaller trips from one side of their province to the other. There were some exceptions, though. Chinese historians recount that Emperor Wu-Ti sent a delegation of 20,000 cavalry to visit the Parthians (modern Iraq) and ended up riding as far as Syria during the early Han Dynasty in 91 BCE, and another similar delegation was sent out nearly 200 years later. The same Chinese historian also reported that the Roman emperor Marcus Aurelius (whom the Chinese identify as "An-tun") likewise sent a delegation back to China. Generally speaking, there is very little evidence of direct contact between Rome and the Far East until Marco Polo's famous venture in the early 1300s. Nevertheless, trade routes persisted from ancient times into the modern era, and with trade comes the cultural diffusion of ideas.

In China, Taoist scholars during the 1st and 2nd centuries devoted hundreds of books in search of a formula for changing lead into gold, which is about 800 years before the subject appeared in Arabic writings in the Middle East. Yet, there is no evidence that Chinese documents ever made their way to the Middle East. There is, however, a great deal of evidence that Arabic scholars of the 8th through 10th centuries were eagerly searching for any information related to alchemy and gathered from any source—written or unwritten. The trade routes between China and the Arabic world collided in Baghdad, which makes the correlation particularly tempting. Such exchanges would not have come from written Taoist documents, but they may have come through orally communicated anecdotes among Indian traders who shared common contacts with the Chinese.

The problem for historians, however, is that there is no evidence in any Arabic writings that alchemy was used for anything other than transmutation; there are no references for using gold to evade death. Yet, the antiaging goal of immortality was the essential purpose behind Chinese Taoist alchemy. That problem might be answered by the fact that the Arabic alchemists were all uniformly Muslim and strongly monotheistic. If someone told tales of Chinese adepts who transformed lead into gold to create the elixir of eternal life and became immortal, a Muslim scholar would likely dismiss all the animistic elements of the story and concentrate on only the more objective scientific elements. If the Chinese tales were convincing enough, then the Arabic scholar would turn to the ancient sources that he trusted and find more viable explanations that seemed to make sense—and perhaps pursue it further using his own science.

We can imagine the same scenario in modern day when we read of ancient Egyptians eating poppy seeds to cure headaches; the ancient texts always included mystical incantations that ask various gods for relief. Modern readers dismiss the incantations because our biochemistry science tells us that poppy seeds contain pantothenic acid, linoleic acid, and diacetylmorphine. It is the codeine and morphine content that triggers the release of endorphins (endogenous opioid peptides) from the pituitary gland throughout the central nervous system that produces a euphoric, analgesic effect to relieve headaches. The correlation that Egyptians noticed between poppy seeds and relief is substantiated, but the incantations and other mystical explanations are easily ignored.

Similarly, if the Muslim scholar saw examples of cinnabar being transformed from bright red crystals into quicksilver mercury and was told that these components might be used to transform lead into gold and eaten to achieve eternal life, the Muslim would naturally ignore the Taoist mysticism and concentrate more on the theory of transmutation. He would search through all the records of recorded science (through Greek and Latin sources) to find more seemly and credible research on the subject.

There is little evidence that the Greeks ever believed in the possibility of true metallic transmutation, and yet that belief was entirely accepted by the Chinese during the same time period that the Arabic scholars began to seriously pursue the topic as a legitimate science. There is no direct evidence of an explicit connection between Chinese Taoism and Arabic alchemy, yet the coincidence is high enough to suggest some sort of informal influence. Taoism's other key influence, however, the quest of immortality, had to find its way to the West through altogether nonscientific means.

THE SPECTER OF IMMORTALITY IN THE WEST

Islam and Fate

Islam does not support the deliberate pursuit of antiaging for its own sake. The central belief of Islam requires man's total submission to God, and so the length and days of his life are determined by God alone. From this perspective, the quest to defy death would seem utterly futile. There are many passages from the Koran that support this presumption by repeating again and again God's ultimate power over life and death (and the resurrection):

> And He alone is the One who gives life and gives death. And to Him alone belongs the alternation of the night and the daylight. (Surah 23:80; see also Surah 2:28, 22:66, and 30:40)

The same point is made even more explicitly in Surah 62:8: "Say to them: Indeed, the death from which you flee shall, most surely, encounter you." There is no history of an antiaging movement among Muslim countries or communities. If Taoist alchemy ever made its way to the Arabic Middle East, we can be assured that the quest of immortality would have been discarded almost immediately.

The Islamic Filter

Islam does not support the deliberate pursuit of antiaging for its own sake. Though the Muslim scholars of Baghdad eagerly pursued the study of alchemy and the possibility of transmuting lead into gold, they did not accept any of the Taoist animism that accompanied the practices. Nevertheless, the Arab writers were still influenced by the folktale culture that pervaded the Silk Road from Taoist China through India and into the Middle East and the Mediterranean. Tales of immortality and the ideals of evading death were woven into the popular stories of the time and were even included among the commentaries of their sacred Koran. Indian mythology speaks of Al Khidr (also named Khwaja Khizr, Pir Padar, or Raja Kidar) as an Indian deity responsible for healing waters. In Islamic tradition, Al Khidr is an immortal being following God's will. There are shrines to Al Khidr along the Indus River in India built by both Muslims and Indian believers. Yet, monotheistic Muslims believe Al Khidr was not only immortal but also deeply Islamic and a reflection of God's absolute power over life and death as well as man's inability to change either.

In the Muslim Middle East, there were no antiaging movements. Yet, the stories of antiaging immortality remained in the literature, even if the Muslim writers refused to accept them. When these same stories found their way to a Christian Europe, which was stimulated by new ideas of Christian humanism and Renaissance hopes of free will and progress, the antiaging movement was reborn. The antiaging movement that began as a product of animistic religion in China would eventually become a science-based movement in early modern Europe.

Toledo and the European Exchange

The chemist and historian Lawrence Principe recounts the very day that Arabic alchemy was first introduced to Christian Europe. It was on Friday, February 11, in the year 1144 when an English monk, Robert of Chester, finished his translation into Latin of an Arabic text titled *On the Composition of Alchemy*.

Robert lived in Toledo, Spain, which had become the forefront of conflict between Christian Europeans and Muslim Moors of Spain during a period roughly parallel with the Crusades in Israel and Jordan along the far eastern shores of the Mediterranean Sea. A generation before Pope Urban II called for French and German knights to help their Byzantine brethren defend the rights of pilgrims to the Holy Land, the Spanish heirs of Christian Visigothic kings had begun a slow process of "reconquering" the lands of Spain from the Muslim Moors who had held control since the early 700s. King Ferdinand the Great inherited a small territory in northern Spain from his father and expanded it considerably. His son, Alfonso VI, continued the expansion southward until he reclaimed Toledo in 1085, which was the first major victory for Christians in Spain in over 300 years. Toledo was the intellectual center of Spain and had been a crossroads of learning for Jewish, Muslim, and Christian scholars since the 900s. Robert of Chester moved from England to Toledo after Alfonso VI reclaimed the city, and he initiated a long period of translating Arabic documents into Latin for Christian study.

In terms of broader chronology, the scholars of Bagdad began translating Greek texts into Arabic beginning in the 9th century. Within 200 years, the Christian scholars of Southern France, Italy, and Northern Spain began translating Arabic texts into Latin by the 11th century. The Arabic versions of the *Romance of Alexander* were only a century old at that time. The massive collection of works by Ibn Sina (known as Avicenna in Latin) were barely 100 years old, while those of Ibn Rushd (known as Averroës in Latin, who wrote on Aristotle) had not yet been written at the time Robert of Chester was translating his Toledo texts into Latin.

The Crusades are often discussed in terms of their violence and intercultural conflict, but like the Arab conquests of the eighth century, the Christian Crusades also triggered significant intellectual exchanges between independent cultures. The scholarly seeds of Renaissance humanism were mostly set in place through the intellectual exchanges that followed the Crusades.

Christian Monotheism and Humanism

The practical content of Arabic scholarship from Bagdad to Toledo translated fairly easily from the Middle East to Europe. Both the Muslims and the Christians rejected animism and polytheism, and they eagerly sought more earthly explanations for the things they saw in the material world. Both the Muslim and Christian scholars were fascinated with the technical information left by the ancients on such subjects as mathematics, astronomy, physics, botany, biology, medicine, and chemistry. Of course, these subjects were not yet categorized in those fields; in the 12th century, they were all collectively known under the universal label of "natural philosophy." Any text that purported to reveal truths about the natural world was collectively known as technical knowledge (from the Greek *tekhne*), while the theoretical subjects were classified by their topics. Specific subjects were rarely distinguished except by practical use. Avicenna compiled a list of everything he knew about healing in his *Canon on Medicine*, which included information on medicine as well as botany, anatomy, and even sociology, psychology, and theology.

One exception was the study of chemistry and chemical reactions, which was still referred to generically as "alchemy" by Robert of Chester. He wrote in the prologue of his translation of *On the Composition of Alchemy* that the subject was entirely new to Europe, which was only partially true. As he interpreted the Arabic text, Robert of Chester categorized alchemy as exclusively the study of metallic transmutation. This was a reasonable conclusion for two reasons. First, Arabic practitioners took great joy in disguising their research under various names so that their secret formulas would remain secret. Arabic scholars were only following the practice of the Greek and Egyptian scholars that preceded them, many of whom were likely hoping to avoid accusations of counterfeiting. And second, the subject seemed (at the time) to be less practically relevant than other subjects dealing with engineering or medicine or mathematics.

In general, none of the natural sciences during the High Middle Ages and early Renaissance (12th through 15th centuries) earned as much respect as traditional philosophy or its cousin theology, which was heralded as the "queen of all sciences," as it focused entirely on the source of all truth, God. Techniques and recipes for various chemicals, dyes, and alloys existed in various manuscripts throughout the European Middle Ages, but when Robert of Chester translated *On the Composition of Alchemy*, the particular subject of alchemy had never been introduced to Europeans before. During the centuries that followed, dozens of other manuscripts on alchemy were also translated, and the subject became increasingly esoteric. It was a favorite field among scholars who liked to tinker in a laboratory with flames and beakers, but the dissemination of their findings remained more or less hidden from the general public. This changed, however, when the scientific revolution placed a greater priority on the practical science than on the philosophy.

Arabic alchemy had no connection to antiaging ideologies or to any quest for immortality on earth. Yet, these European translations of Arabic science books were strongly tied to what would become, over the next few centuries, a rising antiaging movement in Europe. The outside materials influenced European scholars to develop a new sense of humanism—which means, simply, a common consensus that humans can be active agents in the world.

Medieval Priorities before the Renaissance

The European West already had its own legends of the fountain of youth, especially in the Celtic and Gaelic traditions that spread into France and Spain. They did not need the parallel traditions that Islam (in the person of Al Khidr) carried with it from the Far East of China and India, and yet the mixture of both influences would have magnified an already existing mythology. As we discussed in chapter 1 those myths always included some caveats or warnings that made the acquisition of the fountain's properties impossible or inappropriate for humans. There were no systematic antiaging movements in Europe during the Middle Ages prior to the rise of Christian humanism.

Confidence in Progress and the New Fountain of Youth

The rise of Christian humanism during the Renaissance convinced Europeans that conditions in their material world were not always going to be harsh. Because God gave people free will, they did not have to accept the harsh conditions that permeated the earthly realm. They could be improved. With God's help, men could use their knowledge of the natural world to improve living standards, improve communities, and generally make the world a more beautiful place in which to live.

It is sometimes difficult for people in the 21st century to truly appreciate the depth of new optimism that followed the Renaissance. In our modern world, we expect technology to provide solutions for everyday problems as a matter of routine. Yet, this was a new experience for those who were coming out of the widespread political instability of the European Middle Ages. Renewed trade contacts with Arab merchants that arose after the Crusades brought massive wealth into Italy and southern Europe. These new resources, combined with new intellectual perspectives, inspired great confidence that, given enough time, almost any human problem could be overcome.

It is this unshakable belief in progress that reinvigorated the ancient mythology of the fountain of youth. The new intellectual resources flowing in from Arab lands were only the beginning of future promises. If the Arabs had access to such ancient wisdom, what might be found elsewhere? It is in this cultural environment that Christopher Columbus first brought back word of a new passage to the Far East. The discovery of a "new world" only magnified this widespread sense of hope. It is from this Christian humanism that the Spanish court so easily entertained the idea that Ponce de León might actually have stumbled across a very real fountain of youth. Similarly, it is the reason why Christian monks began to reevaluate the lives of antediluvian patriarchs: perhaps God did not forbid men to live hundreds of years; perhaps he wanted man to find a way of regaining such life spans through more healthy life choices. New optimism created a new antiaging movement. Rather than finding the perfect mystical incantation, the new science-based movement focused more on hygiene and medicine by avoiding disease and curing common ailments associated with old age.

CONCLUSION

The idea of finding a magical source for eternal life originates with our most ancient civilizations, and yet these ideas rarely expressed themselves in actual practical movements. In the Far East, Chinese Taoists transformed the myth of a fountain of youth into a practical lifestyle that depended on the discovery of an equivalent elixir of life. Their antiaging movement, however, was religious and mystical in nature and relied on their animistic belief system that did not clearly distinguish between the material and immaterial realms. There was no science behind the movement, and it eventual faded as another more compelling religious system (Buddhism) replaced it. More importantly, it failed to move beyond the Chinese homeland, and though some techniques of alchemy may have traveled along the Silk Road, the larger ideological objects of defying aging never followed suit—at least, not in the form of Taoism.

There were many cultural elements within the Islamic Middle East that could have led to a scientific-based antiaging movement, including the discoveries of Greek and Roman humanists and the monotheistic belief in a single natural order. Yet, the Muslim civilizations lacked the most important belief in free will and independent human agency to create change in the world. As a result, the practical observations of the natural world were reclaimed from ancient Greece and Rome, and even expanded upon greatly, yet they were never employed to make fundamental changes to the human condition. The roots of modern chemistry in the texts of early Arabic alchemists did not lead to a scientific revolution, but instead inspired dozens of individuals to secretly discover their own keys to permanent wealth. The goal of extending the natural life span never entered into the discussion among Islamic scholars.

The confluence of all these elements together in the early European Renaissance could not have been more perfectly timed. The Christian monotheism had matured during the Middle Ages, so when the material conditions began to improve following the Crusades of the 12th and 13th centuries, the intellectual climate was just right for an influx of new ideas. The practical discoveries of the Arabic scholars merged with the free will of Christian theology and produced a new optimism in mankind's ability to change their world. Among the hundreds of new innovations in learning and scholarship, there was a new faith in man's ability to reclaim some control over the length and days of his life.

This young antiaging movement matured as Europe increased its collective knowledge base and expanded its contacts throughout the globe. New direct contacts with China during the 1600s helped restore the prospect of prolonging the human life span to the study of alchemy (which Islam had stripped from it). The alchemy of the modern age did not seek immortality, such as the Taoists monks of China would have desired, but instead pursued the more humble goal of adding significant years to the natural life span. This was not to be gained through mystical incantations nor the discovery of a magical elixir, but instead through the more systematic understanding of the natural forces that operate in the world. This type of understanding not only produced a more consistently refined field of chemistry but also led to the development of all other fields in natural sciences: biology, medicine, botany, physics, astronomy, geology, engineering, and, eventually, the social sciences.

For our purposes, the main importance of the birth of modern science was a new belief that death was not predetermined by nature to occur after a fixed number of years. Nor was it necessarily absolutely determined by God, with no room for human choice or human decision making. This belief in the potential of genuine human progress was essential for the success of an antiaging movement that continues to the modern day. In the next chapter, we will examine the stories of how the early scientists incorporated these antiaging goals into the research that dominates modern science, from evolutionary theory to biochemistry and to our social sciences.

Chapter 3

Enlightened Aging

The sociopolitical changes of the 14th and 15th centuries brought more economic freedom and resources for literary and artistic expression than Europeans had enjoyed through the entire 500 years that preceded. Out of this change came more systematic studies of the natural world, especially in observations of mechanics, in understanding of the shape and structure of the human body, and in those social and political forces that affect daily life. Filippo Brunelleschi, Michelangelo, Leonardo da Vinci, and a host of other artists as well as writers such as Dante Alighieri, Niccolo Machiavelli, and Nicholas Copernicus all studied the way the human world interacted with the natural world, as if it were open to deliberate change. The explosion of work later became known as the Italian Renaissance, which eventually led to the scientific revolution. Historians generally refer to this entire period of transition as the birth of the modern era.

The modern era is defined by the rise of nation-states that gradually replaced the medieval feudal system. Personal relationships between lord and vassal were replaced by our current system of institutionalized governments with impersonal bureaucracies. For the most part, these developments created greater social and economic stability.

The modern era is also defined by a new way of thinking, which we loosely describe as *humanism*—a belief that mankind can make meaningful changes in the world. This new view of the world inspired strong optimism in the future and in man's ability to change conditions that had previously been thought of as unchangeable, including the very length and days of the human life span. The belief in human progress was an essential part of the new science-based antiaging movement.

At first, the humanist worldview reflected strong Christian principles. Human progress must presume individual free will and should be coupled by a confident belief that God wants us to exercise that free will to change the world. Instead of waiting for God to improve human conditions independently, the new Christian humanist believed that God made use of the gifts given to individual people, who then served as his hands on earth. From this philosophical foundation, the early pioneers of science arose. They were mostly deeply religious men, often religious clerics, such as monks, brothers, sisters, or priests.

Over time, however, the religious basis of scientific research shifted. When taken to its logical extreme, the belief that mankind can change the world may lead scholars to challenge God's role in the world entirely. With the start of the 19th century, a new breed of secular humanists argued that man alone was responsible for human change. They doubted any "divine plan" and believed instead that changes in the natural order were either completely random or the product of man's will. From this philosophical foundation, a new form of scholarly atheism arose that saw God as a human invention. Such thinkers were often hostile to the perceived limitations that religious faith placed on individual intellectual freedom.

This secular shift was not quick, nor was it without controversy. It occurred over the span of about 300 years. In the process, the ideology of antiaging became torn between an assortment of supporters and opponents. Some Christian humanists continued to believe that God gave man the tools with which to better his earthly life, including extending the length of his years. Some secular humanists argued that man could almost live forever, if only science were allowed to focus on science alone (and if people rid themselves of such ideas as a holy church and divine providence). There were others who reacted harshly to the rising atheism and questioned antiaging pursuits as if they were inherently secular or even contrary to religious belief.

On the whole, the belief in progress defined scientific discovery, which in turn defined the modern era. The antiaging movement rode the wave of intellectual change with few detractors. This development came slowly and in stages. Yet, throughout the process, a persistent faith and optimism in mankind's ability to improve his earthly conditions propelled the antiaging movement into the mainstream of modern science.

THE BELIEF IN PROGRESS

In 1920, intellectual historian John Bury published the *Idea of Progress*, which argues that modern optimism in the future is a relatively recent phenomenon. The contemporary expectation that science and technology continually improve in positive ways is unique to the modern era and not shared among medieval or even ancient societies. Prior to the 17th century, intellectuals from cultures around the globe believed that the world began as a more perfect place but, for some reason or another, fell to great depths of ignorance and corruption. They usually saw their own time periods as attempting to recover from a lost golden age. We can see this phenomenon in both the 8th- and 9th-century translation movements among the Arabic scholars in the Middle East and the 12th- and 13th-century translation movements among European Christians. Scholars in both Bagdad and Toledo were eager to translate the ancient texts of Greece and Rome because they were links to an older, more knowledgeable time.

Modern students may not think in this way because we tend to assume that older texts are less informed and less accurate than new texts. Yet, throughout the history of Western civilization, from ancient Greece to the Renaissance, most intellectuals believed the exact opposite: they feared that modern books were more likely to be caught up in simplistic intellectual fashions, while the older books were proven by the test of time to be wiser and therefore automatically carried more authority. Until as late as the 17th century, it was rare to find a scholarly book that did not refer back to an ancient authority to justify its arguments (whether it was a real or made-up reference).

Bury argued that the unquestionable reverence for the past changed around the 17th century, when new thinkers began to instead revere their own research. He listed three main changes within the intellectual community that led to this transition: (1) they broke free from their dependency on ancient authorities; (2) they adopted a new purpose for the study of science; and (3) they came to see nature as being guided by unchanging (or immutable) laws. Through small shifts in priorities, modern society became increasingly more optimistic for the future, as people believed progress would continue until the end of time.

Reason versus Antiquity

The preference for modern reasoning over ancient textual authorities occurred because 17th-century intellectuals began to practice and engage in scientific experimentation. Previously, it was often enough just to repeat the conclusions left by an older authority. In the new era, scientists tested the old assertions, and sometimes they found that the old authorities were wrong.

With each new discovery, modern scholars gained a new reason to challenge the infallibility of ancient authors. Nevertheless, their confidence in promoting their own ideas independent of the past grew slowly. Renaissance scholars frequently hid their own arguments behind references to ancient Greeks or Romans because they feared their own reasoning was insufficient to justify breaking from tradition. This had also been very common among Arabic scholars who routinely adopted fake pseudonyms of ancient Greeks to give their contemporary works more credibility. In fact, many of the books on alchemy were credited to scientists (such as Aristotle) who never wrote anything on the subject. Europeans adopted this practice less frequently, but even in Europe, it was not unusual for a modern document to be attributed to an ancient author. The Arabic alchemist Jābir ibn Hayyān (Geber) is listed as having written nearly 3,000 books, which is simply not possible.

The problem with relying on the past authorities is that it discouraged contemporary research, and it encouraged scholars to devote more energy toward finding and translating the old rather than embracing the new. By the turn of the 17th century, this habit had begun to change. Scholars such as Francis Bacon still mentioned the ancients, but his later contemporaries, such as René Descartes, explicitly resisted their presumed authority. The "new science" argued that modern learning should be based on evidence verified through actual experimentation. This new methodology emphasized inductive reasoning rather than deductive reasoning and remains the hallmark of the modern scholarship today.

Difference between Deductive and Inductive Reasoning

The transition from the dominance of deductive reasoning to inductive reasoning largely defines the birth of the modern intellectual history. Deductive reasoning is a logical process that begins with certain presumptions that are assumed to be true, from which all other conclusions are based. Inductive reasoning begins with no presumptions and builds its conclusions from a series of testable observations. Deductive reasoning might be described as "top-down," while inductive reasoning might be described as "bottom-up."

Both forms of reasoning remain important for different sorts of inquiry. For philosophical or moral questions, which consider immaterial truths that cannot be measured, only deductive reasoning is useful because there is no way for quantifying observations to test the conclusions. For the natural sciences, however, inductive reasoning is most useful because it requires testing of material substances that can be measured and manipulated. The purpose of the scientific method is to prove a hypothesis wrong. Success requires a new hypothesis. Failure strengthens the existing hypothesis. This sort of physical experimentation is impossible with moral reasoning, which is why deductive reasoning remains important.

Of the two sorts of reasoning, deductive reasoning provides the most certainty because it begins with a presumption of a truth. At the same time, it is also most liable to challenges because people may disagree on the presumption. By contrast, inductive reasoning may provide more quantifiable evidence, but it leads to less certainty because there is no end to the number of potential tests to challenge a hypothesis. Until the 20th century, both forms of reasoning were recognized as essential to a more complete understanding of truth. Debate over the nature of truth and whether the immaterial realm existed created significant philosophical division. Just prior to the 21st century, some scientists rejected the existence of any intangible reality and therefore rejected the value of deductive reasoning and any metaphysical inquiry as innately "unprovable." Therein lies the underlying causes of the modern conflict between faith and reason.

Science as Utility

The second intellectual shift that promoted the new idea of progress occurred when scholars changed how they viewed the importance of scientific research. In the 13th century, a Franciscan friar named Roger Bacon dedicated his book (titled *Opus Majus* or "Greater Work") to Pope Clement IV and argued that subjects of natural philosophy, such as mathematics, astronomy, physics, and chemistry, were essential for intelligently understanding theology and the Scriptures. In this early Renaissance era, Bacon explained that it was "no diminution but rather an advancement of God's Glory to be versed in the works of his hands."

Bacon took time to explain this point because the popular view held that studying the natural world provided little benefit in the grand scheme of knowledge. Theology was the "queen of all sciences" because it studied God, who was the source of all truth. Anything less was deemed less important. Roger Bacon tried to change this view slightly by justifying the natural sciences as a gateway for better understanding theology. Unlike some of his contemporaries, Bacon embraced the ideal of testing a hypothesis by conducting actual experiments. Yet, he did so with the understanding that scientific knowledge was only useful because it led people toward a greater understanding of God and his role in the world. Bacon was not compelled to make this justification—he sincerely believed it to be true. He and his contemporaries took for granted that studies of the world were less relevant than religious studies, but Bacon also advocated for a new level of respect for natural sciences.

It was not until another Bacon (Francis Bacon) came along in the 17th century that scholars began viewing science as important for its own sake. In 1620, Francis Bacon wrote in *Novum Organum* (*New Instrument*) that the legitimate purpose of science is "the endowment of human life with new inventions and riches." He argued that scientific research leads to "happiness of mankind" and is not limited simply to the more thorough understanding of religious doctrine. Francis Bacon wrote more than 300 years after Roger Bacon, and the cultural priorities had clearly changed. Both Roger Bacon and Francis Bacon were deeply religious men, but 17th-century scholars such as Francis believed God wanted man to pursue scientific knowledge because it led to more fulfilling lives. Science was important because it was useful.

Miracles and Natural Law

Finally, the third intellectual change among scientists was the belief that the laws of nature were unchanging and not subject to variations—even from time to time. This presumption of a single natural order was the hallmark of monotheism in the West, but it did not necessarily mean that the laws of nature were permanently fixed or unchangeable. Islamic society believed that God could (and often did) change the conditions of the world as he saw fit. Christian belief was less flexible. The very plan of salvation presumed that certain laws were always immutable (sin always equals death, and that death always had to be paid, which is why Jesus had to die for our sins). Nevertheless, the church also believed in a providential plan for history, which means that God is actively involved in the world. The basic thesis of St. Augustine's *City of God* is that God used his prophets and his church to bring the rest of the world toward a better understanding of himself. By the time of the early Renaissance, most intellectuals still viewed history as a reflection of that divine plan, determined not by human action but by divine will (Providence). By the end of the Renaissance, the immutability of natural law had become more fixed.

This point is more subtle than it appears because the changes of the 17th century did not really change theology as much as it changed how scientific intellectuals approached it. From one point of view, the immutability of nature may appear to reject divine action: if the laws of nature do not change, then God either cannot or has not chosen to change them. And if God changes them, then the laws are not immutable. Yet, this was never really a part of Christian doctrine. The Catholic Church recounted countless miracles, from the seemingly minor protection of Daniel in the lion's den to the fundamental miracle of the incarnation of Christ in human flesh. Miracles were so common that every saint required at least three of them to be received into the official canon. From this perspective, it could appear that God has frequently made changes to the natural order. Nevertheless, despite the church's strong belief in miracles, it never denied the immutability of natural laws.

This takes some extra explanation. The very definition of a *miracle* is some event or action that is not explainable by natural laws and thus attributable to God alone. That means that miracles can only exist if the natural order of things is unchangeable and immutable. If the natural order was not absolutely fixed, then miraculous events would not be surprising or even remarkable. It is only the certainty that the rules of nature do not change that makes miraculous events so important. For Christians, the belief in miracles is important because it is a constant reminder that despite the natural order of the world, God is still actively involved and still guiding history. Though René Descartes appears to be opposing God's active role in the world with his strong assertion of the immutability of natural law, his conclusions do not follow that path. Like Roger Bacon and Francis Bacon, Descartes was also a deeply religious man who firmly believed in all the tenets of Christianity—including the miraculous.

Early Debate over Faith and Reason

Such subtle distinctions were difficult even for the intellectuals of the 17th century. The mathematician and philosopher Blaise Pascal generally supported René Descartes's preference for inductive reasoning and scientific method rather than depending on ancient authorities alone. At the same time, though, Pascal feared that Descartes's insistence on the immutability of nature could take away from the proper recognition of man's dependency on divine will. He argued that some truths, such as those related to morality and faith, were potentially weakened by the imperfect reasoning of single individuals. Such truths required the authority of a collective body over time, which was guided by divine providence to be protected from error. In these matters, Pascal argued that deductive reasoning was more useful and provided greater certainty than inductive reasoning.

Pascal's arguments were true to Christian teaching, but they did not necessarily oppose René Descartes's theories. Descartes argued that God's mind and motivations were so much more complex than the human mind that it was virtually impossible for man to come close to understanding it. As such, we cannot easily see God's hand in creation, even if we know it defines all of it.

Descartes argued that the practical sciences should be investigated separately from the divine sciences because they relied on substantially different forms of understanding. During the 17th century, these two categories of learning (philosophy and science) were not easily distinguished. The intellectual community debated the issue for some time, with many following Pascal's reasoning. There were others, though, such as Nicolas Malebranche, who argued that there was no conflict at all between faith and reason and heralded the Cartesian method as a necessary intellectual reform.

In the end, the complementary natures of faith and science were generally accepted by leading intellectuals of the 17th and 18th centuries. They recognized that the laws of the natural world were unchanging, and they confidently studied them in the hope of gradually improving the lives and conditions of human society. Scientific research did not weaken moral faith. Nevertheless, the fears of Pascal and other critics were not entirely unfounded. By the 19th century, an increasing number of intellectuals began to argue that faith and reason were altogether incompatible and that reliance on one inevitably undermined the integrity of the other.

Public (Government) Support of Science

On November 28, 1660, a small group of scholars met in England to hear a lecture given by Christopher Wren, a famous architect who had designed more than 50 churches, including St. Paul's Cathedral in London. During the discussions that followed, the group decided to create a more formal society of scholars to better regulate and communicate the massive increase in new knowledge that seemed to be all around them. With the support of King Charles II, the Royal Society of London was formed with the motto *Nullius in Verba* (take nobody's word for it). Based on the scientific method, the Royal Society symbolized the commitment among the leading intellectuals of England to the practical study of science using factual evidence derived from actual, repeatable experimentation. Within a few years, the Royal Society had published a journal titled *Philosophical Transactions*, which remains the world's oldest continuously published journal of science. The new journal introduced the practice of peer review and became a significant vehicle for communicating new discoveries to scholars throughout Europe.

Shortly thereafter, the French Academy of Sciences formed in Paris in 1666 with the support of King Louis XIV. The French counterpart was initially charged with advising the king on scientific matters, but it eventually expanded as a source of intellectual authority in its own right. These institutions, and others that arose in the later century, reflect a collective belief that diligent scientific innovation will lead to continual improvements for individuals and for human society at large. John Bury argues that the idea of progress did not come into its full maturity until the end of the 17th century, and these new institutions demonstrate the official support from the modern states.

The belief in progress greatly changed the antiaging movement. Most previous efforts to prolong the natural life span, particularly in China, assumed that the ancients knew some secret to immortality that had since been lost to the contemporary generation. With the coming of the scientific revolution, the goal of evading sickness and disease and extending the natural life span became a legitimate subject for current research. No longer regarded as a lost secret of the past (dependent on ancient texts and esoteric myths), the antiaging movement placed its hope on the future. Scientific discoveries promised to uncover truths about the human body, its actual (rather than supposed) limitations, and how these conditions might be manipulated or changed to extend human life. This remains the primary guiding principle for such research today.

CHRISTIAN HUMANISM: FROM HYGIENE TO ALCHEMY TO NATURAL PHILOSOPHY

Both Francis Bacon and René Descartes wrote about practical ways that science could promote good health and possibly even extend life. Neither scholar stated explicitly that they expected to live substantially longer than their peers (Bacon died at the age of 65 and Descartes at the age of 54), but they both said there was no scientific reason people should not reach ages similar to those found in the Bible. Moreover, there was no theological reason why the traditional limit of 120 years could not be broken, with some folks possibly reaching 300 or 400 years or even the antediluvian ages of 700 or 800 years. They both believed the stories of men living in far-off lands who routinely lived well past 100. Antiaging was just a matter of mastering scientific knowledge. The secret to a longer, healthier life was in better understanding what science revealed about human hygiene and then applying that knowledge to daily life.

Franciscan Friar Bacon

The earliest texts explaining practical antiaging methods were primarily focused around hygiene and healthy lifestyles. Very early in the Renaissance, during the late 1200s, Roger Bacon wrote a book titled *Preserving the Senses of the Mind from Accidents and Old Age.* In it, he lists all the symptoms of old age, which include gray hair, paleness, wrinkles, weakness of strength, weakness of sight, shortness of breath, and an inability to sleep, most of which are recognizable today. In addition, though, he added other symptoms that clearly reflect the state of medical knowledge of his day: decreasing blood and spirits, abundance of rotten phlegm, filthy spitting, anger, and an unquiet mind.

The latter symptoms reflect the language of an ancient medicine. Bacon relied on the writings of Avicenna and other Arabic scholars who had translated and compiled the texts of ancient authorities 200 years earlier, including Aristotle, Hippocrates, Galen, and other Greek and Roman physicians. According to the Greeks, the world was composed of four basic elements: fire, earth, air, and water. These elements each shared four basic qualities: hot, dry, wet, and cold. Fire was a mixture of hot and dry, while water was a mixture of wet and cold. Similarly, air was a mixture of hot and wet, while earth was a mixture of cold and dry.

Greek medicine simply applied this system to the human body. We all come to life with an abundance of moist internal heat, which is responsible for our early growth and development. Over time, the natural heat within the body consumes the internal moisture, just as a flame consumes the oil. As it does so, the body begins to dry out: hair loses its luster, skin loses it flexibility, and muscle loses its tone and strength. Medical theory argued that disease was a by-product of certain humors (blood, yellow bile, black bile, phlegm), each of which upset the proper balance of moisture and heat in the body. If they created too much moisture, the heat increased to a raging fever, and too little led to aches and premature weakness. Aging and disease, then, were intimately connected.

Bacon's understanding of medical practices was not new, but his use of the information was more unique. He recommended avoiding red meat, because it was more likely to decompose in the body, and places with moist and damp air, because they are likely to exhaust the body's internal heat more quickly. As a good Christian friar, though, he added another layer by arguing that vice and evil thoughts stressed the body's internal processes. The anxiety and disquiet of immorality lead to poor digestion, which leads to putrefied meats, which deprive the muscles of proper nourishment, leading to weakness and a reduction of internal moisture and the natural heat it produces. Therefore, a disordered life leads to frequent disease and early death. Conversely, a well-ordered life will lead to a properly functioning body that resists drying up and growing cold.

Roger Bacon's medical theories closely reflect Arabic theories of alchemy. Most alchemy texts, including the 3,000 or so texts attributed to Jābir ibn Hayyān (known as Geber in the Latin West), relied on the ancient Greek theory of elements. Each metal, such as lead or copper, contained differing proportions of "coolness" and "dryness"—almost as if they were recipes for their composition. The basic theory of alchemy held that some metals were more perfect than others because they contained more perfect ratios of those properties. The secret was to distill the essential properties from common metals to extract "coolness" and "dryness" and then add them back to the alloy to fix, or "heal," the base metal so that it is composed of the new composition of a pure metal.

The philosopher's stone of *Harry Potter* fame originated from an Arabic alchemist named Muhammad ibn Zakariyyā al-Rāzī (or Rasis, in Latin). He believed such a stone would be the one perfect substance that could "heal" all other metals back to their pure states. It was not a coincidence that Arabic alchemists were often also famous as physicians and routinely used the medical terms and phrases from Galen and other Greek physicians as metaphors to describe the process of transmutation.

Roger Bacon borrowed from these same theories when he wrote about the power and effectiveness of various medicines. Each herb or powder was believed to contain the essence of a certain moisture, dryness, heat, or cold. For example, coral, rosemary, aloe wood, serpent's flesh, and bone from a stag's heart were all believed to restore the body's internal moisture. This theory of pharmacology fought disease by restoring the body's proper balance of moisture and heat back to its natural ratio. Bacon devoted his life to alchemy, and he wrote *Preserving the Senses of the Mind* because he believed that if he could understand how medicine healed the body, he might be able to better understand transmutation at all levels—including metals. Almost two-thirds of the quotations used in his book came from a translation of *Secret of Secrets*, spuriously attributed to Aristotle, which is a compilation of Arabic alchemy. In referring to the "secret arts," Bacon wrote of an ancient practitioner "who wisely studied the forces of animals, stones, etc., for the purpose of learning the secrets of Nature, especially the secret of the length of life, gloried in living for one thousand and twenty-five years."

Arabic alchemists never promised to prolong the human life span. Yet, Roger Bacon made the connection through his emerging humanist belief in human agency. The significance of Bacon's book is that he argued that old age might be delayed. Identifying three causes of age—negligence, ignorance, and infection—Bacon claimed that at least two of those are easily treatable through careful living, and the risk of the third can be limited by the first two. Therefore, old age is an accident brought about by a gradual loss of natural heat. The longer that those accidents are avoided, the longer the natural life span becomes—perhaps even to the length attributed to the antediluvian patriarchs.

The older Bacon wrote in *Opus Majus* that "the possibility of the prolongation of life is confirmed by the consideration that the soul naturally is immortal and capable of not dying. So, after the fall, a man might live for a thousand years; and since that time the length of life has been gradually shortened. Therefore, it follows that this shortening is accidental and may be remedied wholly or in part." He did not believe that the traditional limit of 120 years was fixed but rather an unfortunate side effect of evil and sin, which made the world a hostile place to live in. If science could reveal solutions to these age-old problems, perhaps men could regain such previously long lives as Methuselah (969 years), Jared (962 years), and Adam (930 years).

Alchemy in Modern Science

It took more than 300 years for Roger Bacon's book to be translated from Latin into English, and it is relevant that the translation occurred in 1683—just 20 years after the formation of the Royal Society in London and shortly after both Francis Bacon and René Descartes published their works on avoiding old age. Not only had the surname of "Bacon" gained new respect, but hygiene and prolongation of life were very popular subjects in the new age of science and inductive reasoning. The fact that Roger Bacon was also known as an authority on alchemy was not inconsequential.

Most leading scientists of the era, including Robert Boyle, Isaac Newton, and even Francis Bacon (though he loathed to admit it), all studied alchemy as a probable avenue for understanding the underlying unity of the natural world. In this way, the study of alchemy was less about transmuting base metals into gold and more about transmutation itself: the idea that anything (like food or water) could be transformed into something else (like muscle, tissue, or energy) was very appealing. Robert Boyle's alchemy led to his *The Sceptical Chymist* (1661), which theorizes that matter is composed of clusters of particles and that different materials contain different types of clusters. This hypothesis later evolved into the basis of modern molecular theory. The study of alchemy was, essentially, a search for the common elements that allowed for universal transmutation. Such understanding could, conceivably, unlock the secrets of the universe—and perhaps allow sick men to be made permanently well and old men to become young once again.

In 1638, Francis Bacon published *The Historie of Life and Death*, which contains the more explicit subtitle *With Observations Natural and Experimental for the Prolonging of Life*. The book explains the causes of aging and argues that a proper scientific understanding of the human body could allow men to live significantly longer lives. Bacon never mentions alchemy, and considering his political aspirations, he wisely chose not to reveal his study to the public. Nevertheless, beginning in the late 1960s, several historians reexamined his works and private letters and discovered that much of Bacon's underlying presumptions, concepts, and solutions came directly from alchemic theories. For the history of antiaging, Bacon is most significant because he linked together Western ideas of alchemical chemistry with Eastern ideas of alchemical life force. Perhaps most importantly, he then communicated these ideas using a new modern scientific empiricism that broke free from both Arabic transmutation and Far Eastern animism. This modern scientific approach helped to legitimize the study of antiaging and bring it into the mainstream of science.

Bacon's Spirit

Francis Bacon began his book on antiaging by examining the forces that affect the body's exterior. He studied wood, rocks, and minerals and made connections between the factors that cause those substances to decay and those that cause them to be preserved. He reasoned that the human body would be affected in much the same way, and he paid particular attention to the effects of wind, rain, moisture, heat, and cold. He recommended people avoid hot or windy climates and stay nearer to cold and moist.

Bacon followed his study of inanimate substances with an overview of a broad range of plants and animals. Again, he hoped to identify any universal characteristics that could be tied to longer life (and those that might be tied to shorter lives). He studied hardness, shape, size, body temperature, how they obtained their nourishment, and how they reproduced. By examining plants and animals, Bacon concluded that tall trees, elephants, and birds live long lives, but small fruit-bearing trees, small animals, and cold-blooded animals do not. Similarly, he inferred that tall men live longer than short ones; that stronger men live longer than weak ones (due to the firmness of their skin); and that people with black or red hair live longer than those with white hair or skin. Moreover, holy men live longer than philosophers, who live longer than rural dwellers, who live longer than soldiers. In these characteristics, it was the nature of their food (more than their piety) that determined long lives.

Taken as a whole, Bacon concluded that living things differ from nonliving things in their ability to repair themselves. Objects with no life but with firm and dense structure will resist decay for a long time, but they will eventually succumb to wind and heat. Living objects are often softer, yet they also withstand these same forces because they repair themselves. For example, a human hand may become windburned, but after a few days, it will heal. In this way, life itself contributes to longer existence. Bacon recognized that the opposite is also true. Once the life force is spent, the body quickly becomes cold, and there is no longer any ability to repair itself. The once-living objects decompose more quickly than nonliving materials made of stone or wood.

As a Christian humanist, Bacon took for granted that the life force is eternal because its source (God) is also eternal. Life does not die on its own but must suffer from external causes. If cared for properly, Bacon argued that the fire of life "may be eternally preserved." As long as life remains, living bodies should be able to repair themselves forever. Unfortunately, though, Bacon also believed that the life force is both scarce and somewhat fragile. It could be consumed prematurely and is prone to weakening or dying from lack of nourishment or through some external force. The key to prolonging life, then, is to preserve the life force by preventing it from escaping the body and making sure that it is continually nourished.

Most of Bacon's knowledge of medicine came from ancient Greek and Roman theories that were passed along from Arabic scholars. Like Roger Bacon before him, Francis Bacon mostly accepted Aristotle's theory of radical moisture and innate heat as the qualities that keep bodies alive. As the heat cools down and the moisture dries up, bodies become old, and death became unavoidable. Francis Bacon's contribution was the introduction of a new substance called *spirit*. Rather than refer abstractly to a "life force," Bacon regularly called it *spirit*. He believed all the limbs, organs, and other parts of the body are kept moist and warm through the presence of spirits.

Toward the end of *The Historie of Life and Death* Bacon clarifies what he means by *spirit*. He did not mean a soul or some other abstractly divine life force. Instead, Bacon describes it as a "thin, invisible body, yet local, [with dimensions], and real." It is a little like air and water, and yet unlike both. It can be thick, yet it is always invisible. It can replicate itself. It does not consume the body's moisture, but it thrives in it and dies without it. It is from these spirits that youth is contained, and it is from their elimination that people get old and eventually die. It is man's ignorance of the spirit's physical nature that necessitates aging and death.

Taoist Qi in Christian Science

Referring to *spirit* as a physical substance becomes less confusing if we consider Bacon's theories in light of the Taoist idea of *Qi*. In China, the *Qi* was described as "breath," which was meant both literally and spiritually. The difference is that the Taoists explained their antiaging theories in terms of animism and minor gods that spanned the material and immaterial realms, while Bacon explained his theory in terms of physical (albeit invisible) substances that were bound by all the rules of the natural, material world. The fact that these spirits were invisible was unimportant; the air is not visible, yet we recognize it as a very real substance. Bacon was hypothesizing their existence based on observable effects.

What the Taoists described as *Qi*, Bacon renamed as *spirit*. What the Taoists explained as products of immaterial gods and demons, Bacon explained as a physical substance that could be captured, preserved, and nourished (as could any physical object). As spirits are physical substances and not deities, preserving them requires physical solutions: spirits escape through openings in the skin; therefore, Bacon recommended blocking their escape by developing firmer flesh to tighten the pores by applying greasy substances to the skin and by covering all open wounds immediately. These practices keep the spirits in. Rather than suggest incantations to ward off demons or impossible breathing exercises to retain the *Qi*, Bacon's recommendations involved physical solutions. Seek out cold climates with purified air and avoid windy locations that dry out the skin. Eat enough food to provide nourishment to the vitalizing spirit (and aid in self-repair), but also ensure you exercise enough to keep your skin (and pores) firm.

Bacon's antiaging handbook outlines other concepts that seem to have come from Taoist alchemy. When listing ways to perfect the body's ability to repair itself, he describes certain "cordials" that contain spirit-refreshing qualities. Among the most important ingredients of these are flakes of gold, followed by dissolved pearls, emeralds, or other clear gems. Other items, such as unicorn horn, hart's horn, and ivory are less useful but still beneficial. These ingredients do not come from Arabic sources, as Arabic alchemy never suggests the internal consumption of pure things to prolong life. But, they are the hallmark ingredients of Chinese elixirs.

Though Bacon does not refer directly to Taoism, he does discuss Chinese reincarnation in *The Historie of Life and Death*. He calls it *transmigration* and dismisses it "and other heathen heretical opinions" as products of confused reasoning because, as a Christian, Bacon believed the soul is immortal and therefore never requires regeneration. He dismissed the metaphysical culture from which Taoism developed, but he respected their observations.

By modern standards, Bacon's recommendations might seem simplistic, but they were quite scientific compared to East Asian (or even Arabic alchemy) standards. He transformed the concept of *Qi* from its animistic origins and rearticulated it in an empirical context. He could not invoke immaterial gods to explain the source of youth because that denied the reality of the material world operating under its own laws, which he explicitly believed in as both a Christian and a modern scientist. Nor could be speak of "life" or "energy" abstractly because these concepts could not be measured or tested. Instead, he hypothesized that a physical substance existed within the various parts of the body, and it was this substance that enabled flesh to constantly repair itself (and was the distinguishing characteristic between living and nonliving materials). He called that substance *spirit* because it was the closest analog in modern vocabulary.

Francis Bacon and the Seeds of Evolutionary Theory

Another important aspect of Francis Bacon's *Historie of Life and Death* was that it presupposed a connection between all living and nonliving things. His book also traces a relationship between animal biology and human biology. Some of these ideas of material unity came from the premises of Arabic alchemy, which presumed universal characteristics shared by all substances. But Islamic philosophy believed that life was entirely in God's hands and therefore not alterable. The other source of this unifying theory came from Bacon's Christian humanism, which presumed that God made the material world so that man might better understand his creator. This presumption meant that the natural world must reveal (even if hidden) some unifying signature.

For the 17th-century scientists, alchemy was not just about transmutation of metals; it was about discovering common principles of nature. This presumption of commonality eventually led to the theory of human evolution. As early as the 1630s, Francis Bacon never doubted the relationship between animals and humans. He assumed that the relationship was divinely ordained, but it was written into the laws of nature for human benefit. It was the religious convictions of Christian humanism that eventually led scientists to the theory of evolution. Ironically, it was the secularized theory of evolution that eventually led science away from religious convictions.

Vitalism and Mechanism

Bacon's idea of spirits is not entirely different from the ancient Greek physician Galen's theory of "vital forces," but it was applied differently to account for antiaging objectives. In the centuries after Bacon, most physicians retained some belief that a vital force (physical, yet invisible liquid or energy) was responsible for giving life to living creatures. This belief became known, generically, as *vitalism* and remained popular until the early 20th century.

The opposing view is called *mechanism*, and it denies the existence of any such life force and argues that living bodies are nothing more than machines built from and animated by organic materials. The mechanistic view developed later in the 19th century and was initially introduced as a way of examining biological physiology without having to consider the metaphysical implications of a soul. It arose during René Descartes's introduction of the mind-body problem. Later, however, the mechanistic positon became an essential part of a modern atheistic view of biology, as it denied the existence of a soul or spirit for anything, including man. Bacon would not accept such a view and so retained his belief in spirits.

René Descartes and the Mind-Body Problem

Francis Bacon's later contemporary René Descartes is most known for his contributions to philosophy (with his famous *cogito ergo sum*, or "I think, therefore I am"). Like Bacon, Descartes believed that all science should be based on demonstrable principles through evidence-based experiments and inductive reasoning. Unlike Bacon, Descartes went out of his way to dismiss ancient authorities and sought instead to create an entirely new system of learning. His famous quote *cogito ergo sum* is the answer to that quest. He wanted to find a first principle that required no proof (called an axiom) from which he could base all of his later arguments. As if by an epiphany, Descartes realized that the very fact that he was thinking about such things was itself proof that he was a thinking creature. From that point, everything else followed.

Descartes may be most known for his philosophy, but as a practical matter, he wrote considerably more on scientific subjects such as medicine, chemistry, and mechanics. One of the most well-known works during his lifetime was the *Treatise on Man*, which is a practical guidebook on human physiology. Descartes divided the practical sciences into medicine, mechanics, and ethics, and he devoted most of his studies to medicine.

To a large extent, it was Descartes's fascination with prolonging the human life span that drove his medical research. Like Bacon, Descartes was a firm believer that the new empirical approach to science would lead to longer, happier lives. In *Treatise on Man*, he wrote, "I believe it may be possible to find many very sound precepts for the cure of diseases and for their prevention and also even for the retardation of aging." This confidence was based on Descartes's conviction that human life should be examined in the same way that we examine other physical things. Rather than looking at life exclusively in terms of its role within God's plan of salvation, Descartes argues that we should consider it just "as distinctly as we know the various crafts of our artisans," and in so doing, "we might also apply them in the same way to all the uses to which they are adapted, and thus render ourselves the lords and possessors of nature."

It may sound as though Descartes was opposed to religion, but he remained a devout Christian throughout his life. One of his first objectives after discovering the first axiom (*cogito ergo sum*) was to formulate an argument proving the existence of God. Descartes did not intend to remove faith from the study of science, but rather to limit the scientific method to measurable sources of evidence that did not require faith to believe in. He did so as a Christian humanist who believed that God was as real as the natural world, even if he was not explicitly measurable in it.

For modern philosophers, Descartes is probably most known for his book *Meditations on First Philosophy* (1641), in which he argues that the mind and body are distinctly different things. The mind (or what we might call the soul) depends on the laws of God in the spiritual world and exists completely separate from the body. This is different from the body, which exists in the natural world and completely separate from the mind. It is a philosophical mystery to explain how the two separate realms interact, but that was not Descartes's intention. He merely identified the distinction as the "mind-body problem," and he provided mathematical proofs that they were distinct. The manner by which the mind influences the body is left completely at the will of God.

For Descartes, his proof for the mind-body problem provided hope in two ways. First, as the mind was completely separate from the body, theology, ethics, and metaphysical philosophy were also completely independent from the burden of empirical (measurable) proofs that would be required of any natural phenomenon. In other words, God does not require scientific proof for his existence to be understood. Likewise, though, the separation of mind and body also meant that the physical subjects, such as medicine, chemistry, mechanics, also do not require theological justifications for them to be proven true. They are each understood according to their own natures.

Descartes does not answer the mind-body problem. He poses the idea as a way of protecting certain doctrines of religious faith, such as God, the soul, and morality, from "those irreligious people" whom he believed doubted anything that was not explicitly proven with a mathematical formula. He wrote to refute the unbelievers. At the same time, though, Descartes opened the door for two centuries of future debate. How exactly does the immaterial mind effect the material body? If there is no connection, then either there are no exclusively material laws of nature or perhaps there is no such thing as a mind (or a soul).

It is this last conclusion that eventually created a break between science as a reflection of religious faith and science as a reflection of a new atheism. During the 17th century, Christian humanism accepted both science and faith as complementary components. By the end of the 19th century, the two components were seen as contradictory positions. The antiaging movement was caught in the crossfire.

Definition of *Science* in the 17th Century

In the early 17th century, roughly the time of Shakespeare, there were no obvious distinctions between science and philosophy. All learning, knowledge, and wisdom was identified generically as *science*. Those subjects that we call *science* today (chemistry, biology, geology, physics, etc.) were referred to as *natural philosophy*. Those subjects that we call *philosophy* today were referred to as *metaphysics*. At the time, there was little distinction between theoretical, practical, or applied studies. This was, in large part, because most people did not experiment or practice what they wrote about.

Up until the 1800s, theology and epistemology were frequently interwoven into works on chemistry, biology, and mechanics. Scientists were expected to be equally well versed in practical matters as they were in philosophy, literature, and the fine arts. It was quite common for books on scientific subjects, such as chemistry, to include poetry and other light verse as well as references to scripture and ancient philosophers.

An intellectual during the early centuries of the modern era (15th to 19th centuries) was expected to be proficient in almost all subjects. Today, we call such people *polymaths*, which means "someone who is an expert in several fields of study." The professionalization of academia brought an end to these trends. There is so much to know in each field that our modern intellectuals are not expected to know much outside the subject for which they have trained.

THE BIRTH OF SECULAR SCIENCE: FROM OVERPOPULATION TO EVOLUTION AND FREUD

From the start of the early modern era, religion and science were intimately connected by common interests. For the most part, faith and reason shared at least equal validity among most leading intellectuals. The new scientific method provided the mechanism for understanding the world, and faith provided the justification for why the world needed to be studied. During the 15th through 17th centuries, this union remained strong despite the increasing emphasis on empirical evidence and inductive reasoning during the scientific revolution.

Beginning around the end of the 17th century, the unity began to face challenges. New emphasis on inductive reasoning not only stimulated research in the natural sciences, but it also stimulated a broad reassessment of social priorities in general. Leading intellectuals began questioning everything—not just whether the sun or the earth lay in the center of our solar system, but why there should be monarchy as opposed to an aristocracy or a democracy. Scientists and philosophers both applied principles of the scientific method to solve social problems. Historians refer to this broad intellectual movement as "the Enlightenment."

The dynamic tensions that arose from Enlightenment philosophers challenging reigning monarchs threatened the happy union between faith and science, perhaps more than from any other movement. In England, most of the 1600s was marked by a constitutional struggle between aspiring absolute monarchs (James I, Charles I, and James II) and a rising Parliament that demanded equal rights and other constitutional protections. Political conflicts became religious conflicts, and the English Civil War (1642–1651) was as much about the power of the monarchy as it was about the power of dissident religious groups. Those outside of power often blamed the church for supporting those who held power, and growing conflicts over the role of religion in society followed suit.

England and its American colonies experienced their fair share of religious-political conflicts, but, overall, the success of constitutionalism quickly restored religious authority to its traditional place within science and academia. By the time of the American Revolution, the conflict was mostly political in nature, and religious conflict played a very small role. France, on the other hand, had been notoriously resistant to political change during the same 17th and 18th centuries, and this produced growing skepticism of religious authority among French intellectuals. By the time of the French Revolution, almost all of the political reformers vocally opposed religious authority (from the moderate Marquis de Condorcet to the radical Jacobin Maximilien Robespierre) almost more than they rejected monarchical authority. Out of such contests, the previously happy marriage between faith and reason devolved into an unpleasant divorce.

The Secular Progressivism of Marquis de Condorcet

The French aristocrat Marquis de Condorcet was born in France while the English Civil War raged across the channel. He was educated in mathematics at a Jesuit College and was accepted into the French Academy of Science when he was only 26 years old. Condorcet's family was quite prestigious, and he was a favorite among intellectuals who spent their time discussing fashionable ideas within the salons of Paris. He was friends with François-Marie Arouet, the French playwright, philosopher, and natural scientist who wrote under the name of Voltaire. It was from Voltaire and his like-minded acquaintances that Condorcet developed such a strong criticism of religious authority in both civic and personal relationships.

Condorcet was also friends with Thomas Jefferson, who lived in Paris for five years between the American Revolution and the French Revolution. Likewise, he befriended Thomas Paine, whose book *Common Sense* was instrumental in convincing many Americans to shift from reformers to revolutionaries in the months prior to the formal declaration of independence in 1776. When France erupted into its own revolution in 1789, Condorcet was strongly supportive and served as secretary of the legislative assembly. He tended to be more moderate than some of his colleagues, and his version of the French Constitution was eventually rejected in favor of the Jacobin version. After voting against the execution of King Louis XVI, Condorcet found himself out of favor with the more radical revolutionaries and was forced to flee to the rural countryside. Eventually, he was captured and arrested. He died in prison before his scheduled execution, possibly from suicide.

Despite his personal troubles with politics, Condorcet remained intensely hopeful for the future. While he was fleeing from the Jacobins, Condorcet wrote a book titled *Sketch for a Historical Picture of the Progress of the Human Mind*, in which he outlined a broad history of mankind from its earliest phases, when they lived in caves and were little different than the animals, to the present. He divided history into nine stages and identified key innovations of social, political, and intellectual development that had changed the course of civilization.

Condorcet viewed his present day of revolutions as a sort of gateway to a more perfect future, and he believed that in the 10th stage of history, mankind would become masters of nature. All nations would become equal and thereby eliminate the need for war. All social classes would become equal and thereby bring an end to poverty and corruption. And, finally, future scientific discoveries would enable man to overcome his own physical limitations, resulting in an end to disease, aging, and death itself. As he explained,

> Would it be absurd then to suppose that this perfection of the human species might be capable of indefinite progress; that the day will come when death will be due only to extraordinary accidents or to the decay of the vital forces, and that ultimately, the average span between birth and decay will have no assignable value? Certainly, man will not become immortal, but will not the interval between the first breath that he draws and the time when in the natural course of events, without disease or accident, he expires, increase indefinitely?

Condorcet met his own death at the age of 50, in the same year that he wrote those words.

Condorcet was extremely influential in the history of the antiaging movement for two reasons. First, he illustrates the intense hope and expectation of human progress shared among most of the leading intellectual reformers of his time. From such hope came a general confidence that all hurdles will eventually be overcome, even those that are seemingly dictated by nature, such as disease and the human life span. Second, Condorcet also provides an intellectual framework from which the theory of evolution emerges. Such belief in progress necessarily presumes that humans of the past were inferior to the humans of the present, just as the present-day humans will likely be inferior to those yet to be born. When applied to all animal species, the theory of progressive evolution is almost a natural conclusion. Such continuity between plants and animals and humans was already present in Francis Bacon's writings, and it became more explicit as the studies of zoology and human biology developed into more specialized disciplines.

William Godwin as the Radical Optimist

Condorcet was not alone in his intense optimism. Across the English Channel, the philosopher and playwright William Godwin published *An Enquiry Concerning Political Justice* (1793) during the same time that Condorcet was writing his historical *Sketch*. Godwin argued that mankind was already developing an understanding of personal morality that was beginning to render governmental authority and oversight unnecessary. He viewed the French Revolution as an example of individuals overthrowing a government that had grown tyrannical in reaction to growing expectations of individual freedom. The future world would see constant repetition of these revolts until such time as each government gradually faded away and a new, enlightened society emerged to take its place. Almost Utopian in his predictions, Godwin firmly believed that social and political evolution was occurring during his lifetime.

Like Condorcet, Godwin also predicted a time when medical science would progress to such a point that disease would be eradicated, old age would be cured, and death would lose its power over life. The power of the human mind and his intellect would control the forces of nature and the fate of mankind. As the historian Gerald Gruman explained, the late-18th-century optimism and the inevitability of conquering the effects of aging were based on three presumptions: (1) mankind would continue to improve environmental conditions to make the world a happier and more pleasant place to live; (2) future generations would inherit the knowledge (and traits) of their parents, resulting in comparatively rapid change; and (3) advances in medical society would continue unabated until all ailments were solved.

Thomas Malthus: Christian Opposition to Secular Progressivism

These ideas were held with most conviction by those radical thinkers who encouraged and helped facilitate the French Revolution. There were others, however, who equated such progressivism with political radicalism and philosophical atheism. The cleric and political economist Thomas Malthus strongly opposed the optimistic view of human progress and argued instead that the future might become more bleak.

Malthus grew up in the English countryside and then transferred to London around the same time as the Industrial Revolution and its massive influx of workers into the cities. He likened the harsh living conditions of the rapidly increasing urban poor to the plight of animals living in a hostile environment. Animals faced natural checks against overpopulation through starvation, disease, and natural predation. By contrast, human society worked hard to counter such checks, and in his *An Essay on the Principle of Population* (1796), Malthus argues that the rate of human population growth will inevitably offset the rate of food production. When times are plentiful, the population rises, but when resources become scarce, the same population will unavoidably fall into famine and disease. Malthus was not calling for policies that would permit massive starvation, but he did call for increasing the production of public resources.

The progressive optimism of Condorcet and Godwin seemingly ignored the consequences of unchecked development. Malthus added a subtitle to his essay on population that describes the book as an answer to *The Speculations of Mr. Godwin, M. Condorcet, and Other Writers*. At heart, Malthus was arguing against the proposed future where people lived to ages near immortality.

Godwin's answer to Malthus's objections was equally optimistic. He theorized that the minds of future men would become so sophisticated that they "would diminish our eagerness of the gratification of the senses," thereby making sex obsolete and future generations unnecessary. It was a Utopian answer, and the cleric Malthus retorted simply that sexual attraction and sexual relationships were good for mankind and should not be manipulated in an effort to control the population.

More specifically, though, Malthus rejected all three of the presumptions held by Enlightened antiaging advocates. His prediction of recurring famine and disease refuted the assertion that the natural environment of the world would ever be improved to such an extent as to have any meaningful impact on longevity (in other words, there would be no heaven on earth). He recognized that recent breeding practices among pet owners and gardeners proved that some change was possible within a species, but he maintained that there were natural limits to these changes. Malthus explained that you might be able to breed different colors of carnations, but you will never make them as big as a cabbage nor make a potato as large as a house. Finally, he recognized that the natural sciences were improving mankind's ability to control nature, but that sort of progress also had its natural limitations. The human life span was fixed by God or by nature, and no amount of medical discovery could alter that fact.

Malthus did not deny the general theory of progress that was inherent in Christian humanism. Instead, he was rejecting the radical implications of secular humanism to strip the laws of nature from its complementary laws of divine order, faith, and morality. Toward the end of his essay, Malthus writes,

> I cannot quit this subject without taking notice of these conjectures of Mr. Godwin and Mr. Condorcet, concerning the indefinite prolongation of human life, as a very curious instance of the longing of the soul after immortality. Both these gentlemen

have rejected the light of revelation which absolutely promises eternal life in another state. They have also rejected the light of natural religion, which to the ablest intellects in all ages, has indicated the future existence of the soul. Yet so congenial is the idea of immortality to the mind of man that they cannot consent entirely to throw it out of their systems. . . . What a strange and curious proof do these conjectures exhibit of the inconsistency of skepticism!

In other words, Malthus was saying that man needs God to make heaven: he cannot recreate it here on earth (even if his philosophy seems to demand it).

Malthus provided a religious balance to the rising tide of progress, but his overpopulation theory was harshly criticized by people of faith as well as the radical progressives. Certain Christian humanists complained that his picture of the future was too bleak and did not adequately consider that God always protects mankind and provides him with the tools necessary to overcome obstacles. They complained that Malthus did not take into account mankind's ability to devise new technological solutions for new scarcities of resources (through new agricultural revolutions, new methods of equal distribution, etc.). The radicals, like Godwin, criticized him from the opposite position and argued that Malthus was bound by the presumptions of a nonscientific faith. Ironically, Malthus's theories were eventually used most by later scholars who argued for completely secularized scientific humanism, particularly Charles Darwin and Thomas Huxley.

Lamarck's System of Categorization

The political disorder of the French Revolution threw intellectuals in France into great distress, both for those who supported it and for those who criticized it. Some very famous French scholars were executed because of political actions they had engaged in earlier in their careers, including Antoine-Laurent de Lavoisier and his wife, Marie-Anne Pierrette Paulze. Lavoisier supported the French Revolution and was widely renowned for his work in chemistry, including the isolation of 33 natural elements as well as for the introduction of the metric system to the revolutionary government of France (and indirectly to the rest of the world). Nevertheless, Lavoisier was guillotined by the Jacobin government because he had participated in tax farming (tax collecting) during his youth under King Louis XV. The political turmoil that infected French society only increased the tension of other forms of intellectual disagreement.

Jean-Baptiste Lamarck was from a relatively humble family who, prior to the French Revolution, had maintained a long tradition of military service. Lamarck served with distinction at his family's profession but was forced to retire early for medical reasons; he then shifted his attention to studying medicine and botany. He had a gift for organization and eventually published a very popular book that introduced a new system of classification for French plants. This work led to his being hired as a botanist for the king's gardens. During the French Revolution, Lamarck avoided persecution by changing the name of the gardens from *Jardin du Roi* (the King's Gardens) to *Jardin des Plantes* (Garden of Plants), which made the space seem more accessible to the French people. Lamarck was neither a radical nor a monarchist and preferred the neutrality of academic work, but he was not always successful in this pursuit.

Throughout the 1780s and 1790s, Lamarck published extensively on botany and herbology, but when the public gardens and accompanying historical collections were transformed into the French Museum of Natural History, Lamarck was transferred from botany to biology and placed in charge of the "animals without vertebrates." Applying his previous categorization skills to this new task, Lamarck introduced a new system of classification to zoology and continued publishing. During this time, Lamarck made significant contributions to the organization of animal genuses, which continue to be used today, including coining the terms *invertebrate* and *biology*.

At the same time, Lamarck also ventured into other fields, including meteorology, physics, and chemistry. Unfortunately, his resulting book on these subjects, *Hydrogeologie* (1802), was not well received. In part, this was because of the political tensions arising from his colleagues at the museum, especially from fellow zoologist Georges Cuvier. The two men worked together to systematically classify animals (Cuvier was in charge of vertebrate animals), and they organized the specimens in the museum's collection. Cuvier, however, was more politically savvy than Lamarck, and he managed to curry favor with Napoleon's imperial government both as an administrator and as a scientist.

Politics Influencing Scientific Debate

Tension between Cuvier and Lamarck became most pointed over their theories of geological history and the classification of certain fossils. Neither man accepted the rigid creationist account of the earth being formed in six days, though they both unquestionably accepted God's authorship of the world. Cuvier believed that the world had experienced numerous cataclysmic changes that had resulted in mass extinctions from time to time. He pointed to the fossils of extinct animals as proof of the periodic catastrophes that had changed the natural world (including such events as Noah's flood).

By contrast, Lamarck believed in a gradual development in both geology and biology and argued that the fossils were not from extinct animals but from previous versions of animals that are alive today. Lamarck rejected the idea of extinction entirely because it presupposed catastrophic changes and did not recognize how small, yet continual, changes might affect the world. For his part, Lamarck pointed to the examples of gardeners and pet breeders who manipulated strains of flowers and dogs to create a wide diversity of breeds within a very short period of time. What would happen to such changes if the time span was extended to many thousands or even millions of years? Lamarck eventually published these theories in *Philosophie Zoologique* (*The Study of Zoology*, 1809), and he was the first scholar to introduce the idea of biological evolution in a systematic way.

Lamarck faced continual criticism for these theories from Cuvier, which affected his relationship with the French government. One of the turning points in Lamarck's career occurred on a day when Napoleon came to visit the National

Museum. Lamarck attended and brought with him a copy of his book on zoology. One of the professors of the museum recounted that as the emperor passed before Lamarck, "the old man presented Napoleon with a book. 'What is this?' said the Emperor. 'Is this your absurd *Meteorologie* with which you are disgracing your old age? Write on natural history, and I will receive your works with pleasure. This volume I only accept out of consideration for your grey hair. Here!' and he handed the book to an aid-de-camp. Lamarck, who had been vainly endeavoring to explain that it *was* a work on natural history, was weak enough to burst into tears."

Cuvier later used the incident to mock Lamarck in a lecture hall full of students. The ridicule was too much for Lamarck, who was already very frail in his seventies and was slowly going blind. He retired to his home, where he was cared for by his two daughters. He eventually died penniless and dejected by the French academic community. At his funeral, Cuvier used the opportunity to deliver a eulogy that harshly criticized Lamarck and his theories as epic failures.

With no money for a proper burial, Lamarck's family rented a burial plot for five years, after which his remains were removed and subsequently lost among the countless other unknown bones in the catacombs of Paris.

Progressive Evolution

Cuvier believed in cataclysmic change over the course of geological history as well as the special creation of each individual species—not in the seven days outlined in Genesis, but in some fashion according to the wisdom of God as Creator. God created all species at once and then history took over. Similar to Thomas Malthus, Cuvier argued that there are biological limitations to the extent of change that can occur within a species. Dramatic change is impossible. If by chance, through natural heredity, some drastic mutation arose that attempted to change a core component of a species' internal biological system, the animal would simply die, and it would not be passed on. For Cuvier, the biological and geological laws of nature were more or less fixed by God's providential design, and no act of man or accident of chance could fundamentally alter it.

Lamarck did not disagree with God's hand in creation, but he argued that the evidence suggested some degree of constant change throughout history. For whatever reason, God used the evolutionary process of nature to produce man. For both scholars, the fact of God's authorship remained unquestioned, but the means and manner of the authorship were up for debate. For Lamarck, it was a logical conclusion: if we accept that the earth is much older than that accounted for in Genesis (millions of years rather than just 6,000 years), and the fossil and the geological records seemed to suggest that it was, we must also examine the entire process of creation in similarly broader terms. The creation of individual species need not all be accomplished in one day or at the same time. The key to the creation story was recognizing God's ultimate authorship, not the rigid details of how it came about. Lamarck had no difficulty in assuming that the creation of each species could occur over millions of years and yet still follow God's ultimate plan.

More importantly, Lamarck's theory of evolution fit perfectly into the growing intellectual consensus about progress. Lamarck was first and foremost an expert on classification, and it was during his classification of the flora and fauna in the Museum of Natural History that he developed his theories of biological progress. He could have chosen any number of ways of classifying the animals, including size, shape, or physical characteristics. Instead, he chose to organize them according to relative complexity of external structure, internal organs, nervous system, and emotional development.

In this era of intense progressive reasoning, it made sense to presume that the less complex creatures were earlier versions of more complex creatures, with man at the top of the pyramid. Lamarck unquestioningly accepted the necessity of God's hand in each act of creation; he just argued that it occurred first among the lowest organisms, and it occurred frequently. Lamarck explained creation as "spontaneous generation," which happens when inorganic materials become enlivened by a life force to become the most simplistic single-celled organisms. As his example, he pointed to the fact that single-celled organisms cannot survive harsh cold and must die during the winters; yet, every spring, still waters become alive with these simple organisms. From such organisms, all other species emerged. This sort of evolution did not deny the hand of God, but rather suggested a more complex natural system in which God revealed his hand through the process itself. As Lamarck explained, these principles "give a truer and higher idea of the Supreme Author of all existing things, by disclosing to us the simple method that he has adopted for working the wonders of which we are witnesses."

Lamarck began writing on evolution in 1801, which was more than 50 years before the publication of Darwin's famous book *On the Origin of Species* (1859). Yet, it is Darwin (and not Lamarck) who is most often credited as the father of evolutionary theory. The reasons for this are complex and much less historical in nature than they are social and religious. Unlike Condorcet or Godwin, Lamarck's view of historical progress still strongly depended on God to drive each successive transformation. Lamarck's evolution assumed God's involvement in both the direction and extent of biological change, regardless of how slowly it developed. The more radical voices of scientific progressivism rejected this idea because they did not want to accept any limitations that faith could place on human agency (for example, doubting man's ability to make any change to nature at will). Darwin is remembered instead of Lamarck not because he introduced the idea of evolution but because he removed the role of God entirely from its process.

Previous Christian humanists from as far back as Francis Bacon recognized a natural relationship between all created objects, the inanimate to the animate, as well as between animals and humans. Yet, such theories always took for granted that scientific knowledge was valuable because God wanted men to be happy and to improve their conditions in life. As Lamarck explained in his zoology text, the laws of nature are "only immutable so long as it please her Sublime Author to continue her existence . . . with a purpose that is known to its Author alone." Scientists may try to understand how the world operates, but Christian humanists believed it rested with theologians and philosophers to explain why.

In the new secular humanism, the question of why was not only unimportant but could potentially distract scientists from describing natural processes. Charles Darwin effectively removed faith (and God) from science by arguing that the most fundamental miracle of the natural world (the origin and development of life itself) was an accidental by-product of chance alone, with no purpose or intent at all. In this way, man alone was the only possible agent of deliberate change on earth.

Charles Darwin and *On the Origin of Species*

Charles Darwin was the son of an English doctor. His mother died when he was eight years old, and he shifted from medical school to seminary until he finally developed an interest in geology and biology—though he received no formal training in either subject. He became friends with Charles Lyell who wrote *Principles of Geology* (1830), which more systematically applied Lamarck's theory of gradual change to geological history. At the age of 22, Darwin joined a friend on a five-year voyage around the world, traveling westward past the southern tip of Tierra del Fuego.

Though initially enrolled by his father in a seminary for young gentlemen, Darwin had begun to doubt his belief in an active God years before he signed up for his naval adventure. In part, he struggled with the idea that a perfect God could make an imperfect world. Darwin was also heavily influenced by Lamarck's and Lyell's ideas of continual biological and physical evolution. If the world was changing, then at one time it was much less perfect. How could, or why would, God allow such imperfection?

During his voyage, Darwin observed the ichneumon wasp near Rio de Janeiro. The wasp lays its eggs inside living caterpillars to provide food for the larvae as they mature. To human eyes, it is a disgusting process, and the nature of such parasites so disturbed the young scientist that he concluded God would never have intentionally designed such a cruel system of regeneration. It had to have evolved through some other process than by God's divine plan. During the same stop, Darwin and his shipmates became embroiled in physical combat and were involved with an armed suppression of natives in Uruguay. The cruelty against the natives demonstrated by the Spanish ranchers caused Darwin to question the innate goodness of human nature. Perhaps goodness was learned and not natural?

The hardships of his voyages and his lifelong illnesses pushed Darwin closer toward his general skepticism of God and his hand in the world. Shortly after arriving home from his voyage, Darwin married his cousin and set about compiling his notes and observations. He came across the work of Thomas Malthus and concluded that without the rational interference of human ingenuity, the scarcity of resources and constant pressures of overpopulation inevitably created extremely hostile environments for irrational animals. Darwin was particularly sensitive to this idea because he had just lost his young son to scarlet fever; the harsh reality of the natural world seemed ever present.

Also around the same time, Darwin became friends with a new circle of intellectuals at Oxford University led by Thomas Huxley, who was vocally opposed to the political power of the Church of England and to any religious authority in academic science. It was Huxley who coined the term *agnosticism* to describe a belief that recognizes the possibility of God but contends that God has no presence on earth and is thus unknowable by any means. Darwin came to embrace these same beliefs and applied them to his earlier observations on biological diversity. When combined with his belief in the gradual change of geological history and his belief in Lamarck's gradual biological evolution, Darwin formulated a new theory of evolution that completely removed God from the process of creation. He called the process *natural selection*, and he published the fully developed argument in his book *On the Origin of Species* (1859).

Darwin was at home grieving over the death of his son when his theories on natural selection were first presented to the public. His friend Thomas Huxley, however, vocally defended the arguments before the more religious elements of Oxford University. Huxley had his own reasons for doubting the innate goodness of the natural world and the authority of institutional religion. Shortly after their marriage, his wife had been diagnosed with an illness that left her only months to live. The doctors were wrong. She lived another 50 years, but the period of uncertainty was extremely painful for Huxley. Also, shortly thereafter, his firstborn son died at the age of four. Huxley was something of a contrarian by nature, and he made a career out of fighting bureaucratic authority and was very talented both in public debate and in written arguments. He responded to Darwin's critics so forcefully that he earned the nickname "Darwin's Bulldog."

Four years after Darwin published *On the Origin of Species*, Huxley followed it up with his own affirmation of the theory in *Evidence as to Man's Place in Nature* (1863). Throughout his life, Darwin remained elusive and rarely presented his views to the public, except through publications. This was due both to his chronic illnesses as well as to his innate aversion to confrontation. By contrast, Huxley loved confrontation and forcefully promoted the idea of a natural world completely devoid of divine influence. He established contacts with academics overseas, and by the end of the decade, Darwin's theories had become widely accepted among intellectuals who were similarly drawn to secular humanism and its assertion that man and nature are solely responsible for any evidence of earthly progress.

Lamarck's Evolution versus Darwin's Evolution

A common misconception distinguished Darwin's evolution from Lamarck's evolution, which was based on the idea of the inheritance of acquired characteristics (meaning that children can inherit traits that were learned by their parents). Lamarck explained the growth of certain appendages, such as the length of an elephant's trunk or a giraffe's neck, as a result of muscular development during life. He theorized that giraffes began as horses, but through constant stretching to reach high limbs, they had passed along traits of elongated necks to their offspring. Perhaps, more importantly, Lamarck used the theory to explain the loss of certain physical structures, such as a tail (as in the case of most primates) or limbs (as in the case of a snake). If evolution involved continuous reactions to the environment resulting in small progressive changes over a very long period of time, it would be difficult to explain how a limb that used to be useful no longer became so. Just as the excessive use of muscles would lead to inheritable traits, so too Lamarck argued that the lack of usage would also be passed along.

The debate over whether learned traits could be inherited by offspring continued throughout the turn of the 20th century and persisted among biologists as late as the 1940s. Lamarck's primary theoretical contribution was the idea that biological species evolve and change over time, and his theory of learned traits was secondary to this larger idea. Nevertheless, as a result of the debate that spanned several decades, Lamarck's name was permanently associated with the lesser theory. Those who advocated the inheritance of any traits during an animal's lifetime were called "neo-Lamarckians." The discovery of genes and deoxyribonucleic acid (DNA) in 1953 largely ended that debate, with modern biologists staunchly rejecting the idea of inheritance of anything other than genetically defined materials. The force with which the scientists of the 1950s discredited the theory contributed strongly to Lamarck's lesser place in history.

The problem is that Darwin also believed in the inheritance of acquired characteristics. At several points, both in his notes on the subject in the 1830s and in his final publication in 1859, Darwin uses it to explain how some animals may lose certain organs or appendages. Perhaps not as blunt as Lamarck, Darwin argued that the extended use of certain muscles during an animal's lifetime could lead to more developed muscles in their offspring. He cited the development of specialized racehorses as an example. Darwin did not change this theory in his subsequent revisions of the text, nor in his publication of *Descent of Man* in 1871. In fact, the majority of scholars, from Francis Bacon to Ernest MacBride (*Embryology of the Invertebrates*, 1914), presumed such inheritance. After the discovery of hormones by Ernest Starling in 1905, it was popularly believed that the biochemical messengers could change the structure and function of certain organs and muscles. For Darwin, as with Lamarck, the theory of inheriting acquired traits remained secondary to his primary argument for biological evolution outside the will, intent, or influence of God.

The real difference between Lamarck and Darwin lay in the role that God plays in biological evolution. Modern evolutionary biologists who identify Darwin as the "father of modern biology" are not actually pointing to his theory of gradual biological development but are instead referring to his insistence that God played no role in the process. In 1976, the modern evolutionary biologist Richard Dawkins, who also became famous for his outspoken atheism, introduced his book *The Selfish Gene* with the observation that "it was Darwin who first put together a coherent and tenable account of why we exist." Rather than mentioning the theories of evolution, Dawkins explained that "Darwin made it possible" for scientists to answer the meaning of life without having to resort to religion.

Neo-Neo-Lamarckians in the 21st Century

Modern research suggests that acquired traits may be inherited after all. In 2010, a researcher at the University of Copenhagen, Romain Barres, observed that the offspring of rats that were fed high-fat diets were more likely to develop more fat than those whose parents were fed regular diets. Similarly, a neuroscientist from the University of Pennsylvania, Tracy Bale, also identified molecular changes in the DNA of sperm from male rats that experienced unusual stress. They concluded that environmental stresses on the parent may indeed alter the stress response of the offspring. Finally, in 2013, a molecular epidemiologist at KU Leuven University in Belgium, Adelheid Soubry, observed quantifiable differences in the genetic codes between children with obese fathers and children whose fathers were thin.

The underlying theme of the new research is that behaviors learned during adulthood may change the genetic makeup of sperm, which would then be passed along to the next generation. These conclusions remain controversial, but it is clear that the question of inheritance is not entirely closed. Since the 1940s, a new field of epigenetics has studied the various changes to genetic expression that occur without necessarily modifying the original DNA code. Recently, epigenetics has come to include changes of genetic expression that may loop-back to change the genetic structure itself. That latter field is essentially a study of Lamarckian inheritance.

The Legitimate and Illegitimate Children of Darwin

When René Descartes posed the mind-body problem in the 17th century, he hoped to protect the power of faith and religion from the growing empiricism of inductive science. Descartes strongly supported using experimental methods to test theories and build stronger theories. Yet, at the same time, he also believed in the reality of faith and God and his revelations through the church, which required no such physical evidence. His argument simply asserted that the mind (or soul) is distinct from the body, just as the material world is distinct from the immaterial world. Therefore, each realm has its own methods for discovering truth. Descartes was a devout Christian, but he also lived in an era when such faith dominated the intellectual community.

By the time of Charles Darwin, the Enlightenment and its subsequent political instability had already transformed the intellectual community from one that presumed faith to one that innately challenged faith. Huxley argued that faith should have no role in science, and Darwin removed the most difficult obstacle for scientific agnosticism: how do we explain where we came from? Through his theory of natural selection, Darwin argued that mankind arose accidentally through chance reactions with the environment and random variations alone. The Darwin and Huxley argument attempted to solve the mind-body problem by concluding that the mind (or soul) simply does not exist. The material world is a vast collection of material processes, and there is no room in it for an immaterial soul or divine will.

A growing number of scientists welcomed this secular humanism. In 1850, Herbert Spencer initially applied Lamarck's theory of biological evolution to social order and the free market. He argued that the best economic policies are those that include natural competition, which kills off the weaker, less successful businesses while reinforcing the stronger, more successful ones. When applied to philosophy, Spencer argued that ideas ought to live or die on their strength alone and should not be upheld by artificial claims to tradition. It was Spencer who coined the phrase "survival of the fittest," and Darwin used the concept to explain natural selection.

Spencer's sociopolitical theories were so frequently intertwined with Darwin's natural selection that the combined ideology was popularly referred to as "Social Darwinism." Numerous scholars supported the theories, including John Stuart Mill, John Tyndall, and William Graham Sumner (who held the first professorship in sociology). Political policy makers used many of these concepts both in support of and in opposition to governmental laws related to business, social welfare, and labor.

Similarly, Darwin's cousin Francis Galton applied the theory of natural selection to his own studies of aristocratic heredity. In 1869, he published *Hereditary Genius*, in which he argues that intelligence and genius are inherited traits. Galton did not distinguish between congenital and acquired traits but essentially argued that the poor are poor mostly because of their biology. Their natural deficiencies were compounded when the poor married and had offspring when they were unable to adequately provide for their families. This cycle of imprudent marriages led to a continual cycle of urban poverty.

Similarly, Galton argued that wealthy families were successful because of their biological makeup. They typically showed greater restraint in their marital decisions, which led to a continuance of their superior abilities. His theory became known collectively as *eugenics* (a term that he coined). Eugenic theories became wildly popular among intellectuals throughout Europe, England, and the United States. Charles Darwin's *Descent of Man* (1871) was largely written in support of eugenics theory. The ideology spread and resulted in a multitude of eugenics societies whose aim was to discourage "imprudent reproduction" among the lower classes and to encourage more intellectual coupling among the higher families.

Eugenics was popular because it seemed to promise even more progressive development for those who were already smart and well educated. Unfortunately, these theories were taken to their extreme by the German philosopher Friedrich Nietzsche, who argued that certain classes of men were naturally inferior to others and that human society generally supported the weaker elements out of misplaced compassion. Human laws and moral constraints are really just tools to protect the weak from those who are naturally stronger. Nietzsche said those sorts of rules and traditions go against nature. He argued that the superior sorts of people deserve to live outside the traditional rules of society.

In the 20th century, these eugenics ideas found explicit expression in the poli-cies of Adolf Hitler and other dictators who sought to justify their political author-ity. Eugenics was largely responsible for the Jewish Holocaust that occurred during World War II, which resulted in the deaths of nearly 10 million people through the systematic execution of "unworthy" classes. After World War II, the theory of eugenics was understandably abandoned by the intellectual community. Whether for positive or negative ends, the explicit secularization of science held enormous consequences for politics and society throughout the world.

Darwin and Freud Tackle the Mind-Body Problem

Darwin's theory of natural selection provided an answer to the origin of man, but it did not fully answer the mind-body problem. The problem was that Descartes's initial observation that "I think, therefore I am" had yet to be resolved. Scientists may dismiss the soul, or any other reference to a "life force" that animates living beings, but they had a difficult time explaining how and why people think.

One of Descartes's proofs for the existence of God was based on his assertion that man cannot conceive of an idea that he has no experience of. The fact that man even conceives of the idea of God proves that God must have created him with that idea in place. It is called an *ontological argument* and is circular in nature, and yet it also has no obvious refutation except by denying the premise that ideas come from specific experience. This is the heart of the mind-body problem, and though Darwin attempted to dismiss the mind as simply a biological entity, he did not actually solve the problem.

The mind remained a serious difficulty for mechanist biologists arguing that the body is nothing more than organized materials striving to replicate themselves. If that were true, how do we explain mental illness that seems to occur completely independently of physical stress? Within a generation after Darwin, a German psy-chologist named Sigmund Freud introduced a theory of the subconscious. The word *psychology* means "the study of the soul," and it became an emerging disci-pline during the 1870s in Germany and in the United States.

Often referred to as the "father of psychology," Freud is significant because he provided a science-based explanation for emotional and psychological disorders that had no obvious physical symptoms. In *Studies in Hysteria* (1895), Freud argues that most neurosis (mental disorders) can be traced to traumatic experiences that the patient experienced earlier in life but likely forgot over time. He argues that trauma is relative to what a mind already knows, so the experience of the birth canal, or of shifting from breast-feeding to solid foods, or of potty training might seem momentary to adults but could be massively traumatizing for an infant.

Between 1900 and 1903, Freud expanded this theory into a new field that he called *psychoanalysis*, his most famous work being *The Interpretation of Dreams* (1900). Fundamental to Freud's theory is the belief that individuals have no free will; they simply react to the constructs created during the first years of life. The sum of experiences as an infant and toddler determine the personality and emotional reactions later in life. In this way, Freud rejected the idea of an immaterial realm altogether and replaced it with an unknowable psychological realm that he called the "unconscious mind." It is from this unknowable state of mind that all of our concepts of the immaterial come from, including God, the soul, sin, guilt, and so on.

Freud argued that people do not choose to react or feel in one way or another; instead, they respond to the emotional patterns that were determined shortly after birth. In the new psychology, God and religion are mere artifacts of childish ways of thinking that emerge when individuals who lacked a strong fatherly role model as a child later satisfied that need by creating a belief in an all-powerful God. Feelings of faith are a psychological reaction to feelings of guilt and shame, which God promises to cleanse. According to Freud, God is not real but merely a projection of the subconscious mind.

Other psychologists took Freud's determinism and altered the idea for their own theories. The American John B. Watson published *Behavior: An Introduction to Comparative Psychology* (1914) and was followed B. F. Skinner, who wrote *The Behavior of Organisms* (1938) 20 years later. They both established the school of behavioral psychology, which took the rejection of the immaterial realm one step further by rejecting even the subconscious itself. For behaviorists, nothing in human biology, physical or mental, is immaterial. Humans are nothing more than advanced animals that respond to a complex collection of stimuli and responses. There is no free will, no human agency, and no mind-body problem because nothing exists that is not in some way measurable. Conversely, they also argued that if something is not measurable in some way, it must not exist.

For many agnostic and atheistic intellectuals, the new psychology seemed to answer the "mind" side of Descartes's famous problem. Not only was the human body not created by God, but neither was man's identity or even his faith. The idea of God was not planted by God; it was created by man to solve his own psychological deficiencies.

On a logical level, the determinist theory seems to refute the belief in progress because mankind cannot freely choose one alternative over another. Other logical contradictions also arose: How can psychoanalysis help to remedy neuroses that were predetermined by prior experiences? How would a patient ever choose to seek treatment, or successfully accept treatment, unless the decision to do so were already determined by some prior stimulus? Psychological determinism may also undermine the core presumptions of the growing antiaging movement. How can man continue to discover new scientific innovations that break the bounds of natural limitations if he is incapable of breaking beyond his own will?

Nevertheless, the new psychology provided a material answer for that which had always been viewed as an immaterial subject and was great comfort for those intellectuals seeking a scientific order removed from God. The mind-body problem was never really solved or refuted. Instead, the intellectual community no longer found the question as perplexing as it once was. Darwin provided an answer to the "body" portion by saying that man is not substantially different than any animal, and then Freud and Watson provided answers for the "mind" problem by arguing that it is nothing more than an animal reaction to the senses. It really did not matter whether the dichotomy was solved. By the start of the 20th century, most intellectuals had chosen to move on to other questions.

CONCLUSION

In the history of the antiaging movement, Darwin's agnostic approach to evolutionary biology was a watershed moment. In the centuries prior, Christian humanism had promoted the study of science as a means for making man happy and, ultimately, for better understanding God's hand in the world. The systematic pursuit of methods that could cure disease, alleviate the pains of aging, and significantly postpone death were all justified because long life meant more time to fulfill God's plan on earth.

There were many scholars who hoped for antiaging solutions, yet none of them actually sought immortality on earth. The goal of evading death entirely was unique to the Taoist faithful in China, and it did not survive well outside of its animistic homeland. It was not until the rise of certain radical views during the political revolutions of the 18th and 19th centuries that such extreme interpretations reemerged in the West. Fundamentally, Christian humanism believed the heavenly realm was always infinitely superior to the earthly realm. Immortality on earth meant permanent exclusion from heaven, which was almost the very definition of hell. The scholars of the early modern era sought longer lives, not immortal lives.

Figures such as Darwin and Freud changed the intellectual landscape by providing an explanation for scientific phenomenon that had previously been the domain of religion and philosophy alone. They were not the sole cause of its transition, but they and others were symptoms of the new secular humanism. The ideas that used to be limited to minority views among political radicals in the 1790s later became very popular among academics in a wide variety of disciplines in 1970s.

For the antiaging movement, secular humanism allowed scientists to pursue objectives that would have seemed Utopian in prior eras. Researchers uncovered increasingly complex operations in the fields of biochemistry, endocrinology, and pharmacology. Scientific progressivism continued strong into the 20th century, and there were few reasons to doubt the prospect that scholars would overcome almost any barriers of nature. If diseases were cured and the effects of old age treated, why should people die? The atrocities of World War II shook this progressive idealism, but the antiaging movement continued undaunted.

Evolutionary biology became the cornerstone of the modern antiaging movement because it seemed to affirm the theory that mankind had reached the pinnacle of its natural development. The more that scientists understand about evolution, the more likely they will be able to manipulate the environmental conditions that determined original limitations. As we will see in the next chapter, the antiaging champions of the 20th century strove to treat death as if it were a disease and to eliminate it altogether. This would not have been imagined by mainstream thinkers in the era before Darwin.

Chapter 4

Antiaging in the Industrial Age

The 20th century provided the motive, means, and opportunity for a new anti-aging movement based on practical medicine and an intense confidence in its success. American industry promoted a culture of technological and corporate efficiency that spread to all areas of society, inspiring new demands for medical breakthroughs that might cure disease and aging. The intellectual community responded with a pragmatic approach to innovation, which sought continuous discovery, development, and progress for its own sake. As a result, the rate of technological advancement doubled in increasingly shorter periods of time so that the reality of the 1990s surpassed even the imagination of 1890s dreamers. By the year 2000, many biomedical researchers believed the promise of genuine medical treatments for aging and death was just beyond their grasp.

Yet, the path of progress was inconsistent. The intellectual shift that swept the scientific community in 1900 was based on a genuine belief that scientific discovery is always good and that unchecked progress will lead to a better, more humane society. The optimistic faith of the progressive movement took over politics, academia, and the business community. Breakthrough discoveries of germs and hormones promised revolutionary treatments for ailments that seemed impossible to combat only a half century earlier. At the same time, other discoveries in mechanical combustion, explosives, and poisons rendered military combat more lethal than it had ever been. The outbreak of two world wars and a massive economic recession caused even the most optimistic progressives to rethink their confidence in modern technology.

During the first half of the 20th century, scientific research took for granted that science and faith are mutually incompatible areas of discussion. Religious doctrines have no place in scientific research. Yet, the complete isolation of science outside of religion led to horrific political and military atrocities in Nazi Germany, Communist China, and the Soviet Union. For those who rejected faith and religion as archaic inventions of the human imagination, these horrors could not be explained, and the reality of human progress was rejected. For those who retained their religious faith, the innate value of isolated science was suspect. The 1950s saw both an increase in scientific determinism as well as an increase in Christian humanism. Evolutionary biologists who proclaimed themselves avowed atheists seemed incapable of avoiding questions of man's ultimate purpose. Many argued for a new set of moral principles based on evolution alone (without God) to guide society toward more humane practices. Scientific philosophy continued to reject religious interference, yet their arguments often imitated patterns of religious faith.

Intellectual confidence in mankind's ability to improve his living conditions was shaken, but not destroyed, by the horrors of war. New breakthroughs in understanding the endocrine system led to a pharmaceutical revolution during the 1950s and 1960s, and the advent of computing technologies continued to promise innovation in biomedical research. The scientific community broke into two diverging groups: those who no longer believed in human progress and feared the effects of human development (skeptics) and those who had become even more convinced of mankind's ability to make permanent changes to the world and to life itself (neo-progressives). Within the intellectual community, these two sides were more or less evenly matched. Yet, in society at large, the demographic pressures of a growing baby-boomer generation tipped the scales toward the neo-progressives. The youth of the 1960s and 1970s wanted to change the world, and many of them were convinced that it was possible to do so in monumental ways, even if that meant changing the course and direction of human evolution.

The antiaging movement's primary critics were skeptics, who feared that the increasing human dominance in the world could undermine the ecological balance, and religious humanists, who doubted it was possible (or desirable) to create heaven on earth. Yet, the movement found strong support among those neo-progressives who believed evolution had brought mankind to a new threshold of life in which all the old barriers of disease and death were to finally be overcome. It also gained support among the multitude of aging baby boomers facing middle age who were willing to spend a great deal of money on the promise of extending their youthful vitality. By the dawn of the 21st century, the combination of the scientific and popular forces prepared the antiaging movement for unprecedented attention.

PROGRESS AND THE INDUSTRIAL MACHINE

American historians generally refer to the period from 1900 to 1915 as the "progressive era." The dates are fluid, depending on how you define *progressive*, but usually the period starts with the rise of politicians seeking to capture a new urban constituency. Republicans such as President Theodore Roosevelt and President William Howard Taft described themselves as progressives, but so too did Democrats such as President Woodrow Wilson. Cities were booming, and local leaders needed to find ways of solving new urban problems, from sanitation and public safety to housing and public transportation. Change was visible everywhere, and the cultural tone of the times was filled with the promise of continual progress.

The progressive era extended beyond politics, though, and reflected the rapid technological innovations that emerged following the Civil War. In the 1880s and 1890s, a business revolution integrated distribution and efficiency to build transnational corporations of unprecedented wealth. Other technologies in transportation and communication changed daily life as the automobile, telegraph, radio, and moving pictures provided new ways of sharing information, ideas, and entertainment. At the grassroots level, social change was apparent everywhere. The sense of progress that had captured the intellectual community since the 17th century had thoroughly captured popular culture in the 20th century.

Progressive politicians heavily relied on university scholars to lend their expertise to solving the social problems of urban living. Community neighborhoods were studied by sociologists; law enforcement practices were reformed by criminologists; programs for the urban poor were initiated by social workers; and public health was protected by new agencies regulating food and drug safety. Public education for both youth and adults became a national priority. In the process, the scientific community became less theoretical and more pragmatic.

William James and Pragmatism

Charles Darwin and Sigmund Freud effectively removed God from science and biology and created a new contest between faith and reason. Darwin's contribution went largely unchallenged, and the debate over evolution continues to be framed in those terms today. Freud's contribution, however, was not equally satisfying. Darwin's evolution reflected the idea of human progress, but Freud's scientific determinism did not. If man had no free will, how could he change his conditions or his life? A third figure, William James, whose career spanned medicine, psychology, and philosophy, provided a more satisfying solution for progressives looking for a new intellectual approach to the problem of free will. During his lifetime, William James's influence and popularity was challenged only by Charles Darwin.

William James was the son of an eccentric theologian who socialized with other unconventional American writers, such as Ralph Waldo Emerson, Henry David Thoreau, Louisa May Alcott, and Walt Whitman. He grew up in a household that believed in God and yet rejected most religious institutions of his time. His brother, the famous novelist Henry James, described himself as a "realist" and continued to criticize organized religion throughout his life in his own writings. For his part, William James wanted to believe in God, but he found it difficult to reconcile his faith with the increasingly popular scientific determinism. After graduating from Harvard Medical School in 1869, James faced an emotional breakdown that stemmed from a sense of life's meaninglessness. If Darwin were right, and there was no intention behind life, then what was the reason for living? James was momentarily suicidal, but he eventually drew himself out of his depression by reading the philosopher Charles Renouvier, who argued for individual free will. James concluded that the decision to believe in free will was itself an act of will. Likewise, his decision to be happy or to find personal meaning was equally his will.

In the years that followed, William James taught physiology at Harvard, but he quickly moved into the emerging discipline of psychology. He offered the first psychology classes in the country and eventually wrote *The Principle of Psychology* (1890), which served as a foundation for later research in the subject, including the introduction of the nation's first psychology laboratory. James soon shifted his interest from psychology to philosophy, and together with Charles Sanders Peirce, he founded *pragmatism* as a new philosophical school of thought. He published a number of books on the subject, including *The Will to Believe and Other Essays in Popular Philosophy* (1897) and *Pragmatism: A New Way for Old Ways of Thinking* (1907). James's classes were always filled to overflowing, and his ideas were hugely influential on later scientists such as Albert Einstein, Niels Bohr, and Bertrand Russell.

The essential element of pragmatism was that it restored the possibility of free will to philosophy, and it provided a pathway for religious belief within a world-view that was inherently secular humanist. James tackled the mind-body problem by arguing that ideas (the mind) are only meaningful if they result in practical changes. Individuals should measure truth according to whether the idea works and not according to an abstract standard. As such, he believed that philosophy ought to be geared toward specific actions. He did not reject the mind, but he believed that the pragmatic impact on the body was all that really mattered.

This theory of pragmatism satisfied both the atheists and the people who yearned to reconcile their scientific empiricism to their personal faith. James did not argue that there is an immaterial realm or that God exists. Instead, he argued that a personal belief in God gives meaning to people's lives; therefore, the meaning is real, and their belief is real. Truth is defined by the choice to believe. Conversely, for those who did not believe, they could find meaning in some other source. As long as the idea is meaningful to each individual, the idea is real. Philosophical consistency was not important to James.

Pragmatism provided an intellectual foundation for the continuance of progressive hope. With free will, mankind could still use science to change his conditions (rather than remain bound by them). William James was opposed by some religious thinkers, such G. K. Chesterton and Henri Bergson, both of whom believed that the immaterial world is as real as the physical world, regardless of whether we believe in it. They argued that truth is defined by those standards and not by our own. Bergson in particular criticized pragmatism as a way for scientists to mask their religious convictions (or atheism) as a scientific conclusion without the need for following traditional philosophical methods (or consistency). Nevertheless, for the modern scientist bent on discovering all that science has to offer, William James provided a convenient compromise.

New Science: Germs

Meanwhile, the academic community was making tremendous breakthroughs in medical science. During the 1830s, the Italian biologist Agostino Bassi researched the causes of Italy's failing silkworm industry. The prevailing theory of the time was adapted from Georges Louis Leclerc de Buffon's and Jean-Baptiste Lamarck's theories of spontaneous generation, which argued that sometimes new life spontaneously emerges on dead materials. If that were true, there was nothing to be done about treating the silkworm disease. Bassi devoted 25 years to the subject and eventually discovered that the disease is carried by microscopic organisms that spread from creature to creature through physical contact. Treatment consisted of removing the infected worms and isolating them from the healthy ones. Bassi is credited with saving Italy's silkworm industry.

Ten years later, the French biologist Louis Pasteur built upon Bassi's research to study the process of fermentation in the hope of saving his country's failing wine industry. His contemporaries believed fermentation occurs spontaneously through internal transformations of elements within the wine. Pasteur managed to identify several microorganisms responsible for the process and helped to prevent the spread of diseases through "bad wine" by simply heating the liquids to a temperature that kills the bacteria (up to 100 degrees)—a process that we now call *pasteurization*. Later, Pasteur applied the same theory of invading microorganisms to combat farmyard diseases and eventually developed an anthrax vaccine for herd animals in the 1880s. As early as the 1860s, Pasteur's research directly influenced Joseph Lister, the British surgeon who used the ideas to develop antiseptic practices to kill germs during internal operations. He discovered that the survival rate of amputations using such practices rose from 55 percent to 85 percent.

The field of bacteriology was then formally launched by Robert Koch, the German physician who studied the anthrax cycle and discovered the bacteria responsible for cholera and tuberculosis. He earned a Nobel Prize in Medicine in 1905. By the end of the 1880s, these men had proven that most diseases can be attributed to a specific microorganism, and that microorganisms can be studied independently in a laboratory. Given enough research into their life cycles, the weakness of each microorganism might be discovered, leading to eventual cures. The germ theory provided great hope for those who believed that aging and death are mostly the result of increasing diseases.

New Science: Steroids and Everlasting Youth

The idea of microorganisms (germs) being responsible for disease led other researchers to theorize that there are other microscopic chemical compounds that operate within the human body. One of the major questions of the day was how the internal organs manage to work in harmony with each other when they are all physically separate. About midway through the 1800s, French physician Charles-Édouard Brown-Séquard conducted extensive research on the nervous system and discovered that the spinal cord is primarily responsible for the transmission of information related to sensation and feeling from the outer parts of the body to the brain. Brown-Séquard theorized that the information is passed along by means of a special chemical, which he had yet to isolate. He suspected that the chemical had its origins in the sex organs and developed a theory that connected sexual maturity with aging and death.

Brown-Séquard was an extremely prolific researcher who contributed more than 500 articles to the field of medicine. He taught at the École de Médecine in Paris and at Harvard Medical School in Boston. He also worked as a respected physician in London and New York City. Toward the end of his career, however, Brown-Séquard seriously jeopardized his reputation with the introduction of a new theory on the prolongation of life. In the late 1880s, he presented a paper to the Biological Society of Paris that claimed he had discovered the "elixir of life."

Based on his belief that the master chemical responsible for sustaining all the organs of the body is contained in the sex organs, Brown-Séquard theorized that life is maintained and animated by whatever it is that the sex organs produce. Similar to Francis Bacon's theory of spirits, he thought the vitalizing force was physical and might be isolated in the same way that microorganisms can be isolated from various diseases. He noted that sexual vitality is directly connected to the life cycle: youths maturing into adults became sexually active, and as they lost their sexual vitality, so too they lost their youth. Brown-Séquard concluded that if science isolated the substances from the sexual organs, perhaps age could be deferred indefinitely.

The "elixir of life" was composed of tissues extracted from the gonads of a variety of living animals, including guinea pigs, dogs, lambs, and so on. The animals were sedated while Brown-Séquard used a syringe to extract materials, which he then pulverized together in a mortar and filtered multiple times into a serum. He injected that serum into his own body as a test subject in the hope of revitalizing himself. According to his own accounts, the injections gave him more energy. He was in his seventies when he began this research, and after only a few days of taking the injections, he found he could work longer days in the lab and stand for longer periods of time without resting. News of his results spread around the world, but the scientific community was more skeptical. More than a few cases surfaced of toxic reactions when others tried to replicate the procedures. Perhaps more damning, however, was the fact that Brown-Séquard himself died about five years after his initial presentation, at the age of 77.

In hindsight, we now know that Brown-Séquard was only half wrong. It is true that the sexual organs produce a substance that is directly related to increased energy and vigor. Today, we know it as the hormone *testosterone*, and it is the primary source of anabolic steroids illegally used by athletes to enhance performance. It does indeed help to stimulate muscle growth and endurance if used in conjunction with specialized training practices. Unfortunately, later researchers required 40 pounds of bull testes to produce just 20 milligrams of viable material, so the small doses created by Brown-Séquard were likely not effective. He felt more energetic because he wanted to feel energetic.

Brown-Séquard was not without his influence. Within a decade or two, his theory of special chemicals that communicate between organs was confirmed by a British physician, Ernest Starling, who eventually coined the term *hormone* to describe the chemical messengers that travel through the bloodstream and the nervous system to relay information throughout the body. Just as each disease was suspected of being caused by a particular microorganism, researchers started searching for the particular hormones that were unique to each organ. This research took most of the 1920s, 1930s, and 1940s to complete, but the result was a revolution in endocrinology. By the end of the 1950s, drug companies had learned how to synthesize these chemicals, producing a subsequent revolution in the pharmacology industry.

New Science: Germ Cells

Around the same time as Brown-Séquard, the German zoologist August Weismann introduced a theory of "germ-plasm." Weismann was heavily influenced by Darwin's theory of natural selection and studied the possible pathways of development between single-celled organisms and their more advanced mammalian cousins. His research had a lasting impact on both biomedicine and on the antiaging movement. Specifically, he studied single-celled life-forms and concluded that they are immortal. Individually, they divide and replicate, but collectively they do not appear to change or age. They do not exhibit any symptoms of *senescence*, which means the loss of vitality related to aging. Unless acted upon by some outside force (such as an accidental change in environmental conditions), Weismann concluded that single-celled organisms do not die naturally.

As more advanced animals all exhibit senescence, Weismann concluded that the onset of aging and death must have been introduced to life-forms through the process of natural selection. In an early essay titled "The Duration of Life" (1881), Weismann explained, "I consider that death is not a primary necessity, but that it has been secondarily acquired as an adaptation." He argues that the human life span is therefore determined by the need for reproduction. If an individual dies before he or she has reproduced, the species may become extinct. Likewise, if the individual dies before the young are capable of caring for themselves, the species may also falter. Yet, after the young successfully reach the age for reproduction, the parents are no longer necessary. The longer people live, the more likely they are to succumb to some sort of affliction (illness, disease, or other). Death, therefore, was introduced by natural selection as a means for clearing away the previous generation so that the newer generations can best thrive.

This evolutionary explanation for death held both positive and negative implications for antiaging. On the positive side, if Weismann were correct and the existence of death was added to life-forms as a chance reaction to environmental conditions through the process of natural selection, it might be theoretically possible to live without death. He wrote, "It must be admitted that we can see no reason why the power of cell-multiplication should not be unlimited, and why the organism should not therefore be endowed with everlasting life."

The negative aspect of the evolutionary acquisition of death is that any alteration of human senescence would require scientists to overcome the combined pressures of the natural environment. Weismann theorized that the bulk of human cells have limited capacity for cellular replication because they are only intended to protect the germ cells up to the time when they can reproduce. The soma (body) cells evolved to be a protective container for the germ (egg) cells and are more or less disposable, as they face the harsh conditions of the natural environment.

Most cells of individual bodies are prone to wear and tear, which eventually leads to senescence and death. The life of the species, however, continues indefinitely through the reproduction of each subsequent body. Extending individual human life would therefore take substantial biomedical intervention to increase the soma cell's capacity to reproduce.

Metchnikoff—Death Should Not Be Frightening

Although Weismann was relatively cautious in his predictions, there were others who were solidly optimistic. The deputy director of the Louis Pasteur Institute in France, Élie Metchnikoff, believed that extending the human life span was possible and inevitable, given the current state of scientific discovery. Metchnikoff, who was born in Russia, was personally invited to the French institute by Louis Pasteur. He made a name for himself by studying the cell's natural ability to fight off disease through the use of phagocytosis, which is a process by which foreign substances and hostile microorganisms are engulfed by living cells and destroyed or consumed. Metchnikoff's work on cellular immunity earned him a Nobel Prize in Medicine in 1908, and he is sometimes called the "father of natural immunity."

Like many of his contemporaries, Metchnikoff could not resist applying his scientific knowledge to the field of philosophy. In 1904, he published *The Nature of Man*, which is essentially a summation of progressive thought from that time. In it, he argues that, throughout history, man has been predisposed by natural selection to view his natural world with hostility and pessimism. Life is filled with hardship, struggle, disease, old age, and death. Yet, recent discoveries in the field of the biological sciences had opened up new reasons to be optimistic. Metchnikoff's research into the cell's autoimmune reactions gave him hope that most diseases could be eradicated through proper research. As old age is mostly a result of wear and tear caused by disease, he also believed that old age could be radically limited through proper care. If those two fears were addressed, death would eventually lose its meaning. He did not predict immortality, but he believed the life span could be extended long enough that its eventual end would be embraced as a natural event. With such biomedical breakthroughs, Metchnikoff believed that everyone would have a chance to embrace life for its own meaning and not as a constant flight from disease and death.

A few years later, Metchnikoff expanded these ideas in *The Prolongation of Life* (1908). He had compiled all the current research of his time to create this practical guidebook for extending human life and ensuring meaningful existence. Using current theories of microorganisms, hormones, autoimmunity, and evolutionary theory, Metchnikoff opened his book by explaining that almost all diseases are the result of specific microbes invading the body. Borrowing Weismann's assertion that death is not necessarily natural, Metchnikoff then argued that old age is not natural but reflects symptoms of a long-lasting disease. White hair, weakened muscle tissue, and the loss of energy are all symptoms of a constant war between invading diseases and phagocytes trying to protect the body. Over time, the normal wear and tear of the conflict leads to senility and death.

Metchnikoff argued that natural selection resulted in the creation of a variety of organs in the human body that served a particular use against a particular threat in the natural environment at a particular period in history. Unfortunately, as the environmental conditions changed, those organs remained intact because there were no reasons to be rid of them. These legacy organs added to the resource load that taxed human vitality. Metchnikoff believed the stomach and the large intestine had really been designed for herbivores, but when mankind evolved into flesh-eating animals, these organs were less suitable. The result was that human-kind carries around more fecal matter than is good for the body. The microorgan-isms that feed off the putrid matter in the large intestines spread throughout the body, forcing the autoimmune system to constantly fight their toxins. Over time, he argued, the struggle exhausts the body's resources, and it slowly breaks down into old age and finally death.

The solution, therefore, for extending human life is to fight the microbes that dominate the vast cavities of the large intestine. Metchnikoff suggested ingesting countermicrobes from acidophilus to strengthen the phagocytes and delay the wear and tear from the autoimmune reactions. He also suggested avoiding red meat, eating more yogurt (or other foods with probiotics), and avoiding foods that cause constipation. With some proper precautions, individuals might be able to retard the effects of old age immediately.

By treating old age and death as if they were a disease rather than a natural end to life, both Weismann and Metchnikoff opened the door for later scientists to discover ways of "curing" the disease. For most of the early 20th century, antiaging researchers held these theories as ultimate objectives for goals set far in the distant future. There was less hope for immediate results in the short-term, but there was constant hope that these objectives might eventually be met through long-term scientific discovery. In this way, the purpose of biological sciences could be found in practical results and not through intangible objectives of faith and religious conviction.

THE CHALLENGE TO PROGRESSIVISM

American historians generally set the end date for the progressive era as 1915, which is just about the time that war erupted in Europe. Initially, the conflict was seen by most Europeans as a necessary release of political tensions that had been building since the end of the last century. They believed it would result in a short war and an adjusted (or corrected) balance of power. In fact, however, World War I lasted four years in Europe, primarily because both sides were more or less evenly matched by military technology. Over the course of the war, 16 nations mobilized 65 million soldiers with machine guns, motorized artillery pieces, airplanes with high explosives, and poisoned gas, leading to 8.5 million deaths and 21 million wounded. The use of poison gas was especially troublesome to medical scientists who witnessed the deliberate use and effects of aggressive microorganisms against other humans. The collective optimism of progressivism was challenged by the obvious reality that scientific innovation could be used just as easily to destroy life as to preserve it.

The culture of progress was further assaulted by the failure of the victorious nations to find an equitable peace that would lead to more democratic principles for world governance. Woodrow Wilson's dream of a League of Nations ruled by law and not by force crumbled under the weight of a peace treaty, which seemed to reward the already powerful empires of England and France and unfairly punish their competitors of Germany and Austria. The United States rejected the treaty and the League, not once but twice, out of fear that it would be used to sustain a system of alliances based on a constant threat of military retribution. The 1920s were marked by twin forces promoting cultural reform (through the Eighteenth and Nineteenth Amendments) and undisciplined vice (through the Jazz Age, beer wars, and a booming financial economy). When the economy collapsed during the 1930s and dictators took over the bulk of European governments, the intellectual community faced a difficult challenge in finding progress and enduring cultural success from mankind's recent innovations.

World War II provided the greatest assault on the spirit of human progress because it demonstrated horrific abuse of evolutionary theory and secularized philosophy. Adolf Hitler's eugenics programs were implemented with totalitarian efficiency, but they were not unique. Since the time of John Galton, Herbert Spencer, and the publication of Darwin's *Descent of Man*, eugenics theory had become fashionable among most leading intellectuals. It reflected the natural by-product of progressive thought by applying scientific objectivity to human relations. Like breeders of prize racehorses, the best elements of society were encouraged to be highly selective in their breeding practices, and governments were encouraged to provide incentives for equitable unions and disincentives for less desirable ones. Quite apart from Germany, eugenics societies also popped up in England, France, and the United States. In the United States alone, the American Eugenics Society boasted members from academia, industry, and politics. In the 17 years between 1905 and 1922, 18 states passed laws designed to limit "irresponsible breeding" of criminals and other "feebleminded" members of society. The Supreme Court upheld these laws in *Buck v. Bell* (1927), in which Chief Justice Oliver Wendell Holmes justified the forced sterilization of a woman with the words, "Three generations of imbeciles are enough."

Adolf Hitler's regime implemented these enlightened principles with grotesque efficiency, resulting in the systematic murder of nearly 10 million individuals who were deemed unworthy and threats to the social order. For decades, many progressive scientists had encouraged their colleagues to break free from religious traditions that placed man as a unique creature endowed by God with special purpose and gifts. They argued instead that man was nothing more than a complex animal that should be studied without regard to moral or theological expectations. Unfortunately, the horror of Nazi Germany did exactly that. The Nazis stuffed other humans into cattle cars and slaughtered them like unwanted herd animals. Images of piled bodies following the liberations of concentration camps in Poland screamed an insult against humanity and further illustrated the larger cost of the war.

In six years of conflict, 45 nations had become directly involved in the fighting, resulting in 15 million soldiers killed and 25 million soldiers wounded on the battlefield, with another 45 million civilians killed off the battlefield. Almost 100 million people lost their homes and were forced to move elsewhere. The extent to which science and technology were used to destroy human life and human civilization suggests that man's greatest obstacle is not the natural environment but his own decision making. Perhaps nature is more at risk from man than man from nature.

Reinhold Niebuhr and the New Christian Humanism

During the era of the two World Wars, much of the intellectual community was torn between a desire to keep science and technology free from religious oversight on the one hand and an equal desire to see social progress toward goals that were traditionally viewed as religious ends (peace, justice, and goodwill toward men). Blunt atheism seemed too harsh in light of recent totalitarian governments, but orthodox religion seemed too restrictive in light of modern science. A new sort of Christian humanism was needed to find a balance between secular science and religious conviction. Within the intellectual community, the liberal Protestant minister Reinhold Niebuhr gained great influence.

Niebuhr wrote more than a dozen books and countless essays. He advised policy makers in the U.S. State Department and was greatly regarded by professors in almost all academic fields. He described himself as a "Christian realist" and argued that society was better because of its faith. He applied pragmatism to theology and concluded that faith provides hope to mankind, and without faith the belief in human progress is lost. In his 1949 book, *Faith and History*, Niebuhr argues there is no difference between simple faith and "blind faith"—if you possess a little, you believe in all of it, and most people hold some belief in an unseen immaterial realm. Science provided mankind with the knowledge of the world, but it was faith that made use of it. Using an analogy of a man behind the wheel of a car, he explained that it was science that brought about knowledge of how to create the vehicle and how the parts of the vehicle worked. It was from the lessons of faith, however, that man learned how to drive with caution, in a way that conforms to the safety and well-being of the community. Humanity needs faith to ensure social order.

The new Christian humanism differed from its previous iteration because it was much less "Christian" and more "religious minded." Niebuhr was a Protestant minister, but he focused more on the ecumenical ties that bind all faiths together (such as Judaism and Christianity) than the specific theological doctrines that may separate them. In this way, his lack of orthodoxy gave comfort to some intellectuals who may have preferred agnosticism but opposed its political and moral implications. Scientists and other intellectuals embraced Niebuhr's theology because it did not require much but still provided a way of keeping both faith and science in the same philosophy.

Julian Huxley and *Religion without Revelation*

Other intellectuals also found inspiration from Reinhold Niebuhr, even those who steadfastly maintained their agnosticism (or atheism). The central message of the new Christian humanism was that there is a core set of religious principles that ensure human progress. Without these, the atrocities of Hitler or Stalin might seem almost inevitable, and human progress would always be in doubt. Niebuhr's arguments, however, were so broadly based that they were conducive to any religion—which meant that they were also conducive to no religion. Following this line of thought, Thomas Huxley's biologist grandson Julian Huxley wrote a number of books arguing for a new religion without God at all. He called it a "religion without revelation."

Like his grandfather, Julian Huxley strongly supported Darwin's theory of evolution, including all of its secular implications of a world completely removed from God and divine purpose. Yet, like Niebuhr, Julian was also traumatized by the horrors of world war and came to strongly believe that mankind needed to agree on some basic principles of social justice and moral order. Following World War I, he wrote *Religion without Revelation* (1927) in an attempt to restore some sense of moral order to a modern scientific world. After World War II, he repeated the call with the 1950 essay "New Bottles for New Wine," which makes the same basic argument. Julian Huxley firmly believed in the necessity of a new consensus that extended across national borders. He strongly supported the United Nations' *Declaration on Human Rights* and became the first director of the United Nations Educational, Scientific and Cultural Organization (UNESCO).

Huxley argued that religious faith is beneficial to society, even if it is contrary to his scientific faith. His younger novelist brother, Aldous Huxley, held a more cynical view of the world, which is reflected in his 1932 novel *Brave New World*, in which the future is controlled by a tyrannical government that uses drugs and other technologies to continually pacify an unambitious public. For Julian, though, the future held great promise, and he remained steadfast in his progressive optimism.

In the early 1950s, Julian Huxley explained, "In our Western World the myth of progress has now fallen on evil days. It was attacked by many writers on the grounds that the idea of progress cannot be reconciled with the retrogressions of Fascism and Nazism and the horrors of the recent war." He continued with the observation that "the patient labors of the students of evolution, whether stellar evolution, biological evolution, or social evolution, have revealed that progress is not myth but science, not an erroneous wish-fulfillment, but a fact . . . [and] the scientific doctrine of progress is destined to replace not only the myth of progress, but all other myths of human earthly destiny. It will inevitably become one of the cornerstones of man's theology." Julian Huxley's optimism came from a new way of interpreting evolution.

According to Darwin's theory, each species evolved according to its reaction to environmental conditions, which resulted in promoting various characteristics during sexual reproduction. As long as species remained dependent on nature, they would continue to change. Since before the dawn of the scientific age, mankind had slowly become a master over nature. As Huxley explained, "The human species is now the spearhead of the evolutionary process, the only portion of the stuff of which our world is made which is capable of further progress."

For Huxley, this meant that man can choose the manner by which he continues to evolve. He believed religious faith emerged as a coping mechanism to explain the mysteries of the world, but as man revealed the science behind each mystery, he no longer needed a traditional religion. Instead, he should consciously seek out all the benefits that traditional religion provides and then apply them to a new atheistic faith based on scientific progress.

Following the pragmatic philosophical approach, Julian Huxley explained, "If we wish to work towards a purpose for the future of man, we must formulate that purpose ourselves. Purposes in life are made, not found." He added that in the new science-based religion, mankind should stop putting "off the responsibilities that are really his on to the shoulders of mythical gods or metaphysical absolutes." In the postwar world, Huxley believed that the first responsibilities were to find a common consensus on social justice and the proper balance between state support and individual liberty. Once civil order is maintained, science will be able to achieve unparalleled discoveries, including overcoming such traditional enemies as disease, old age, and death.

George Gaylord Simpson and Progressive Skeptics

Other evolutionary biologists were less optimistic than Julian Huxley. George Gaylord Simpson was a paleontologist at the American Museum of Natural History who studied the migration patterns of large mammals from many millions of years ago. He applied evolutionary theory to explain the changes he found in both the flora and fauna collections and engaged in on-site archeology in South America to further his research. After the war, Simpson became a professor at Columbia University and published a book on the social implications of Darwin's evolution titled *The Meaning of Evolution* (1949). Unlike Huxley, Simpson found no place in evolutionary biology for progress. In his words, "It is a childish idea—but one deeply ingrained in our thinking." He explained, "Progression merely in the sense of succession occurs in all things, but one must be hopelessly romantic or unrealistically optimistic to think that its trend is necessarily for the good."

Part of Simpson's opposition to the idea of progress arose as an unavoidable implication from life evolving without any sense of divine purpose. Apart from the pragmatic usefulness of religious morality, Simpson argued that there is absolutely nothing "real" about it at all. Evolution is cold and unmoved by sentiment, compassion, or free will. Biological organisms simply adapt to conditions; they do not choose to evolve up or down. Our very definitions of upward or downward

The History of the Earth in 24 Hours

It is difficult to fully appreciate just how long a billion years is, yet evolutionary theory uses that unit of time frequently. One way to make the context more meaningful is to set the history of the earth within the framework of a 24-hour day. Within that ratio, the earth was completely lifeless until sometime between 4:00 a.m. and 9:00 a.m. (about 740 million to 1,840 million years), when the first organic molecules must have formed. Scientists theorize that it was not until 2:00 p.m. (nearly 58 percent of earth's history, or 2,635 million years) that the first ingredients of organic molecules formed into the first single-celled algae. At that point, life seems to have accelerated. Organisms that were capable of sexual reproduction appeared around 6:00 p.m., with seaweed, jellyfish, and trilobites appearing during the last half hour before 9:00 p.m. Plants appeared on land just before 10:00 p.m., and dinosaurs roamed just before 11:00 p.m. The first mammals appeared at 11:30 p.m., and humans emerged a little more than a minute before midnight.

According to evolutionary theory, for more than 91 percent of earth's history, there was no life outside of the oceans. The time between life on land to the present represents just over 0.08 percent of the total time since the earth was formed, or just over 2 hours and 8 minutes of a 24-hour day. Half of that time was devoted to the origin of dinosaurs. Evolutionary theory usually speaks in terms of billions of years, but as a ratio of the entire process, mammalian life only represents 21 minutes, or 0.0145 percent, of a 24-hour day—just 200 million years. Modern humans may not have witnessed very much at all of the entire span of earth's history, but they have been present during a little more than 3 percent of mammalian evolution—which is about 45 minutes if mammalian history were converted into a 24-hour day.

progress are meaningless to life. From this perspective, Simpson argued that for all practical purposes in terms of progressive hierarchy, mankind is no different from a tapeworm. They both adapted to environmental conditions and thrived as a result.

In part, Simpson's view is also a reaction to the eugenics arguments that preceded World War II, in which leading scientists argued that mankind is at the top of the evolutionary ladder. Tyrannical governments used the theory to justify forced hierarchies between humans and encouraged selective breeding toward an ever-higher goal as both necessary and good. Following the Nazi Holocaust, such conclusions were obviously offensive. Rather than blaming the absence of common religious moral restraints for these ideas, Simpson blamed the arrogance of an "anthropocentric" definition of progress.

Silent Spring and Deep Ecology

Initially, World War II caused many former progressives to question whether man is at the top of the evolutionary ladder. After a generation had passed, skepticism found fuel from other sorts of biological injustices related to the natural environment. The conservation movement emerged at the same time as industrialization began to alter the physical landscape during the late 1800s and 1900s. For the earliest pioneers of this movement, such as Theodore Roosevelt and John Muir, the goal of conservation was to preserve the wilderness because its natural beauty is a treasure that should not be wasted before future generations had an opportunity to admire it. Conservation was more of a reaction to the ugliness of industrial sprawl than it was about ecology. The conservation movement changed just around the time of World War II, after the Wisconsin forester Aldo Leopold introduced the concept of wildlife management as a separate discipline in biology. In his work, Leopold stressed the importance of biological diversity for both privately owned farms and pastures as well as for government-owned lands. The idea of environmental ethics implies that human development is not acceptable if it comes at the cost of environmental integrity.

The new ecological worldview inspired science writers of the 1950s who were already questioning the reality of human progress. During this same time period, the pharmaceutical industry underwent a revolution of biochemical understanding that resulted in a constant stream of new medicines, drugs, and chemicals intended to improve daily life. Penicillin prevented infections, cortisone helped to reduce swelling, and the tranquilizer meprobamate altered mood swings. By the end of the decade, scientists had discovered an anabolic steroid capable of inhibiting conception, which meant that a simple oral pill could prevent pregnancy.

Unfortunately, the rising drug culture also led to some tragic deaths. The drug thalidomide was designed as a non-habit-forming sedative, but it was later shown to cause serious birth defects when taken by pregnant mothers. By 1962, the United States had passed the Food, Drug and Cosmetic Act, which added a host of regulatory controls over the pharmaceutical industry as a public safety measure.

Also in 1962, nature writer Rachel Carson published *Silent Spring*, which warns of the impact of dangerous chemicals on the environment. Immediately after the war and throughout the 1950s, Carson had written books on the mysteries under the sea and the interrelationship between birds and fish and other oceanic life. By the dawn of the 1960s, Carson had become more concerned about how chemicals affect the environment. She was particularly concerned by the effects of dichlorodiphenyltrichloroethane, or DDT, which was a pesticide widely used to kill a variety of insects.

The chemical was recognized as an insecticide by Paul Hermann Müller in 1939 and used as an antimalaria and antityphoid tool during World War II. Müller earned a Nobel Prize for his lifesaving discovery in 1948. Yet, Rachel Carson argued that DDT not only killed insects but left a lasting impact on an entire chain of organisms, including plants, birds, animals, and even humans. Not only did the indiscriminate killing of insects alter the animal populations who fed on them, but the poison accumulated in animal tissues, resulting in secondary diseases. Carson's book was a national best seller and inspired a wave of public support for more stringent environmental regulations, including the eventual formation of the

Environmental Protection Agency in 1970, and the federal ban on consumer use of DDT in 1972.

In part, the new environmental movement reflected growing skepticism in human progress. Evolutionists may debate whether man represents the pinnacle of human evolution, but the new sensitivity to ecological balance suggested that humans may be unavoidably detrimental to other organisms. In 1972, Norwegian philosopher Arne Naess introduced the idea of "deep ecology," which is a worldview that seeks to fundamentally alter human society to better accommodate other plants and animals that share the same environmental system. Though he supported short-term solutions such as recycling and pollution controls, Naess proposed long-term solutions in which mankind restructured society so that its interests were kept in equal priority with the interests of other life-forms.

Though Naess never described himself as misanthropic (against humanity), his theories were used by numerous public advocacy groups that saw humanity as an inherent threat to the global environment. Such groups as Zero Population Growth contend that consumption of the earth's resources by an increasing human population disturbs the ecological balance. Other groups, such as Earth First, engage in proactive demonstrations to limit human development and lessen the ecological presence in the world. Such arguments not only question the idea of human progress but also assert an alternative theory of human devolution. From the perspective of such worldviews, the prospect of prolonging human life or potentially avoiding human death would not be seen as progress but as an ecological disaster.

THE RETURN TO PROGRESSIVISM

Cultural awareness may have challenged the sense of human progress as a biological certainty, but, ironically, it also promoted the goal of social and political change. One of the other effects of World War II was a boom in new births. From 1945 to 1946, the number of new babies increased 25 percent, from 2.8 million to 3.5 million, and this rate of population growth continued for more than a decade. As a result of this "baby boom," the 1960s was dominated by a disproportionately large group of youths between the ages of 18 and 25. Their sensitivity to political and social problems greatly accelerated the civil rights movement and also led to further increases in antipoverty programs. Public reactions to intentional and unintentional consequences of economic, social, and technological progress largely defined the decade.

Many of the new community action programs and public advocacy groups of the 1960s may have appeared to be pessimistic in nature. Environmentalism, feminism, and anticapitalism all suggest that, if left unchecked, humanity tends toward repression and abuse. Yet, these movements also presumed that public action might make a difference. Baby boomers joined marches and protested social conditions because they felt that they could make a positive change if they worked together. This optimistic outlook differed very little from Julian Huxley's advocacy for a new global consensus on peace and human progress.

Evolutionary biologists may have debated larger questions of human progress over the course of millions of years, but most of the social activists of the 1960s and 1970s believed that human society could change for the better if enough people cooperated in the effort. The horrors of World War II may have threatened the optimistic outlook within the academic community, but the youthful idealism of the baby-boomer generation ensured that the popular belief in human progress remained strong. The academic community was not unaffected. Many of the ideas that arose during the 1890s reappeared with new scientific expressions in the 1970s.

Baby Boomers and Gerontology

The 1960s opened with a renewed scientific interest in old age and the possibility of deferring death. In part, it may have been a result of the growing baby-boomer generation that was just reaching its late teens. The pressure would not have been from the boomers themselves, but from their parents, who were increasingly interested in the future world that the boomers would inherit. One such father, Robert de Ropp, was an English biochemist who migrated to the United States immediately after the war. At the age of 45, he wrote *Man against Aging* (1959), which was one of the first books on gerontology.

After outlining the symptoms of aging, which included both benefits (intelligence, wisdom, caution) and detriments (weakness, forgetfulness, senility, eventual death), de Ropp explained that there were really only three areas of scientific research devoted to aging. The first area included research into the biological problems associated with aging and how medicine might be used to delay their effects. The second area included research into the clinical problems of aging and how to treat the diseases once they affect the individual. The third area related to social problems associated with aging and focused on ways of making society more helpful for the aged. In light of the booming generation that was just then reaching maturity, de Ropp concluded that these fields of research were extremely important and yet currently underdeveloped and requiring more attention.

The second and third fields of gerontology were more practical by nature. Doctors should research ways to treat older bodies, and governments should look into better ways of keeping senior citizens involved in the community. The first field, however, was more speculative; it dealt with the very old dream of antiaging. It was exciting in its purpose but not often viewed as a practical subject. For his part, Robert de Ropp was not very hopeful that science would discover a solution to old age. In his 1959 book, he wrote that death is "inexorable, inevitable, inescapable. It is as much a part of life as is growth and development, the descending portion of the great arc of which growth and development are the rising portion. Living things can no more escape aging than a stone, thrown in the air, can escape falling back to earth."

For all his pessimism about antiaging goals, de Ropp was nonetheless very influential in the movement. His attention to the deficiencies of gerontological research inspired action in the academic community. In 1960, there were no institutions dedicated to any of these three areas of research, and there was almost no research money. The situation changed relatively quickly, though, and before the decade was out, several medical universities had introduced special fields in gerontology. In 1974, the National Institute on Aging was formed under the umbrella of the National Institutes of Health. By that time, the baby boomers were beginning to enter their thirties, and issues of aging had grown more important. Though medical care and social welfare remained important, the truly exciting areas of research lay in the dream of evading age and avoiding death.

Rebirth of Weismann

Bernard Strehler wrote *Time, Cells, and Aging* in 1962 as a progressive answer to the growing number of skeptics in this field. He framed his book around a synopsis of August Weismann's evolutionary theories on the germ and soma cells, beginning with a definition of life in biological terms. Strehler, like Weismann, argued that life is defined as any set of chemical systems capable of reproducing themselves. This definition rejects the notion of soul, spirit, or other life force—life is purely mechanical and is defined by biochemical interactions. Strehler added a point, though, by saying that these chemical systems also "make use of energy and matter from their environment to produce more of themselves."

The difference between Weismann's argument and Strehler's is that in the time between 1906 and 1962, biochemists had discovered deoxyribonucleic acid (DNA) and had a better understanding of chromosomes and the process of genetic inheritance. His explanation in *Time, Cells, and Aging* brought Weismann's argument up to date.

In addition, Strehler is most famous for incorporating the concept of entropy into biochemistry. Thermodynamics is a branch of physics that studies the interrelationships between heat, matter, and energy. The first law of thermodynamics states that energy cannot be created or destroyed in a closed system. The second law of thermodynamics (entropy) states that some amount of energy is always lost when moved from one state to another or from one system to another. The basic idea is that energy does not multiply on its own, and unless it is replenished from an outside source, energy is always gradually lost through action over time. Strehler used the concept of entropy to explain aging.

The idea was not completely original. Strehler essentially adopted Francis Bacon's theory of aging (itself modified from Aristotle), which argued that life is based on inner heat and moisture. As we age, we lose the heat and moisture, and our organs eventually lose their vitality. Bacon believed that life is animated by physical spirits that inhabit the muscles and organs. Strehler did not believe in vitalism, so instead of spirits, he argued that living objects are animated by simple energy gained from the surrounding environment through some sort of ingestion.

Single-celled organisms find and absorb fuel directly from the matter that is around them. But, these organisms are also vulnerable to changes in their immediate environment and are prone to die from any number of natural accidents. As a defensive measure, most multicellular organisms developed protective layers around themselves (the soma cells, or bodies) to protect their more fragile replication systems (the germ, or egg cells). For these more complex creatures, food must pass through the body to reach the replicating cells. As the organism loses its ability to replenish its internal energy through outside fuel, the body will die, along with its internal replicating system. Fortunately, by that time, the organism's germs cells have already passed on through replication, and the organism lives anew in a different body.

From a strictly mechanistic definition of life, it is only the replication of the germ cells that really matter to the long-term life of the organism. In strict terms of evolutionary biology, the outer shell that is created and replaced from each individual to another is meaningless.

These theories are in direct contrast to Christian humanist or other vitalist theories. Typically, we think of ourselves as individuals, with personal identities and human thought. In short, we usually define the uniqueness of life by the uniqueness of each person's soul. If our soul leaves the body, we are dead, even if the body continues to pump blood and oxygen to the brain. In the mechanistic views of Strehler and Weismann, human identity and emotional uniqueness have nothing to do with the basic function of life, which is simply to replicate.

This seems rather depressing for those "outer shells" who have evolved the ability to think and ponder about philosophy (humans, that is). Yet, Strehler was a progressive. He used these biological theories to argue that the future of even the individual bodies was ultimately hopeful. Like Weismann, he believed that death of the body was an adaptation that evolved as a reaction to a harsh environment. Instead of letting the accidents of the world kill the germ (DNA) cells, the organism periodically lets its temporary body suffer the bulk of the accidents, while the DNA is safely passed on to another carrier body. For Strehler, that meant that there is no biological reason why the body could not continue, through the use of technology, to resist natural accidents and ultimately avoid death. In 2001, Strehler explained, "My simple view is that aging is those things that go wrong when cells lose their ability to divide. . . . If we could replace our cells as rapidly as they deteriorate, we could probably live very long, if not indefinitely."

After hearing news of Strehler's death in 2001, the director of the Alzheimer's Disease Research Center at the University of Southern California, Caleb Finch, wrote that Strehler's book "inspired me as a graduate student, and huge numbers of other scholars and scientists to take this new field of biogerontology seriously." Back in 1960, the disillusionment that followed the World Wars had pushed some elements of academia into a pessimistic worldview that questioned progress, the future, and even life itself. Yet, the new baby-boomer optimism needed more promise of hope. For many young evolutionary biologists, Strehler provided a pathway for meaningful discovery. His book provided inspiration for a generation of gerontological researchers who saw the potential of unlocking the genuinely monumental secrets of life and death.

Dawkins and *The Selfish Gene*

Scientific atheism and genetic determinism can be tricky for progressives because they suggest that human free will is more or less inconsequential to the basic progress of evolution. In essence, it assumes that life has no innate meaning. This was the same struggle that led William James into suicidal despair in the 1870s. At the same time, that struggle led William James to the conclusion that pragmatic philosophy allows students to separate what they are unable to prove from what they want to believe. During the 1950s, young evolutionary biologists may have thought that life had no innate meaning, but that did not prevent them from inventing their own meaning as an act of free will. That was the essence of Julian Huxley's conclusion when he proposed creating a new religion out of evolutionary science. He wanted the modern world to intentionally choose a meaning for life based on brotherhood and goodwill. In the 1970s, such pragmatic philosophy took on new expressions and energized the progressive antiaging movement once again.

In 1976, a young zoology professor named Richard Dawkins published *The Selfish Gene*, which is a mixture of biological and social commentary. On its most obvious level, Dawkins provides a layman's explanation of evolution using essentially the same concepts as Wiesmann and Strehler. He explains how the most important function of life is for the genes to find ways to keep reproducing. From that perspective, he describes each organism (including man) as a "survival machine." The particular vehicle (or body) that the genes are wrapped in are of less importance than the long-term survival of the replicating genes.

The title *Selfish Gene* was intended to convey two points. First, it argues that evolution occurred at the genetic level and not at the level of the genetic packaging (the body). The gene is innately selfish because our DNA does not aspire toward anything more than avoiding danger and reproducing. Any other trait or characteristics that mankind exhibits (such as altruism) comes from cultural learning and not from any innate predisposition. Second, the title implies that, from a biological perspective, life is nothing more than continuous genetic replication, which means that any question about the transcendent meaning of life is inherently futile.

Dawkins rejected religion and faith, but he believed strongly in the power of individual free will. Beyond the biological issues, one of his main purposes for writing the book was to argue that society should choose for itself what sort of moral altruism to endorse and support. In the book's conclusion, he explains that "even if we look on the dark side and assume that individual man is fundamentally selfish, our conscious foresight—our capacity to simulate the future in imagination—could save us from the worst selfish excesses of the blind replicators. . . . We have the power to defy the selfish genes of our birth." Dawkins believed that human life is more or less accidental, with no innate meaning, but he was not a biological determinist.

Dawkins argued that our genetic predispositions do not provide any guidance for morality or altruism. He begins his book by explaining that "one of the dominant messages of *The Selfish Gene* . . . is that we should not derive our values from

Darwinism, unless it is with a negative sign. Our brains have evolved to a point where we are capable of rebelling against our selfish genes. The fact that we can do so is made obvious by our use of contraceptives." His point is that our genes only seek replication, and yet contraceptives are a deliberate rejection of our natural desire to replicate.

Dawkins did not believe in a soul or in any divine plan for mankind, but he did not want to abandon hope in mankind's ability to affect significant changes, not only in politics but in evolution itself. He was an avowed atheist who devoted much of his time speaking on the need for atheists to be more proactive in their advocacy for removing all remnants of religious thought from education and public forums. At the same time, he recognized the value of altruism and social equality. Like Julian Huxley before him, he believed that if mankind were to arrive at any sort of shared principles, it had to do so deliberately and without relying on traditional definitions of faith, religion, or the supernatural.

In terms of strict biological evolution, Dawkins was not really progressive because he did not believe that any one gene set was particularly better or more developed than another. At the same time, his belief in individual free will meant that mankind could determine its future and perhaps even change the course of evolution. In his final words, Dawkins explained, "We are built as gene machines, . . . but we have the power to turn against our creators. We, alone on earth, can rebel against the tyranny of selfish replicators." This change in thinking was essential for any future antiaging movement to take hold within the community of evolutionary biologists.

CONCLUSION

The science behind the modern antiaging movement is mostly propelled by evolutionary biologists, biochemists, and gerontologists who actively study the mechanical process of the human body in search of some way to delay or avoid senescence. The changing outlooks and philosophies of such scientists play a significant role in the seriousness and legitimacy of the effort to prolong human life. By the end of the 20th century, most of the dominant voices within the field of evolutionary biology believed that humans had no souls and that there was no such thing as life after death. As such, one of the historic obstacles to pursuing immortality on earth was removed because there was no fear that anything would be missed by not dying. For others with less clearly defined views of spiritual life, the attraction of the antiaging movement is less about avoiding death and more about maintaining consistent health.

False Dichotomy between Faith and Reason

The belief in human progress suffered a great deal as a result of the two World Wars, but it reemerged in a slightly different form in the youthfulness of the baby-boomer generation. The progressives of the 1900s may have included both Christian humanists and secular humanists; both sorts believed that there was a higher and more transcendent end that the world was progressing toward. Mostly, their definition of progress was philosophical in nature, and that is why both the Christian and secular humanists often shared the same language and values when describing the future of mankind.

In the 2000s, progressivism had changed. No longer linked to the language of the previous Christian humanist tradition, contemporary postwar secular humanists framed the future of mankind in terms of human choice and collective consensus. Scientific research as well as human behavior became more frequently justified according to pragmatic results and individual preference rather than by transcendent standards of morality. Hope for the future, though, remained strong. Rather than following Julian Huxley's dream of a new sort of morality based on scientific religion, the new progressives hoped for more worldly objectives: longer life, eradication of disease and poverty, and eternal youth and vigor.

This pragmatic materialism alienated some, though not all, of the Christian humanists. They feared that secular humanism had permanently altered the natural sciences and especially those fields that tend to deny specific purpose for mankind, such as deep ecology and evolutionary biology. A false dichotomy between faith and reason intensified and impacted the antiaging movement significantly by forcing it to the side of atheism and agnosticism.

Some of the more fundamentalist Christian groups oppose biological evolution precisely because of its association with atheism, and in so doing, they also reject scientific efforts to use technology to prolong the human life span and avoid death. In some cases, these groups are also distrustful of traditional medicine altogether and prefer alternative homeopathic solutions instead. This opposition is often welcomed by those scientists who are openly atheistic; they dismiss the religious-based criticisms as anti-intellectual and antiscience. For these sorts of secular progressives, the antiaging movement provides a promise of practical salvation as a pragmatic alternative to an immaterial heaven. A third middle ground of more traditional Christian humanists still recognize the intrinsic value of scientific discovery, but they remain unwilling to let science define or alter their faith. For this latter group, the antiaging movement is supported when it seeks to improve the quality of life on earth and is generally opposed when it seeks to evade death as the ultimate objective.

A Pew Research poll from 2013 indicates that about 60 percent of religious Americans believe advances in antiaging medical technology are good because they allow people to live healthier lives. The same poll indicates that only about half that number (30 percent) support using such technology to extend life to an average of 120 years.

The Fear of Aging and Death

Antiaging science and technology of the 21st century is mostly moved forward by those scientists who remain skeptical of life after death and who tend to doubt that anything exists outside the material world. Within the popular culture, though, there are a host of other less philosophical reasons why people may support the antiaging movement. Those who love the pleasures of youthful vigor will likely support anything that extends youth and delays death. One of the effects of a more secularized society is that people often do not think about such final questions as the meaning of life and what happens after death. Instead, the focus is more on entertainment, exciting experiences, and more immediate gratification. In this way, the prospect of eternal youth is more appealing than the traditional satisfaction of wisdom and accomplishment promised in old age.

Hollywood movie stars and other cultural icons promote youth and beauty as goals in themselves. As communication technology increased in the latter half of the 20th century, so too did the power and influence of the entertainment industry's ability to define power and beauty. Beauty is young and vibrant, and often not natural.

Several opinion polls conducted by women's magazines in 2010–2012 indicate that most Americans would undergo plastic surgery if it was an economically viable option for them. In some cases, as many as 70 percent of women wanted such surgery. The number of teenage girls undergoing plastic surgery increased 28 percent from 2011 to 2012. The invention of social media seems to have played a role in these decision-making processes. One study reveals that the number of women who wanted plastic surgery increased 31 percent after viewing unfavorable pictures of themselves posted on the Internet. In another poll, 35 percent of women aged 40 and over believe plastic surgery should be free and included under any national health care plan.

In addition to a growing desire to look young and beautiful, there also seems to be a correlation to the decline of religious faith and the fear of getting old and suffering debilitating handicaps before death. A 2001 study conducted by Victor G. Cicirelli indicates that those who do not believe in life after death are more likely to fear death. For those who do not necessarily fear death, they may fear the suffering that might accompany the process of dying. Another Pew Research poll in 2013 notes that 60 percent of Americans do not want to live past age 90, and 30 percent do not want to live past age 80. For most of these respondents, their hesitancy is based on a fear of running out of money and not being able to care for themselves in the manner they are accustomed to. The other major fear is that age-related diseases will cause suffering and dependency on others.

Despite the general fears of old age and dying, a 2014 Pew Research poll indicates that most people are optimistic about scientific and technological progress; nearly 60 percent believe that dramatic and substantial changes will occur before the year 2065. Of those that are more pessimistic about the future, the most common explanation is their fear that science will alter human DNA in an attempt to make future generations smarter, healthier, or more athletic. Another related fear is that technology will lead to implants or some other device that will make it unlikely for individuals to disconnect from the vast communication networks that tie people together. These two innovations also happen to be core objectives of the antiaging movement among natural scientists. Progressives of the 21st century may support antiaging tools, but they remain less convinced of the value of transhumanist technology that recreates human capacities and may overcome long-standing obstacles such as death.

The 20th century began with an unchallenged hope for the future that included a presumption that human life would improve. By the end of the century, that hope had suffered some tarnish. Yet, the incredible developments of biomedical technology, combined with the popular demand for tools to retain youthfulness, kept the fundamental hope of the antiaging movement alive.

In the next, and final, chapter on the history of antiaging movement, we examine the scientific progress and debates surrounding the Human Genome Project and its impact on public and private support for finding ways of radically extending life well beyond the traditional 120-year limit.

Chapter 5

Antiaging in the 21st Century: From Theory to Practice

The antiaging movement took on new dimensions of credibility and popularity with the onset of the 21st century. For centuries, the dream of prolonging human life had served as a long-term objective for intellectuals and scientists, going as far back as Francis Bacon in the 1200s. Usually, though, this dream was treated as a dream only; the practical recommendations were often more limited. Leading medical experts debated the probable effects of their treatments on the quality and length of the human life span, but mainstream scientists rarely allowed themselves to be caught promising specific results from specific methods and treatments. Those scientists who did make such claims were pushed to the periphery of academia. Since the 20th century, respectable scientists have tried not to make practical claims about immortality that cannot yet be proven true.

This trend of hesitation changed as the year 2000 approached. In part, the change in tone reflected the promise of a new burgeoning millennium and all of its expected technologies. In part, it also reflected the growing market for new solutions demanded by an aging baby-boomer population. Finally, it was the by-product of a slow shift from a Judeo-Christian worldview to a more secular outlook that questioned the traditional definition of life after death. Growing intellectual agnosticism combined with a popular culture fixated on retaining youthfulness, and both provided a theoretical foundation for a new, practical antiaging movement. In the 21st century, doctors wrote hundreds of books explicitly promising increased quality of life as well as a radically extended natural life span.

Amid this cultural popularity, the antiaging movement also benefited from a biomedical breakthrough called the Human Genome Project, which promised new answers for many long-standing medical questions. Why do some people become vulnerable to diseases and others do not? Why do some people live long lives and others do not? For decades, doctors theorized that certain diseases and age-related problems were genetically related. Almost every field of medicine, from immunology to cardiac care; cancer research; and essentially all age-related research of gerontology saw hope in the unraveling of the human DNA sequence. The excitement of potential discovery tempted many scientists to make predictions that they would have strongly resisted even a few decades earlier. More noticeably, the marketing for antiaging treatments flooded media outlets: television, radio, magazines, and the Internet.

The popular success of such bold claims among some antiaging advocates stirred controversy within the scientific community. Researchers in traditional geriatric medicine were fearful of the comparison between their "legitimate" research and the "sensational" claims of popular antiaging medicines sold online. For many traditional gerontologists who limited their research to age-related diseases (rather than curing death), their field had only recently achieved recognition as a legitimate research discipline. The National Institute on Aging (NIA) was formed in 1974, but it only received a tiny fraction of the funds sent to the larger National Institutes of Health (NIH). This priority began to change in the 1990s as rates of dementia, Alzheimer's, and other age-related diseases increased with the aging baby boomers. The proportion of NIA funding increased by a factor of 150, and the field as a whole enjoyed greater attention and scrutiny from federal policy makers. Some of these traditional gerontologists feared that the popular, and often sensational, claims of antiaging remedies sold online or over the television might tarnish the reputation of a discipline that had only recently been embraced by mainstream medicine.

By 2002, an open war of words had erupted between the traditional gerontologists and the antiaging researchers who were sometimes derogatorily referred to as "immortalists." The debate waged for almost a decade through articles in academic journals and speeches at medical conferences, with many books written on both sides. The public rarely read the academic journals and rarely heard the conference speeches, but they became increasingly aware of the discussion—and the immortalists seemed to be winning the day. Many popular antiaging books found a mainstream audience, and public awareness of potential antiaging remedies increased. The market potential of rejuvenation and medicines that might extend life attracted heavy investors from private industry who banked on the growing demand.

The fears of the traditional gerontologists were premature. By the end of the century's first decade, the market for both antiaging remedies as well as the more traditional geriatric research objectives had both increased. Investment in senior care facilities, Alzheimer's research, and cancer prevention dominated the health industry. In terms of medicine, 10 of the top 15 prescriptions were written for age-related diseases such as high cholesterol, Type II diabetes, and arthritis. The debate between antiaging proponents and traditional gerontologists gradually quieted after both sides realized that the public attention raised by the conflict increased the positive image of the scientific community at large. Today, the antiaging dreams of enduring youthfulness and prolonged life spans are deeply entrenched in both popular culture and the scientific communities. Moral and ethical considerations arise on occasion, but they no longer determine the course or direction of the movement.

ANTIAGING TECHNIQUES OF THE 1970s, 1980s, AND 1990s

How exactly can we achieve longer life spans? Scientists use animals (rodents and insects, usually) to study the effects of certain foods and behaviors on longevity. Typically, a research study involves two groups of animals: treatment and control. The treatment group is given something or has something taken away from them. The control receives no treatment. After extended observations of the effects on both groups, the average life span of the treatment group is compared to that of the control group. The average life span of a rodent or fruit fly is so much less than that of a human that it allows researchers to evaluate multiple life cycles over a relatively short period of time. Based on the assumption that rats and other animals often share similar genetic systems with humans, scientists use the data from their research to make recommendations that can be applied to human diet or exercise.

The trick in finding a research-based method for extending the human life span is to find and isolate the right variable. For much of the 20th century, researchers focused on the traditional variables of diet and exercise. Hundreds of studies conducted from the 1950s to the 1970s manipulated levels of protein, fat, carbohydrates, vitamin E, antioxidants, minerals, and other self-selected diets in an attempt to isolate the one factor that contributed to long life. Other studies examined various forms of exercise or other environmental stimulants. If researchers discovered the same general trends over a variety of different animal species (rats, roundworms, fruit flies, etc.), there was greater support for the conclusion that the treatment would also be successful in extending human life.

Dietary Restriction

By the late 1980s, research into the role of nutrition and diet in determining average life span culminated in a massive research project on dietary restriction. The two authors of the study, Roy Walford and his doctoral student Richard Weindruch, not only compiled all previous research on nutritional deprivation but also compared the average life spans of multiple animals—from rats to spiders. They devoted more than a decade to gathering the research, long after Walford had ceased being a student and continued on as a colleague. Together, they compared their findings with other correlational studies of life spans of people living in different cultures around the world, with varying traditions of food intake. They also studied the medical histories of patients with low-calorie lifestyles, including anorexia patients.

After many years of research and multiple papers, the two scientists concluded that reducing caloric intake by as much as 20 percent of that traditionally recommended could lead to substantially longer life spans. As long as the diets were generally nutritious and the subjects did not suffer from malnutrition, the research suggested that decreasing caloric intake could potentially double life expectancy. Without committing themselves to specific predictions, the authors suggested that a carefully prescribed restricted diet could result in a new average life expectancy for humans of between 110 and 115 years, and possibly quite longer.

The authors used evolutionary theory to explain the results. The theory of natural selection rests on the presumption that all living organisms continually face a hostile environment, such as the problem of gathering enough food to survive. Each organism develops defense mechanisms to survive long enough to reproduce and pass their genes along to the next generation. From this beginning, Weindruch and Walford concluded that some of an organism's best defenses are activated only when they are placed under noticeable environmental stress. When confronted with restricted access to food, life-forms tend to respond with enhanced repair and protective processes, and their metabolic systems become more efficient at processing nutritional sources. They extended their research over multiple species to determine (or demonstrate) certain common reactions shared across the genetic spectrum. If they could prove that all organisms demonstrate these common reactions, that would indicate the phenomenon was an artifact of evolutionary development and was not limited to only a few types of animals. Taking the logic one step further, they argued that once these natural reactions to dietary restriction were proven to be evolutionary in nature, scientists should expect humans to react in much the same way as any other species.

Weindruch and Walford made a convincing argument, and throughout the 1990s, the dietary restriction model became extremely popular among antiaging researchers. A host of antiaging manuals published their results as the "only proven solution," and it was frequently cited as one of many methods for retaining youth. Companies that sold dieting supplements often summarized the conclusion that less weight resulted in longer, healthier lives, and the dietary restriction research served as a major reference source.

Yet, the popularity was relatively short-lived; by the start of the 2000s, the dietary restriction model had begun to lose some of its prestige. One factor was that the long-term effects on humans remained unknown. Despite their claims of evolutionary causation, the effects of dietary restriction were not equally demonstrated in all species and were not easily demonstrated in human studies. Part of the problem is that the average human life span is near 80 years, and so it is impossible for the effects of the model to be accurately measured in such a short period of time. Some short-term studies were conducted on healthy men and women, but the results were generally inconclusive. In 2007, the National Institute on Aging funded a study of dietary restriction on nonhuman primates (the Rhesus monkey), which suggested some positive effect on the reduction of age-related diseases. Yet, there were no significant differences in average life span.

The negative side effects of dietary restriction were perhaps more significant to the decline in popularity: lack of energy, lack of concentration, and lack of motivation. These effects were more pronounced in humans than in other life-forms because of their advanced mental faculties. Most of the negative side effects of the model were psychological, including despondency, depression, and a tendency for binge eating. The effects suggested that human physiology may not respond to

Roy Walford and Richard Weindruch

Roy Walford died in 2004 of ALS (better known as Lou Gehrig's disease) at the age of 79. He had been living on a diet of 1,600 calories per day for more than 15 years. Before his death, he attributed his disease to the toxic environmental conditions that he had suffered while living in a self-contained terrarium in Arizona called BioSphere-2. Walford firmly believed in the effectiveness of dietary restriction until the day he died.

Richard Weindruch, Walford's student, is still living as of 2016 and works as the director of LifeGen Technologies, which he cofounded in 2009. It specializes in researching the expressions of genes found in fat deposits in an effort to identify the elements that may be responsible for aging. His company and research were bought by Nu Skin Enterprises, which markets a variety of nutritional and cosmetic supplements designed to promote antiaging.

dietary restriction in the same way as rats or mice, which have limited cognitive development. That may mean that the doubling of life span found in rats will not carry over to humans. In addition, there were some basic questions about whether the treatment regime was worth the cost. If the price of a substantially longer life required constantly living at near-starvation levels with impaired cognitive abilities and unpredictable fluctuations in mood and motivation, it might be better to live a shorter life with greater potential for happiness.

Dietary restriction continues to be featured in contemporary antiaging handbooks, and there are numerous private antiaging treatment centers that incorporate the method in their prescribed plans. Yet, for the most part, the hope of radically enhanced life extension does not rest in nutritional models. To some extent, the popularity of the model suffered from the emergence of other competing antiaging treatments, which also appeared around the turn of the millennium and seemed to be more technologically complex: hormonal treatments, designer steroids, and genetic manipulation.

Hormonal Manipulation

In the broad picture, modern animal studies do not differ substantially from the methods used by such classical physicians as Galen or Hippocrates. Even in ancient times, the doctor would administer a treatment of some sort, watch the results, and then either continue or discontinue the treatment based on the outcome. In the modern era, the primary difference is that evolutionary theory enables medical scientists to use animals instead of humans to test treatments, and the observable results are recorded numerous times in aggregate and measured with instruments with significantly greater precision. The recommendation from such modern studies rely on more observable data to support their potency, but the general process of trial and error with recorded results is largely the same as it was in ancient times.

A critical drawback of using animal-based laboratory studies to identify environmental factors that may affect human life span (including nutrition, exercise, or stress) is that the research is almost always correlational in nature. Scientists subject an animal to various conditions and then measure their effects. These effects are mostly external: Did the animal contract a disease? Did the animal lose strength or become vulnerable to other maladies? How long did the animal live? What was the effect on weight, blood counts, and other measurable characteristics? Typically, the results are summarized with statistical generalizations in an attempt to identify patterns of effects. At best, these studies report a correlation between the extent of the environmental factor and the most common characteristics that followed. These sorts of studies cannot explain with much precision what is actually happening inside the animal to produce these results.

There are other forms of studies that strive to find causal explanations of processes inside the organism. Most often, these studies focus on biochemical reactions conducted outside the body (known as *in vitro*, or "in the glass") and try to identify how such processes would operate inside the body (known as *in vivo*, or "within the living"). This in vitro approach to medicine developed slowly throughout the early the 20th century as scientists uncovered the biomedical processes of the human endocrine system. The endocrine system coordinates the functions of the organs in the human body by sending out various chemical compounds through the bloodstream to regulate the broad range of biochemical reactions needed to sustain life, which we call our *metabolism*. Through a combination of hormones and enzymes, the endocrine system sustains a vast network of interdependent chemical reactions that operate at the cellular level to tell each organ when to start, stop, or vary their rate of functions. Hormones are specialized chemical compounds that affect the permeability of cell membranes, govern the rate of chemical reactions (including cascading chains of reactions), activate or inhibit enzyme systems, and influence the functions of genes at the chromosomal level. In short, the endocrine system is the process that explains how the human body lives and does what it does.

Biologists discovered the theory of hormones and the interrelated endocrine system around the turn of the 20th century, but it took decades to identify the chemical components of various hormones produced by each vital organ. After the chemical structure of each hormone was identified, researchers began working on ways of synthesizing them outside of the human body (in vitro). This was a major leap in internal medicine; if researchers could identify the breakdown in the chemical communication system that each organ depended on, they could simply add the missing chemical and potentially restore proper functioning. If the pancreas failed to produce the necessary insulin to regulate the body's blood-sugar levels, the liver, brain, muscle tissue, and other critical organs of that system would also be affected. Doctors could prescribe artificially synthesized insulin to partially correct the faulty pancreas and thereby also correct the related problems in the brain and liver. Diabetes is directly related to diseases of the pancreas, and most diabetes medicines involve some degree of insulin manipulation. This approach to medical research is more causal than correlational. Scientists identify the reaction in the lab (in vitro) and then replicate it in the body (in vivo). There are still elements of correlation, as the results of each new compound are tested and correlated in actual use. Nevertheless, the scientific understanding and explanation of how the medicine is working is more deeply understood.

The theory behind hormone-based pharmaceuticals was known by the late 1930s, but it was not until after World War II that pharmaceutical companies discovered how to economically synthesize these chemicals as forms of medical treatment. The first hormone treatments were developed during the war years with the artificial synthesis of cortisone, which is an anti-inflammatory hormone produced by the adrenal glands. Doctors began regularly prescribing cortisone to treat rheumatoid arthritis as early as 1949. The drug was first produced by the Merck Pharmaceutical Company after it was isolated and synthesized by Philip Hench and Edward Kendall, both of whom earned a Nobel Prize for their discovery the following year. A second hormone that was artificially synthesized around the same time was the female sex hormone progesterone. When combined with another female sex hormone, estrogen, the resulting treatment could prevent conception by convincing the female body that it was already pregnant. The drug became the first oral contraceptive and eventually became known simply as "the pill." It was first developed in 1957, but it did not receive FDA approval as a contraceptive until 1960.

Between 1950 and 1960, dozens of new drugs were developed to offset hormone deficiencies, resulting in treatments for a multitude of ailments, from hypertension to psychosis. Tranquilizers became easily accessible and heavily prescribed, as were asthma inhalers and treatments for blood disorders. Technological advances in microscopes, chromatography, radioimmunoassay, and enhanced X-ray scanners such as computerized tomography (CT) provide more sophisticated tools for isolating and synthesizing more complex drugs. The related fields of antibiotics, pain relief, and cancer treatment experienced similar growth. In the 1960s, the pharmaceutical revolution swept the field of medicine as physicians relied more heavily on pills to solve common ailments. Though the subfield of antiaging medicine was not a priority among most practitioners, the potential for finding a chemical-based solution to the problem of aging remained a constant dream.

Anabolic Steroids and Male Strength

Most of the earliest drug treatments were synthesized biochemicals called *steroids*. Steroids refer to a chemical structure that is shared by most of the "messengers" found in the body, including cholesterol (sometimes referred to as the "master steroid"), cholic acids, and hormones related to sexual reproduction and adrenal functions. When most people think of steroids, they usually think of the performance-enhancing drugs used by athletes to gain a competitive advantage. However, steroids are also found in most anti-inflammatory drugs, such as those used in asthma inhalers, as well as in all birth control prescriptions.

Nevertheless, anabolic steroids do build up tissues and will improve performance. The most common anabolic steroid family comes from the male sex hormone testosterone, which was first isolated and synthesized in the 1930s. At the time, it was almost immediately identified as a possible tool for boosting soldier's strength and performance. Historical rumors suggest that the Nazis used testosterone experimentally to boost the strength of their storm troopers during the war, but it is not clear whether the research ever resulted in practical use. What was clear was that by the end of the war, testosterone was recognized as a potential chemical tool for magnifying strength and endurance.

At the war's end, in 1945, the popular science writer Paul de Kruif published a book titled *The Male Hormone*, which tells the story of his personal experiences taking testosterone as a dietary supplement. He was 55 years old and had a long history of both scientific interest and physical prowess. After a year of taking the drug, de Kruif reported significant gains in muscle improvement, endurance, and in his general energy levels. He felt testosterone was the secret to maintaining manliness and youthful vitality. In his words, "It's what makes bulls bulls," and de Kruif promised he would "try to renew my aging tissues with testosterone as long as I can."

The Potential of Steroids and Performance Enhancement

Paul de Kruif was a scientist turned journalist who specialized in a sensational narrative style that often placed drama over facts. It is difficult to understand precisely where de Kruif obtained his testosterone, and it is quite likely that he simply heard about a clinical trial conducted by Herman Bundesen on a group of soldiers returning from the field. Rather than taking the drugs himself, it is more likely that he generalized the results from Budesen's program and personalized all the positive conclusions into his own life narrative.

Despite Paul de Kruif's claim of taking oral doses of testosterone supplements with no side effects and instant results, the actual development of the male hormone took more than a decade to produce. The first officially synthesized precursor to testosterone was methandrostenalone, which was developed and sold by Ciba Pharmaceuticals in 1958. Legally, the hormone was only approved for the treatment of hypogonadic conditions where weight gain was needed, such as osteoporosis and dwarfism. In practice, however, the drug was used almost immediately for performance enhancement among weight lifters and professional bodybuilders. The prospect of adding male characteristics of strength and endurance to athletes who already had such characteristics meant they could potentially double their "maleness" and become twice as strong with twice as much endurance.

Unofficially, the first accounts of testosterone used by athletes emerged in the early 1950s as the Soviet weight-lifting team began sweeping international competitions. In 1952, the American Olympic weight-lifting coach, Bob Hoffman, became suspicious of some sort of illegal supplement after the Soviet team walked away with seven Olympic medals (three gold and three silver). Two years later, while in Austria, Hoffman and the team physician, John Ziegler, took one of the Soviet trainers out for drinks at a local bar and managed to extract the secret. The Soviet lifters were using a form of testosterone. The Soviet trainer claimed that the results were good but that the athletes complained of urinary problems and a host of other side effects.

Ziegler went back to the United States and began working on his own variant of testosterone, hoping to have fewer side effects. After a few years, he managed to synthesize methandrostenalone and sold the patent to Ciba Pharmaceuticals, which marketed the compound under the name Dianabol. Despite the official indications for the drug, Ziegler immediately started giving it out to the weight lifters who worked out at his gym. When combined with a specialized training regimen, Ziegler found rapid results as his test subjects won a series of international competitions.

News of the drug spread within the athletic community, and by 1962, trainers in the National Football League had begun giving their players Dianabol during practice. Over the course of the next two decades, more than two dozen variants of anabolic steroids were developed. Evidence of steroid use emerged in Major League Baseball and among athletes in cycling and track-and-field competitions. Incidents of suspected abuse prompted the International Olympic Committee to officially include anabolic steroids on the list of banned substances, which also included amphetamines, stimulants, narcotics, and tranquilizers. The committee had no viable means of testing for the drug, but it was officially prohibited. Medical historian William Taylor vividly recounted that by the end of the 1970s, anabolic steroids had become so common that "on Southern California beaches bodybuilders wore T-shirts that read, *Dianabol, the Breakfast of Champions.*"

In theory, anabolic steroids provided a competitive advantage because they artificially magnified the strength that accompanies youthful vigor. In practice, however, the effects are usually limited to muscle development alone and do not similarly enhance joints, cardiac health, or the central nervous system. A 23-year-old athlete who multiplies his or her muscle mass by three or four times places three or four times as much stress on his or her joints and an even greater proportion of stress on the heart muscle and on other organs of the body. Negative side effects became apparent early on. A group of football players for the San Diego Chargers approached their trainers in the 1960s and voiced their concerns that the "little pink pills" they were taking might result in shrunken testicles and long-term liver damage. After a team meeting, the use of the steroids was cut back. In other sports, the usage was not so easily controlled, and athletes began reporting liver damage, cardiac stress, and harsh emotional and psychological mood swings.

Anecdotal instances of young athletes dropping dead from cardiac arrest circulated among the professionals. As early as 1967, John Ziegler admitted that he did not realize the potential for drug abuse among athletes who self-medicated at 10 and 20 times the recommended schedule. He became a vocal opponent of anabolic steroids and "categorically condemned" their use by athletes for performance enhancement. By 1980, the International Olympic Committee had implemented tests to identify steroid abuse among their athletes. Officially, anabolic steroids were never legally permitted for use as a performance-enhancing drug.

Ergogenic versus Therapeutic Use

The public remained largely ignorant of the widespread use of anabolic steroids and other chemical-based performance enhancers among athletes until the early 1980s. The International Olympic Committee tested athletes for the 1980 Olympics held in Moscow, and not a single competitor tested positive. As far as the public was concerned, international sporting events were mostly unaffected by chemical supplements, and the competition remained a matter of training and personal fitness. In fact, the methods used for drug testing in 1980 were woefully inadequate. By that time, the delivery methods for testosterone included gels and films that were applied topically as an ointment (or as a patch) directly above the targeted tissues and suspensions that were injected directly into the targeted muscles. As long as the athlete had stopped taking the drugs prior to competition, the Olympic testing methods of 1980 were incapable of detecting testosterone.

The situation changed in 1982, when new methods were developed to identify unnaturally high levels of testosterone in a person's system. These testing methods were first used at the 1983 Pan-American Games held in Caracas, Venezuela, and the world was shocked by the results. When news of the new test reached the coaches, an unusually large number of athletes chose to stay home at the last moment. After the first day of the games, when winning athletes were tested immediately after the competition and found to have steroids in their system, the scandal captured headlines throughout the world. Almost immediately, there was a rash of "illnesses" at the games, and dozens of athletes chose to go home rather than face the inevitable testing. When the games were over, 19 athletes from 10 countries had been disqualified—resulting in 23 medals being passed along to the next competing athletes. More than a dozen Americans left the games voluntarily.

The public was both alarmed and fascinated by the use of steroids in these competitions. They were alarmed by the sheer number of incidents of abuse, but they were also fascinated by the fact that the drugs really did enhance performance. At first, the public seemed more alarmed, especially by the potential side effects that steroids may cause both to the legitimacy of athletic competition as well as to the health and safety of the athletes themselves. Yet, relatively quickly, observers displayed a quiet fascination at the results. After years of dreaming of magic pills that increased human abilities, the record-breaking results of steroid use proved such pills were possible. Every year, athletes ran faster, jumped farther, lifted heavier, and broke speed and distance records in almost every sport. If drugs were responsible for these achievements, the prospect of using drugs to overcome other natural limitations became equally possible.

In 1984, Robert Goldman and Ronald Klatz published a book with the sensational title *Death in the Locker Room: Steroids, Cocaine & Sports*. It is mostly narrated by Robert Goldman, who was an athlete who held multiple world records in strength training, including the most consecutive sit-ups and the most handstand push-ups. He begins the book with a graphic account of his bodybuilder friend who is dying of a rare liver cancer, which he ascribes to the use of steroids. Goldman spent years collecting scientific research on steroids and combined it with his anecdotal stories of athletes in a wide variety of sports who used, abused, and suffered from the effects of performance-enhancing drugs. After conducting his research, Goldman wrote, "*I can state unequivocally that drugs, especially anabolic steroids, have no business in sports*. Anabolic steroids bestow few benefits, and none that are worth the terrible risks of taking them."

Goldman and Klatz were careful to distinguish the difference between the ergogenic use and the therapeutic use of anabolic steroids. *Ergogenic* refers to the use of any drug for the purpose of gaining a competitive advantage. *Therapeutic* refers to the use of any drug intended to address a deficiency or otherwise heal the effects of disease. In 1984, Goldman and Klatz recognized the potential for the therapeutic use of steroids for patients who suffered from osteoporosis, severe burns, pituitary dwarfism, breast cancer, and certain cases of anemia. The authors also recognized that there were instances when athletes required specific medicines to treat damage from excessive exercise. In these cases, though, the purpose of the treatment was therapeutic to treat a particular medical disorder. They argued strongly against using any ergogenic drugs to enhance natural conditions for normally healthy individuals. The potential for anabolic steroids or other hormone use for healthy adults was not considered a viable option.

American Academy of Anti-aging Medicine (A4M)

Despite the negative press for anabolic steroids and other ergogenic drugs in athletic competitions, the rate of use increased throughout the 1980s and 1990s. Traditional steroids such as testosterone and its variants were replaced by more sophisticated steroid analogs that provided very specific performance benefits with limited unintended side effects. Ironically, much of the motivation for these innovations arose from the need to create new designer drugs that were undetectable by existing drug tests. There was an invisible race between illicit researchers responding to the demands of elite athletes needing a competitive edge and those legal researchers who were trying to develop new ways of detecting each generation of ergogenic drugs. For the most part, the drug testers were always handicapped by the fact that they had to react to the new steroid after it was already secretly introduced and in place for several seasons. The result was a proliferation of steroid use rather than a decline.

For the antiaging movement, these innovations among ergogenic researchers provided a new avenue for chemical solutions to combat age-related weakness. Testosterone is an age-related hormone that follows a natural life-cycle curve. At young ages, testosterone is barely present in boys who are still growing. As they reach the age of sexual maturation, their testosterone levels increase, as do their secondary sex characteristics: voices change, muscles develop, and they begin to sprout facial hair. The increase in testosterone levels tapers off when men reach their late forties, at which point the levels begin to decline. Beginning around age 60, the sex-related hormones diminish, and adult males begin to lose their strength and endurance. They begin to gain fatty tissues and otherwise show the signs of age. It was precisely these trends that caused people like Brown-Séquard and Paul de Kruif to view testosterone as a potential fountain of youth, or elixir of life, to maintain youthful vigor into advanced ages.

The obvious success of anabolic steroids to enhance the vigor of male youth in competitive sports was not ignored by researchers who were themselves reaching middle age. Even the staunch opponents of anabolic steroids began to change their definitions of "therapeutic use." In 1990, Daniel Rudman published a research study in the *New England Journal of Medicine* that examined the impact of human growth hormone (hGH) on healthy middle-aged adults between 60 and 80 years. After a year of observation, the research team discovered that the treatment group had lost fatty tissue, increased their lean muscle mass, and exhibited tighter skin. The study held significant implications for antiaging, and it was immediately cited by research companies that were already selling other ergogenic drugs for athletes. Human growth hormone is not a testosterone variant, but because of the difficulty of detecting it, elite athletes had already begun using the drug as a substitute for traditional anabolic steroids. Rudman's study opened new opportunities for ergogenic treatment and for physicians willing to supply a booming demand.

Robert Goldman and Ronald Klatz were among the first researchers to change their views of how steroids and other traditionally ergogenic drugs might be used for older adults. If young athletes could gain an advantage by adding biochemical supplements of youthfulness, then why not apply the same advantage to older adults who may actually be experiencing diminished testosterone levels? In this case, the therapeutic use would not be limited to well-known diseases such as osteoporosis or pituitary disorders. Instead, by treating age and death like diseases, the use of anabolic steroids would constitute a legitimate treatment option for maintaining wellness.

With this reasoning, Robert Goldman and Ronald Klatz formed the American Academy of Anti-aging Medicine (A4M) in 1993. At the time, Goldman did not have a medical degree, but he earned one in osteopathy later from a school in Belize. Klatz already had a degree in osteopathic medicine and served as the association's first physician, though he was not a medical doctor (the two both received permission to practice as medical doctors in 2007 but were not allowed to prescribe medicine). Goldman provided skill in promotion and organization, and Klatz provided a certain credibility. The stated mission of A4M is "the advancement of technology to detect, prevent, and treat aging related disease and to promote research into methods to retard and optimize the human aging process." More specifically, the association asserts that most of the signs of aging can be treated with advanced medical technologies, resulting in increased life span and overall better quality of life.

Though A4M does not endorse any particular life-extension technology, it does serve as a clearinghouse for any antiaging technologies and provides certification for physicians wanting to specialize in "antiaging medicine." Goldman and Katz collaborated on dozens of books, but this time they were not warning about the abuse of ergogenic drugs. Instead, they were promoting the benefits of new hormone-based medicines to ensure healthier lifestyles and longer life spans. The two were especially hopeful of the power of hGH, but they also promoted hormone replacement therapies of estrogen, testosterone, and other anabolic steroid precursors as well as a host of herbal and dietary supplements. They wrote numerous books on the subject, with titles such as *Stopping the Clock: Why Many of Us Will Live Past 100 and Enjoy Every Minute!* (1996); *Grow Young with hGH* (1997); *Anti-aging Medical Therapies* (1997); *Ten Weeks to a Younger You* (1999); *Brain Fitness: Anti-aging to Fight Alzheimer's Disease* (1999); *The New Anti-aging Revolution: Stopping the Clock for a Younger, Sexier, and Happier You* (2002); *The Science of Anti-aging Medicine* (2003); and *121 Ways to Live 121 Years and More!* (2005), and each has numerous reprints. Ronald Klatz claims to have coined the term *antiaging medicine*, and A4M is routinely cited as the first medical association of the new antiaging movement. By 2012, A4M boasted 26,000 members in 110 countries and was hosting annual antiaging conferences around the world.

The Gerontological Reaction

In 2016, the A4M membership base includes scientists, researchers, and practitioners, with 85 percent holding medical degrees. The association also provides certifications for antiaging and regenerative medicine for physicians and certifications for antiaging health practitioners as well as nine other certifications for subjects such as brain fitness, lifestyle coaching, and advanced metabolic endocrinology. Certifications begin with the purchase of a training manual for $600 and involves taking a 120-question multiple-choice exam followed by a 40- to 60-minute oral exam. A4M also provides five-day online workshops for $5,000. The association claims to have certified more than 60,000 doctors and practitioners worldwide, yet A4M is not recognized by the American Medical Association (AMA). Indeed, the field of antiaging medicine is not recognized by the AMA as a legitimate subdiscipline.

A4M is very effective in mobilizing a concerted market reaction to growing public demand. Nearly one-third of the American population (75 million) is categorized as "baby boomers, having been born between 1944 and 1964. By 2000, this generation maintained the highest per capita living expenses ever ($46,000), enjoyed annual discretionary expenses of about $8,000, and was responsible for about 80 percent of all luxury travel and almost half of all luxury cars sold. More than any other period in history, the maturing baby boomers emerged during a time when the largest share of society also held the largest amount of available money to spend on priorities that reflected their own interests.

These priorities focused heavily on fitness, cosmetics, and antiaging. The number one cosmetic enhancement in 2002 was Botox injections (nearly 3 million procedures), which deaden facial muscles to reduce signs of wrinkles. Health club memberships grew from nearly $20 billion in 1994 to over $67 billion in 2009, with 10 million new gym memberships every year. The market for hormone treatment centers reached $800 million in 2000 and grew to more than $122 billion in 2013. Over 60 percent of adults age 60 and over were regularly taking daily nonprescription supplements of some kind. When these markets are combined with dietary supplements, nontraditional herbal remedies, and age-related prescription drugs, the overall antiaging market is measured in the hundreds of billions of dollars.

As the 21st century dawned, there was a great deal of money to be made in any number of antiaging remedies, supplies, and programs. The flood of new marketing campaigns from nonphysician amateurs or non-AMA-credentialed private enterprises inspired a harsh reaction from those academic researchers who studied gerontology as a practical medical discipline. From the start, critics from within the geriatric research community had voiced concern at the growing antiaging marketplace. Shortly after publishing his study on the effects of hGH, Daniel Rudman warned, "This is not a fountain of youth," and explained that "the aging process is very complicated and has many aspects." Other researchers came out in vocal opposition, including Leonard Hayflick, Bruce Carnes, and S. Jay Olshansky, each of whom has contributed significant research that is often cited by other antiaging champions. For most of the early 2000s, the three men wrote a series of articles criticizing A4M and the entire field of popular antiaging medicine as "quack medicine."

In 2001, Olshansky and Carnes published a book titled *The Quest for Immortality*, which warns the public against commercial treatments that claim to extend the human life span. The two researchers recognized that significant progress has been made in curing disease and protecting against childhood mortality, which has increased the average life expectancy. Yet, they also argued that there was no scientific evidence that the human life span was actually increasing or ever could be lengthened. The following year, Olshansky presented "silver fleece" awards to those organizations and business that made "the most outrageous or exaggerated claims about human aging." The first organization to be presented with the award was A4M for "leading the lay public and some in the medical and scientific community to the mistaken belief that technologies already exist that stop or reverse human aging" as well as for creating "an alleged medical subspecialty and accreditation in anti-aging medicine, even though there are no proven anti-aging medicines in existence." Two years later, Olshansky bestowed the award on Robert Goldman and Ronald Klatz personally for their line of products that "use clever hype and pseudo-scientific mumbo-jumbo to convince consumers that 'nutraceuticals' and 'cosmeceuticals' can alter the aging process." Goldman and Klatz responded with a $120 million defamation lawsuit, and Olshansky countersued. After several years of wrangling, both sides eventually dropped their suits.

Despite the strong opposition to the irresponsible marketing claims of antiaging enterprises trying to take advantage of the aging baby-boomer population, the academic research community did not reject the idea of antiaging science. In fact, both Carnes and Olshansky made it clear that they personally believed that science may at some point be able to alter the biological process of aging. As Carnes explained in 2004, "It's unfortunate that so much anti-aging quackery is surfacing just when scientists are making substantive progress." Likewise, Olshansky explained, "I'm a strong supporter of anti-aging research." But he added, "It's my job to protect public health, and inform the public about the truth of what we know and what we don't know." In their book *The Quest for Immortality*, the two authors explain, "The life extension industry begins with a grain of truth but quickly gets mixed with a tablespoon of bad science, a cup of greed, a pint of exaggeration and a gallon of human desire for a longer, healthier life—a recipe for false hope, broken promises and unfulfilled dreams." The grain of truth that the authors refer to is not in hormone treatments that impact the endocrine system, but in something even smaller. It is the promise of genetic manipulation at the cellular level that most captured the attention of antiaging researchers in the 21st century.

PATHWAY TO THE HUMAN GENOME PROJECT

After exploring how the endocrine system might be manipulated though chemical therapies involving artificially synthesized hormones, enzymes, and other supplements, scientists began looking even deeper into the functioning of the human metabolism. The endocrine system relies on a fixed architecture that is governed by genetic blueprints, which tell the body which chemicals to synthesize, which to turn off, and generally how to create and maintain the human metabolism. During the 1970s and 1980s, as researchers gained greater understanding of the complex biochemical interactions that occur continuously within the body, many came to regard the genetic encoding as a sort of "master key." Certainly, there were many external factors such as smoking, overeating, or exposure to other toxins in the environment that had a great impact on life span. But, assuming those elements were under control, the remaining factors of the human metabolism were determined by each person's genes. As the technology developed to allow for more systematic understanding of gene expression, even the most serious gerontologists began to hold out hope that almost any aspect of human life could be enhanced, including the very rate of aging and the inevitability of death.

Leonard Hayflick and Cell Division

One of the more popular theories of aging that emerged during the 1960s and 1970s was that cells simply lost their ability to divide and fell into senescence (or cell death). The idea that aging and death are related to a cellular vitality can be traced back to Weismann's germ theory from the 1890s. Over the course of the 20th century, the theory was mentioned periodically by gerontologists trying to understand the root cause of aging. Weismann's research suggested that single-celled organisms were more or less immortal in that they could perpetually replicate themselves without end. As such, it was some evolutionary cause that made the soma cells of larger organisms incapable of eternal reproduction and therefore susceptible to death. As proof of this theory, Alexis Carrel began an experiment in 1908 in which he managed to create and maintain a culture of heart cells from a young chicken that ended up surviving 34 years. The theory was that individual cells are immortal by default and only die when confronted by harmful external factors such as insufficient nutrition or adverse environmental conditions (heat or cold).

In 1958, Leonard Hayflick began comparing cancer cells with normal human cells in an attempt to isolate the factors that cause cancers to form. In the process, he extracted lung cells from fetal tissue to create a clean, healthy cell sample to serve as a control group. During his research, Hayflick realized that the lung cells routinely stopped dividing after about 50 doublings. He knew the cells had not died because they continued to take in sustenance, but they no longer divided. They just got older. In 1961, Hayflick published his findings and began a new research track that examined the maximum number of divisions of various cell types. He found that fetal cells divide more often than adult cells, and certain species divide more than others. His research established what later became known as the "Hayflick limit," which refers to the maximum number of times that a cell can divide.

Beginning in the 1960s, gerontologists began to theorize that the life span of each organism is determined by its Hayflick limit. The cells of mice usually double between 14 and 28 times, the cells of humans double from 40 to 60 times, and the cells of the very long-lived tortoises experience over 100 doublings. Later research from the 1970s and 1980s suggested that different types of cells within the body also have different life expectancies as well as different Hayflick limits. Blood cells seem to live short lives and replicate frequently, while other cells found in blood marrow do not seem to have any limits at all. Neuron cells in the brain and the cells of the heart muscle do not replicate at all, but neither do they seem to die. Cancer cells also seem to have no replication limits, nor do they seem to die naturally.

Up until the late 1990s, there was no clear understanding of why some cells live longer while others die early or why the limits of division vary from cell to cell. This mystery provided both hope and despair for gerontologists. The hope lay in the fact that the unknown quantity might be discovered and thereby manipulated to allow for unlimited cell divisions, possibly resulting in unending life. The despair lay in the fact that the limitations may be genetically determined, which means that they are less likely to be alterable.

Genes and DNA

A little more genetic background is necessary to understand how or why cells divide. Scientists have known since the mid-1800s that our physical characteristics are contained in our genes. After growing and charting the characteristics of more than 10,000 pea plants, an Austrian monk named Johann Gregor Mendel discovered that genes come in pairs (one set from each parent) and are inherited as distinct units, which means they do not require the presence of other genes to be passed on. He also discovered that sometimes alternate sets of genes pass from one generation to the next, but only the dominant set will be expressed in a physical characteristic. Mendel had no advanced technologies to see or identify genes; he simply cataloged the expressions of differing traits found among his pea plants.

Mendel's understanding of genes was little understood at the time that he published his results in 1865, but genes became more important as scientists used new microscopic techniques to observe different stages of cell division. In the 1880s, the German biologist Walther Flemming observed things that look like tiny fibers, or threads, that change during cell division. He stained the materials to make them more visible and drew pictures of the complete cell division process. In this way, he discovered that the threads, which he called *chromotin* (later named *chromosomes*), split lengthwise during division so that the opposite pairs would find matches and create exact duplicates. The process of cell division was called *mitosis*, and this provided a theory to explain how genes were carried from one cell to the next.

Within a decade, another Germany biologist, Theodor Boveri, used Flemming's research to study reproduction. He helped to distinguish the number of chromosomes in various cells and recognized that when the sperm chromosomes joined with the egg chromosomes after fertilization, only one set remained. This provided a more detailed explanation of the process that Mendel had described only generally. In 1902, American biologist Walter Sutton was able to more precisely identify the number and shapes of 11 distinct chromosomes. His research provided a single coherent explanation of Mendel's theories of inheritance, though it was another decade before Thomas Morgan cataloged the characteristics of thousands of fruit flies to demonstrate the connection between chromosome division and the inheritance of specific traits.

It took nearly 50 years to be able to identify what the threadlike fibers are that make up each chromosome. When American biologist James Watson and English chemist Francis Crick discovered the double-helix shape of DNA in 1953, researchers were able to better identify the chromosomes' chemical makeup and how many there were. Each chromosome is made up of a single long DNA molecule, which is about 3 inches long, but it is so tightly wrapped together that it looks like tiny threads under a microscope. Using more advanced technology, Joe Hin Tjio and Albert Levan reported there are exactly 46 DNA strands to form 23 chromosome pairs in human cells (each pair consisting of single DNA strands inherited from each parent). Later research revealed that each species has a different and distinct number of chromosomes.

It was not until the 1960s that scientists were able to identify genes within the DNA strands. Each DNA strand is composed of billions of nucleic acid pairs called *nucleotides*. These form the basic building blocks of each DNA string. Mendel's genes are made up of a series of nucleotides, and the host of genes are strung together in specific locations along the 23 chromosomes. The entire set of DNA strands is called the *genome*. There are only four different types of nucleotides, yet there are more than 3 billion pairs, which means that the expression of each gene is really determined by the order of the nucleotide pairs. Because these molecules are so small, it is impossible to physically distinguish one base pair from another; it required more advanced microscopy technology with more sophisticated tools of chemical analysis than available at the time.

In 1975, Frederick Sanger discovered a process for sequencing the nucleotide pairs that make up the DNA strings. This discovery earned him a second Nobel Prize in 1980. It provided a critical jump in genetic research because the sequencing process opened the door for potentially mapping the entire human genome.

The Telomerase Enzyme and the Cell's Natural Counter

Three years after Sanger, Elizabeth Blackburn, a biochemist researching the DNA sequence of a single-celled organism, discovered that the ends of the chromosomes are made of simple repeating DNA sequences. After examining other organisms, she found similar characteristics in them, which suggested that the chromosomes of all animals contain simple repetitious DNA segments at their ends. Working with Jack Szostak, Blackburn later theorized that those simple DNA segments, called *telomeres*, protect the chromosome ends from being damaged. In the same way that someone might cut a piece of string longer than needed, the chromosomes use the telomeres to create a little extra DNA sequence to ensure the active portion of the chromosomes remain undamaged during replication.

Shortly thereafter, in 1984, Carol Greider identified an enzyme called *telomerase*, which seemed to provide the template for making the telomere sequences. In plain language, the enzyme telomerase allows cells to create more telomeres. Later, another researcher in Edinburgh, Howard Cook, used a newly developed tool for determining the length of the telomeres and discovered that certain types of cells contain longer telomere lengths than others. At the time, Cook assumed the telomere lengths were determined by tissue type alone. In 1990, however, Greider and two other researchers, Calvin Harley and Bruce Futcher, realized that there is a correlation between telomere length and cell aging. Telomere length was shorter in cells taken from older people and longer in cells taken from younger people. The length of the telomere varied with certain kinds of tissues, but it also became clear that they shortened as cells divided.

Greider and her colleagues developed a theory that seemed to explain the differing Hayflick limits from various kinds of cells. Each cell type contains differing amounts of telomerase, which determined telomere length. Each time the cell divides, a portion of the telomere is lost, thereby making it work as a sort of counter for cell division. In normal cells, when the Hayflick limit is reached and the telomere reaches a certain shortness, the cell usually enters senescence (death). In some cases, where the telomerase enzyme is present, the chromosome maintains long telomeres because the telomerase enzyme helps to replace the telomeres, no matter how many times the cell divides. For these cells, there is no Hayflick limit, and the cell is essentially immortal. Greider, Blackburn, and Szostak each shared a Nobel Prize for their discoveries in 2009.

The presence of telomerase does suggest the possibility of unlimited cell division and, thus, unlimited life span. In practice, the elongated telomere often results in faulty DNA replication, leading to the creation of cancer cells. More often than not, it is the surviving cancer cells that are immortal. This discovery led to a host of tempting possibilities: were telomeres intended to prevent tumors from forming? If so, then removing the telomerase might help in fighting cancer. At the same time, would appropriately applied telomerase help to trigger a rejuvenation of older cells to become younger? If so, this might be a possible antiaging solution. The problem with either solution is that this process occurs simultaneously in millions of cells. It is almost impossible to find a chemical solution that guarantees that only the right kinds of cells receive the immortality while still allowing the wrong kinds of cells to die.

Nevertheless, the discovery of the relationship between telomeres and cellular aging was extremely exciting for antiaging researchers, especially as it happened around the same time that researchers were beginning the decade-long quest to completely unravel DNA through the Human Genome Project. The possibility that a genetic code might be responsible for the length of each cell's telomere meant that gene manipulation might allow scientists to program the DNA encoding to properly assign cellular senescence when it was necessary and to defer it (or deny it altogether) when it was not. As William Clark wrote in *A Means to an End* (1999), "Completion of the Human Genome Project early in the next century will eventually make it possible to identify each of the key genes involved in human aging. We will then be able to dissect senescence and aging at a level never before possible."

The Human Genome Project

From the start of Mendel's garden of peas, the idea of potentially identifying and isolating every possible human gene seemed like a natural end for hereditary science. Yet, in Mendel's time, it would have been dismissed as seemingly impossible. The dream did not become practical until the structure and nature of the DNA molecules were understood and the tools and technology for identifying various nucleotide sequences were developed. Those elements did not fall into place until the 1980s, when computing technology provided a practical means of sorting and sequencing 3 billion pairs of genetic nucleotides.

A project of this scope required multiple research facilities working simultaneously and in conjunction with each other. It also needed sophisticated technology and places to house them. In short, the project required billions of dollars, which was funding on a scale that could only be arranged through governments. The U.S. Department of Energy was the first to attach itself to the idea of mapping the human genome, which was initially marketed as an opportunity to develop safeguards against genetic mutation following potential radiation disasters. The following year, in 1988, Congress authorized a joint research group through the

National Institutes of Health (NIH) and the Department of Energy to develop a feasibility study. One of the original discoverers of the chemical structure of DNA, James Watson, was chosen to lead the new Office of Human Genome Research, which eventually morphed into the National Center for Human Genome Research (NCHGR).

The original project in 1990 proposed a series of 5-year plans, with a projected completion date of 2005 (15 years later). The first 5-year plan was mostly devoted to creating the tools needed for sequencing. During this period, the project was opened to researchers in Great Britain and the Medical Research Council of the United Kingdom also dedicated funds and materials to the project. The rate of technology improved faster than expected, and a second 5-year plan was announced 2 years early in 1993. It focused on developing and perfecting sequencing techniques by unraveling the genome of one or more simple organisms as practice. At the same time, a second research thread of the project was launched to discover the genetic makeup of various cancers and other diseases. In addition, new research labs were opened in other countries around the world, including France, Germany, Japan, and China. An Internet site was developed so that researchers could upload all the raw data as soon as it was obtained, thus ensuring that the results would not be hoarded (or possibly patented) by a single research cohort. The Human Genome Project was truly a collaborative effort using resources around the globe.

The third and final 5-year plan was announced in 1998. At this time, most of the tools were already in place, and some elements of the human genome had already been sequenced. The news was published in *Science* magazine, and excitement over the project's potential spread among both academics and the popular press. During the same year, at least two other private companies announced they would begin their own efforts to unravel the DNA code, but only Celera Genomics made any significant progress. As a private corporation, the company was quite open about their intention to file for patents on the genetic sequences they discovered that could lead to medical treatments.

This spurred a race between the publicly funded and openly accessible research of the Human Genome Project and the privately financed proprietary research of Celera Genomics. The competition created natural incentives on both sides and captured a great deal of public attention. For three years, more than 2,800 researchers at 20 institutions around the world worked on sequencing, and in 2001, both Celera Genomics and the Human Genome Project announced approximately the same results at approximately the same time. The public project immediately published its findings for about 90 percent of the sequence. The final 10 percent was completed and published in 2003.

The final race was a tie, but as a practical matter, Celera Genomics had demonstrated greater efficiencies. The government-funded project took 13 years and $3 billion, whereas the Celera Genomics project took only 3 years and $300 million. Admittedly, much of the technology that Celera relied on had already been developed by the time they started. Nevertheless, Celera also developed their own techniques of sequencing (called the "shotgun" method), which proved much faster

Statisticians and Biologists

Biology used to be considered less math intensive than engineering, physics, or chemistry, but that is changing. Modern structural biologists and geneticists work closely with statisticians to analyze trends within large amounts of data. Most professional articles published on genetics-related topics include biologists and at least one statistician.

Since the advent of the Human Genome Project, statisticians have become essential for creating the necessary tools for understanding extremely large amounts of data. The human genome contains more than 3 trillion nucleotide pairs, and those genetic sequences produce an untold number of phenotype expressions. The information found in a DNA sequence has little value if it is not somehow related to a particular set of expressions. Researchers try to isolate particular gene sequences with particular expressions by comparing large populations that share similar characteristics. For example, to isolate the genes related to color blindness, researchers would collect the genome sequences of several thousand people who all share the same color-blind traits. Then, their genome sequences could be compared to another population of several thousand more patients who do not have those color-blind traits but who may share several other common characteristics. By comparing the two groups in aggregate, scientists may be able to determine differences that could help isolate the genetic sequences related to color blindness.

Unfortunately, the resulting databases of comparative genome sequences can include several quadrillion (1,000,000,000,000) pieces of data. It is not physically possible to compare that amount of information with any precision. To manage the data, statisticians create special algorithms to find trends that may indicate relationships within the data that would otherwise be lost in a sea of numbers. It is almost impossible to study genetics without the aid of highly trained mathematicians to develop tools for interpreting the information.

than the method originally developed by Sanger in the 1970s. In the end, after the sequencing had been completed and some basic discoveries published, Celera donated much of its data to the same GenBank that is openly accessible to researchers around the world. The net result was that many observers concluded that though government funding is deeper, private firms are often more nimble and efficient in conducting research—including such massive projects as this. By 2015, dozens of private firms around the world were providing the service of individual genome sequencing for anyone who desired it. The entire process takes only a few days and costs around $1,400. In 2016, Ancestry.com began marketing limited DNA sequencing procedures to determine family origins for only $99.

The Aftermath of the Human Genome

When the Human Genome Project was initially launched, biologists had calculated that there were about 100,000 human genes. This number was based on an estimation of the number of protein combinations needed for human metabolic function. In 2001, with 90 percent of the sequencing complete, scientists were surprised to discover that the actual number of genes was closer to 30,000. Two years later, when the sequence was entirely complete, the final number of genes was adjusted downward to about 20,000. It became clear that the expressions of human traits potentially required the combination of multiple genes, and the various genetic combinations meant that, at a practical level, each gene could serve multiple functions.

The discovery of a smaller number of human genes was a disappointment for some antiaging researchers. The potential for multiple purposes from common expression of various genes created an added difficulty to understanding the practical meaning of particular nucleotide sequences. There are more than 3 billion nucleotide pairs, and if each pair were a letter, the grouping of those letters would create a word for each gene. Yet, it turns out that the same words could be used multiple times and in multiple ways. Each gene is expressed in a particular cell, as the unique ribonucleic acid (RNA) strands trigger the creation of particular proteins needed for that cell. Though the entire DNA genome exists in every cell, the cells of each organ have very different functions. Only that part of the DNA sequence related to that cell function is ever expressed in any given organ. That means that even within the same organ, the RNA transcription process could potentially utilize any number of genetic sequences that differ not only according to type but perhaps also according to various stages in the life cycle. A cell may rely on one combination of genes to create certain proteins that activate functions of the cell at a young age and then shift to another combination of genes to create other proteins that trigger other effects at a later age. Unless every combination is recorded, tracking the complete list of genetic functions is extremely difficult.

In part, some of the confusion about the potential of the human genome arose from the expectations of what each gene represents. Mendel originally cataloged only the visible traits when he traced the heredity of his plants. He identified sets of these traits and set down laws of inheritance, which include the principle of segregation, the principle of independent assortment, and the law of dominance. These generalizations, however, refer to the physical expression of collected traits called *phenotypes* (such as eye color, ear lobe length, skin tone, etc.) and not to the biochemical combinations that define those traits. The Danish biologist Wilhelm Johannsen coined the term *gene* in 1909 to describe those traits.

Even in Johannsen's time, the idea of a gene was mostly tied to the phenotypes (or physical traits) or the biological functions of an organism. There was still no understanding of DNA or the biochemical building blocks that make up the DNA molecules. After the 1960s, the modern definition of gene changed to refer to a particular sequence of nucleotides along their vast DNA molecule chain, yet it is common to make the simple assumption that a single chemical gene is responsible for a single phenotype (physical trait). Mendel's laws of inheritance still apply for the outward expression, but they may not hold the same reliability at the biochemical

ANTIAGING IN THE 21ST CENTURY

level. In practice, each gene may be responsible for only a tiny function or a part of a characteristic in the human body. More likely, there are numerous genes that are responsible for more complex characteristics.

After sequencing the human genome, the next step in genetic research was to identify the expressions of each gene and gene combination. This step is the most difficult and may likely take a very long time to complete, possibly a century or more. There may be only 20,000 genes, but there could potentially be billions of expressions from the multitude of genetic combinations. Given the vast amount of data in the genome, most of the research involves statistical generalizations taken from aggregated correlations between particular genes (or gene combinations) and particular characteristics. It is only after thousands, perhaps millions, of genome maps have been correlated together with the life histories of actual patients that scientists will begin to identify dependable patterns.

The statistical approach to genetic research creates a problem for antiaging advocates who were hoping to find an "aging" gene that could be conveniently turned off at will. Correlative studies require a long time when life expectancy is included as one of the factors. Other antiaging characteristics may be exceedingly difficult to identify even with the genome map because they operate unseen and are known only by their effects. For example, how can scientists isolate the triggering process that cells use to identify when to let telomeres shorten (thereby limiting cell replication) and when to allow for unlimited cell replication (thereby allowing for immortal cells)? Other difficulties arise for characteristics that all members of a population share, which is especially common for certain physical signs of aging. How can scientists isolate the decreasing production of testosterone, or hGH, or other anabolic steroid traits when everyone experiences the same effects? How can scientists correlate various life histories to identify particular gene combinations when all members of the study group carry the same genes? Nevertheless, most contemporary genetic research is necessarily published as correlational data. A significant number of people with gene "X" have a greater than average likelihood of exhibiting "Y" trait. Causal research that can state with certainty that gene "X" always leads to "Y" trait remains a distant goal.

The irony is that one of the initial advantages of pursuing a genetic approach to antiaging was that the biochemical nature of the process of genetic expression implied greater certainty. If a chemist mixes reagent A with reagent B, the same chemical reaction should always occur. Chemistry is not supposed to have variable results. Yet, given the size of possible genetic combinations relative to the immense number of possible expressions, plus the extreme difficulty of watching the actual process of gene expression in real time (in vivo), that type of chemical certainty remains elusive. For the pessimist (or realist), the prospect of identifying or manipulating these genetic traits seems exceedingly unlikely, if not impossible. For the progressive optimist (or idealist), the mystery only remains to be discovered. In the end, some elements of the antiaging movement became more realistic about finding immediate solutions to curing aging, while others became even more hopeful that the solutions may someday be discovered.

The Ageless Woman

Richard Walker studies individuals with rare diseases that seem to slow down the aging process. In 2009, Walker published an account of his research on a teenaged girl who did not appear to age past her toddler years. He heard about a 12-year old girl named Brooke Greenberg who still looked as if she were a little more than a year old from a television show and contacted the family. He gathered family histories and tried to identify the cause for the condition, which he and the girl's physician simply labeled Syndrome X because it was hitherto unknown. The girl eventually died of respiratory issues at the age of 20, and yet she never seemed to age past the toddler stage. Due to the publicity of the case, Walker came in contact with seven other cases of children with very similar conditions.

Collaborating with the researchers at Stanford University, Walker collected genome sequences from all the children and 27 family members. The goal was to compare the sequence of the nonaging toddlers with a control group of regularly aging children to identity any anomalies. The research was published in 2015. It concluded that the development of internal tissues (blood and other organs) appeared to be normal, and only the external appearance remained young. Even for this small group of 30, the tests did not reveal any clear genetic marker.

The Prematurely Old Man

In 1886, the English physician Jonathan Hutchinson came across a six-year old boy who resembled an old man, with balding hair, wrinkles, and other age-related conditions. A decade later, his colleague Hastings Gilford came across another patient with similar characteristics, and he published a report on the new disease in 1904, which he named *progeria* (which means "prematurely old" in Greek). Since then, researchers often refer to it as Hutchinson-Gilford syndrome. It remains extremely rare, but more than 100 cases have been reported. Most patients die around age 16 from arteriosclerosis, but some have been recorded to have lived as long as 26 years.

In the 21st century, the antiaging researcher Michael Fossel has studied Hutchinson-Gilford syndrome as well as other disease that appear to accelerate the aging process. His goal is to study the genomes of afflicted patients to isolate the genes that may be responsible for aging. If there is a hyperactive sequence that may be responsible for accelerating aging, it is possible that suppressing that (or a similar) sequence may help to decelerate aging. Fossel is also studying the correlation between accelerated aging and shorted telomere lengths in afflicted patients.

Still others began to place much less reliance on genetic causation for solving the problem of aging. There was another cohort of gerontologists who never believed that aging was determined by genetics. They believed death was a consequence of a buildup of cellular waste or possibly a by-product of the gradual wear and tear of cellular tissues. In either case, these researchers never believed that there could be any genes that cause aging because aging is an unavoidable side effect of living in a physical environment. Needless to say, these skeptics were never among the antiaging advocates.

THE WAR BETWEEN ANTIAGING AND LONGEVITY

The Human Genome Project did not solve the practical problems of curing aging, age-related diseases, or death. Yet, the popularity of the antiaging movement was undaunted by the absence of an easy "aging" gene in the DNA. From the perception of public opinion, the very fact that scientists were able to unravel such a complex mystery as the human genome was sufficient proof that more achievements awaited in the future. The commercial sector specializing in antiaging treatments, supplements, and related products increased significantly. Marketing companies used the prospect of future medical breakthroughs to advertise current products, resulting in billions of dollars in profits.

The increase in popular antiaging marketing campaigns had the opposite effect on more than a few academic scientists who were well aware of the limitations of the Human Genome Project. Of most concern were advertisements that claimed to reverse or slow aging, especially when the researchers who studied the subject intimately knew there is no scientific support for the claim. Such conflict between opportunistic charlatanism and legitimate science is fairly common and is not limited to the modern era. The real source of tension was between legitimate researchers who had genuine disagreements over whether it was possible to find practical solutions to aging or death. In one camp were the realists who saw no viable scientific means for slowing down or reversing the effects of the aging process. In the other camp were those idealists who recognized that no solutions were currently available, but like the progressive antiaging advocates of the past, they genuinely believed that some solutions were possible.

It was the debate within the scientific community that made the popular antiaging marketplace so troublesome. The presence of the entrepreneurs who seemed to be taking advantage of the baby boomers' demand for eternal youth only amplified the problem between the realists and the idealists. The realists do not believe that the human life span can be extended. Quality of life may be improved, but the length of our days is more or less fixed. The idealists believe that the life span is flexible and might be extended with proper scientific discovery. The credibility (and hope) of both sides was challenged by the popularity of so many non-science-based commercial products. In many cases, the most vocal opponents of the charlatans were those who truly believed in the eventual potential of life extension.

Radical Antiaging

It can be difficult to distinguish between those scientists who believe that the natural life span can be extended, and those opportunists who take advantage of the cultural credibility of scientific discovery to make money. In both cases, the leading figures usually claim to be scientists, and they both make similar arguments about how science will result in the radical extension of life. Typically, "radical extension" means that the human life span will be increased to 200, or 400, or even 1,000 years. In some cases, radical antiaging gerontologists argue that death itself is an optional end and not biologically necessary.

One criterion for distinguishing legitimate scientists from popular salesmen lay in the credibility of the scientific research and the degree to which they engage in the "scientific discussion" that is waged in scholarly journals through peer-reviewed research. Publishing a book is not enough to establish professional credibility because many of the profit-based antiaging clinics maintain their own presses, and other popular trade publishing houses are guided more by potential sales than by scientific rigor. Almost all amateur antiaging gurus have books to sell. Credibility usually requires the consistent publication of scientific research in peer-reviewed journals. Another criterion to consider is the degree to which the researcher is associated with for-profit antiaging institutions. Are they spokesmen for a particular product or service? There are a great number of credible gerontologists that fulfill both criteria and who also believe in radical life extension. We consider only three to demonstrate the spectrum of researchers.

Michael Fossel

Michael Fossel is a clinical professor at Michigan State University and a practicing doctor at a local hospital. His research interests related to aging began when he studied children suffering from a rare disease known as Hutchinson-Gilford syndrome, which is a condition that appears to accelerate the aging process. Patients usually die at an age of 12 or 13, though they show physical symptoms of being in their extreme old age. Fossel wrote several articles for the *Journal of American Medical Association* in the 1990s on the relationship between telomere length and aging. He concluded that Hutchinson-Gilford syndrome was a result of children being born with unusually short telomere lengths, which caused their cells to enter senescence early. Fossel's research is considered mainstream, as is his theoretical approach to the discipline.

Fossel initially believed that the human life span was fixed, but after Carol Greider's discovery of the telomere and telomerase connection, he changed his opinion. Beginning in 1997, Fossel published a series of books that explore the potential of telomerase for radically extending human life. These include *Reversing Human Aging* (1997); *Cells, Aging, and Human Disease* (2004); *The Immortality Edge: Realize the Secrets of Your Telomeres for a Longer, Healthier Life* (2010); and *The Telomerase Revolution* (2015). For many years, he served as the founding editor of the *Journal of Anti-aging Medicine* (later titled *Rejuvenation Research* and edited by Aubrey de Grey), which is a peer-reviewed journal specializing in aging research. Fossel's motto for the journal was, "The question is not 'will we extend healthy life?' but 'when and how?'" He had ties with commercial biotech consulting companies, including TransVio Technology Ventures, and he founded Telocyte in 2015, which is biotechnology company that uses telomerase to treat Alzheimer's disease. Fossel is a highly sought speaker, with more than 70 appearances on international media venues and an equal number of invited lectures where he explains the potential for modern science to overcome previous obstacles to extending human life span.

Stanley Shostak

On the other side of the spectrum is a biologist who is known for being highly critical of the field of biology and especially its emphasis on genetics as the master key to human metabolism. Stanley Shostak is a biologist at the University of Pittsburgh and has written more than 80 articles and several books on the evolution of death and life. In *Death of Life* (1998) and *The Evolution of Sameness and Difference* (1999), Shostak provides a philosophical critique of the current state of the field of biology and genetics. He was very critical of the Human Genome Project for placing such emphasis on DNA as the primary key to answering problems of aging, disease, and metabolism. Rather than an "evolutionist," Shostak described himself instead as a "devolutionist" because he believed that DNA is as influenced by changing environmental conditions during life as it is by its hereditary history.

He followed with another book titled *Becoming Immortal: Combining Cloning and Stem-cell Therapy* (2002), in which he argues, "Immortality is closer than you think." Based on the conviction that modern living conditions can be manipulated to facilitate immortality, Shostak then examines the political and cultural implications that follow when immortality becomes common. Some of his more speculative conclusions include halting the aging process at a level just before sexual maturity (age 11 or so) and the colonization of other planets through long-term interstellar flights. In his 2006 book *The Evolution of Death*, Shostak continues the theme of inverting evolution to argue that senescence has itself evolved. He suggests that adding the self-renewing cells of embryonic tissues may lead to rejuvenation.

Shostak is one of many scientists that believe in a concept called *transhumanism*, in which humanity evolves to include more enduring capacities through a combination of biological and technological innovations. It is not unique to the 21st century. In the 1950s, Julian Huxley first introduced the concept in an essay titled "Transhumanism," in which he concludes, "The human species can, if it wishes, transcend itself—not just sporadically, an individual here in one way, an individual there in another way, but in its entirety, as humanity. We need a name for this new belief. Perhaps transhumanism will serve: man remaining man, but transcending himself, by realizing new possibilities of and for his human nature." Shostak is definitely not part of mainstream gerontology, but neither is he in any way affiliated with promoting antiaging products or services. He is academically inclined to the reality of radical life extension.

Aubrey de Grey

Perhaps the most highly publicized proponent of radical life extension is Aubrey de Grey. He serves as the chief science officer of a California-based research institute, which he cofounded, called Strategies for Engineered Negligible Senescence (SENS) Research Foundation. He made headlines around the world when he proclaimed that the first person to live to be 1,000 years old is alive today, and the quote was immediately repeated by a host of other antiaging advocates in both academic and private enterprise. In a 2015 interview, Aubrey de Grey explained that he does not believe in immortality per se: "The first thing I want to do is get rid of the use of this word *immortality* because it's enormously damaging. It is not just wrong; it is damaging. . . . It means zero risk of death from any cause—whereas I just work on one particular cause of death, namely aging." Nevertheless, when asked about the odds that a person alive today would be able to indefinitely avoid the diseases and ill effects of old age, de Grey answered, "Probably about 80 percent."

In some ways, Aubrey de Grey shares similarities with Robert Goldman and Ronald Klatz of A4M, in that he began his career in a field unrelated to biology. He was in charge of software development for the Cambridge Genetics Department where his wife worked as a biologist. He wrote a book titled *The Mitochondrial Free Radical Theory of Aging* (1999) around the time of the Human Genome Project and earned a doctorate in gerontology from Oxford as a result. Like Goldman and Klatz, Aubrey de Grey is quite skilled at promoting the market potential of the antiaging movement, and he also created an institute that provides consultation services for antiaging products and regimens. He is frequently seen on television outlets and is a speaker in high demand, noted for his characteristically long beard and his willingness to claim that death is potentially curable.

The primary difference between Aubrey de Grey and Goldman and Klatz is that Grey has published in numerous peer-reviewed journals. Admittedly, many of his articles were written in response to criticism and most were published in journals for which he serves as editor; yet, they are peer-reviewed, and the research was often clinically based. His conferences include respected gerontologists that both agree with and oppose his theories.

Aubrey de Grey cofounded the Methuselah Foundation in 2003, which provides funding for antiaging research. One of its grant awards is the Methuselah Mouse Prize, which goes to researchers who can substantially increase the longevity of mice. Three awards have been given out. At the time, de Grey wrote, "Contrary to what one might conclude from the popular press, anti-aging drugs do not yet exist. . . . A drug that rejuvenates aspects of the aged body but does not increase life expectancy is an anti-frailty drug, not an anti-aging one." Yet, he formed the foundation because he believed "scientists are on the threshold of the development of genuine anti-aging drugs—pharmaceutical and genetic therapies that, jointly, can rationally be expected to postpone and even reverse age-related degeneration in humans, thereby markedly extending healthy lifespan." In 2009, de Grey formed the SENS Research Foundation, which "works to develop, promote, and ensure widespread access to regenerative medicine solutions to the disabilities and diseases of aging."

De Grey's willingness to make sensational predictions has prompted suspicion from other members of the academic community. In February 2005, de Grey's

Methuselah Foundation joined researchers at the Massachusetts Institute of Technology (MIT) in offering a $20,000 prize for any molecular biologist who could demonstrably prove that the research goal of SENS was "so wrong that it is unworthy of learned debate." Three of the submissions were published in MIT's *Technology Review* journal, along with de Grey's rebuttals as well as the challengers' responses. The judging panel did not find enough evidence to award the prize, but they nevertheless concluded that "SENS does not compel the assent of many knowledgeable scientists; but neither is it demonstrably wrong." Later in the year, de Grey wrote an article in *EMBO*, a prestigious journal of the European Molecular Biology Organization, criticizing the pessimistic view of the gerontological community for rejecting the goals and objectives of SENS research. In response, a collection of 28 biogerontologists (including Steven Austad, Bruce Carnes, and S. Jay Olshansky) signed a letter that "each one of the specific proposals that comprise the SENS agenda is, at our present stage of ignorance, exceptionally optimistic." As usual, de Grey responded to the criticism with his own rebuttal. For the most part, de Grey is not dismissed as a charlatan, but he is criticized for being overly confident in antiaging potentials.

More Moderate Prolongevity

In contrast to the proponents of radical antiaging, a sizable proportion of biogerontologists might describe themselves as supporting the moderate goals of prolongevity. The term *antiaging medicine* had, for some gerontologists, become so tightly linked to sensationalism of both the market-focused A4M as well as Aubrey de Grey that they resisted using the term in their writings. Instead, they argued they were promoting the prolongation of healthy living. This group of researchers is more easily distinguished from the market-based promoters because they tend to resist making any claims of extending the human life span. At the same time, they also avoid concluding that the human life span is permanently fixed. For the most part, they believe in the potential of scientific discovery but remain convinced that the pace of discovery will continue to be relatively slow and will not immediately result in life extension.

João Pedro de Magalhães

João Pedro de Magalhães leads the Integrative Genomics of Ageing Group at Liverpool University in Great Britain and has written more than 50 articles and participated in genome sequencing of bowhead whales and naked mole-rats. His specialty is in using computer modeling and other statistical tools to compare the genomes of animals and humans, and as such, he is responsible for the maintenance of several online databases containing these sorts of data. De Magalhães focuses on animals with exceptionally long life spans in an attempt to find the genetic markers that may explain slower rates of aging.

De Magalhães is probably most representative of a group of moderate scientists who are convinced that life extension is possible but doubtful that it can be achieved at radical levels in our lifetimes. In a 2014 article, he explains that "curing aging is scientifically possible and not even the most challenging enterprise in the biosciences." Following de Grey's optimism, he continued by saying, "Developing the means to abolish aging is also an ethical endeavor because the goal of biomedical research is to allow people to be as healthy as possible for as long as possible." In contrast to de Grey, he also adds, "There is no evidence, however, that we are near to developing the technologies permitting radical life extension."

Steven Austad

Steven Austad is a researcher of cellular and structural biology and served as interim director of the Barshop Institute for Longevity and Aging Studies, which specializes in geriatric research. Austad is the author of numerous articles and books, including *Why We Age* (1997) and *Handbook on the Biology of Aging* (2010). He later joined S. Jay Olshansky and Bruce Carnes in their efforts to expose the lack of scientific foundation for claims made by amateur antiaging companies and was especially critical of Robert Goldman and Ronald Klatz's A4M. He also rejected Aubrey de Grey's predictions that scientists might someday find a cure for death.

Yet, Austad also believed that the natural life span is not fixed. In 1999, while attending a gerontology symposium, Austad explained to a reporter that the first person to live to be 150 was already alive. The interview prompted his friend S. Jay Olshansky to make a bet. They each put $150 into a fund that would mature in the year 2150. If no one had reached the age of 150 years prior to that date, Olshansky's descendants would inherit the fund. If someone had, then Austad's descendants would. The wager drew media attention and helped tie Austad and Olshansky together as friendly competitors.

S. Jay Olshansky

S. Jay Olshansky is a sociologist at the University of Chicago, where he specializes in evolutionary and biological theories of aging. He is not a physician or a clinical researcher, but Olshansky has devoted decades of research on statistical analysis of trends in human aging and their implications for public policy in a field referred to as *biodemography*. He has authored more than 100 articles on the subject and several books, including *The Quest for Immortality* (2002), which he wrote with fellow biodemographer Bruce Carnes. After surveying recent scientific developments in the field of antiaging research, the two argue that the recent significant increases in average life expectancy are primarily due to the removal of childhood diseases. They do not believe that life expectancy will continue to increase much beyond age 85 because that would require significant breakthroughs in the biology of the aging process itself. In 2002, Olshansky and Carnes did not believe that was at all likely.

Olshansky is included on the list of moderate prolongevists because his position on the subject has evolved over the course of the decade into the 2010s. Around the time that he published *The Quest for Immortality*, Olshansky was most concerned with exposing the marketing claims made by amateur antiaging companies.

During the same year (2002), Olshansky, Carnes, and Leonard Hayflick (source of the "Hayflick limit") organized a group of 51 scientists to sign a joint "Position Statement" on antiaging products, which they published in the *Scientific American*. They followed the statement with a subsequent article in the same journal titled "No Truth to the Fountain of Youth." In it, they explicitly warn, "No currently marketed intervention—none—has yet been proved to slow, stop or reverse human aging, and some can be downright dangerous. . . . Anyone purporting to offer an anti-aging product today is either mistaken or lying." The three authors followed up these articles with the annual Silver Fleece awards intended to expose the "quackery" of "spurious antiaging medicine."

Despite his strong opposition to spurious claims made by antiaging marketing campaigns, Olshansky still retained a general openness to the possibility that science may someday find a solution to medical aging. Following his famous bet with Steven Austad, the two began promoting an initiative that would involve substantial government funding, $3 billion a year, to be directed to finding a biochemical solution to arrest the process of aging. In 2015, Olshansky published *Aging: The Longevity Dividend* (2015), which presents the initiative as a sustained argument.

Later that year, both men met with officials at the U.S. Food and Drug Administration (FDA) to pitch a long-term study of 3,000 elderly people to test a new potential antiaging drug called *metformin* (see chapter 12). The unusual aspect of this proposal was that the group promoting the clinical trial included all academics and was unconnected to a pharmaceutical company. If successful, the drug would be sold as a generic treatment at a price of a few cents per dose. The research was based on the discovery of a genetic variant identified as IGF-1, which may have some connection to aging.

At the time, Olshansky clarified, "We're not arguing—and we've never argued—that we're trying to achieve life extension. . . . We'll probably live a little longer if we succeed, but that's not the goal. The goal is the extension of the period of healthy life." Though Olshansky is certainly not associated with radical life extension, he nevertheless still believes that the human life span is variable and that science may hold the key for extending it, even if only a little at a time.

Fixed Life Span Gerontologists

Since the start of the Human Genome Project, most of the excitement behind research in biogerontology has been related to studying the process of aging and potentially discovering the key to slowing it (or possibly even reversing it). Yet, during the height of the genome sequencing race, there were some researchers who remained unconvinced that aging could ever be slowed or in any way altered. These folks believed that science may successfully make life more comfortable by removing the effects of the most common age-related diseases, but material decay is unavoidable. The aging process cannot be altered.

The idea of a fixed life span is certainly not new. It was the default presumption up until Weismann and others, around the turn of the 20th century, suggested that death is an evolutionary development and not natural to the cell. This ray of hope, however, was seriously challenged by Leonard Hayflick, who discovered that most cells have a limited number times that they can divide. Once the limit is reached, the cells enter into senescence, and the aging and dying process begins. Those cells that escape this natural limit typically end up causing damage in the body and morph into cancer cells. For this reason, Hayflick was vocal in his criticism of 21st-century antiaging marketing schemes, and that is why he so frequently signed on to Olshansky's position papers. Michael Fossel and others placed great hope in the potential of telomerase to circumvent the natural Hayflick limit. Yet, Hayflick's theory argued that those cells that avoid the natural limit usually end up as cancer cells. Other researchers, including Aubrey de Grey, also argued that adding telomerase to artificially lengthen telomeres would likely lead to cancer. (Clearly, Aubrey de Grey believed there are other ways of avoiding the natural end of aging.)

The fixed life span biogerontologists are not necessarily pessimistic in their outlook. As the immunologist William Clark explains in his 1999 book *A Means to an End: The Biological Basis of Aging and Death*, "The bottom line is that everything we know about maximum possible lifespan in animals generally, and about evolution, suggests that true human maximal lifespan will not likely change in the absence of some sort of natural or man-made disaster." This is contrary to the technological sort of optimism commonly found in the antiaging movement, but Clark foresaw a future of increased comforts. Rather than postponing the final day of death, the advances of medical research will more likely shorten the final dying process. Clark ends his book with a sort of mixed hopefulness, saying, "As senescence-related disease causes of death are gradually eliminated . . . average lifespan will increase at the population level, but as individuals, our major organ systems will gradually grow weaker until we simply expire. More and more death certificates will read 'died of natural causes.' This is not a bad goal in itself."

Clark was not alone in this perspective. A large number of practitioners of geriatric medicine have similar views. They come in contact with elderly people in their practices every day, and though the pains of age-related conditions are obvious, there is not necessarily a sense of despair or loss among the patients. Many of the guidebooks that stress the objective of "living well" in old age develop the same point. A medical practitioner and professor at the University of North Carolina, Nortin Hadler, wrote several books warning patients to avoid unnecessary treatments that promise to alleviate and extend life. In *Rethinking Aging* (2011), Hadler wrote, "Although aging and dying are not diseases, older Americans are subject to intense marketing in the name of 'successful aging' and 'long life,' as if both are commodities." His point is that patients are not only overprescribed, resulting in nationally inflated medical costs, but they are also being encouraged to avoid the value found in the process of aging itself. For those who believe in a fixed life span, death is not necessarily an evil to always be avoided.

While some gerontologists who believe in a fixed life span are not pessimistic, there are others who are. Caleb Finch is a highly respected gerontologist at the Leonard Davis School of Gerontology at the University of Southern California, and codirector of the Alzheimer's Disease Research Center on the same campus. He has written more than 475 articles and several books, including the standard *Handbook of the Biology of Aging* (1979); *Aging: A Natural History* (1995); *Chance, Development, and Aging* (2000); and *The Biology of Human Longevity* (2007). Finch argues that genetics only plays a small part in the aging process and that other environmental conditions play a more determining role. Though he recognizes the value of medical advances that control disease, Finch argues that the modern world actually presents more toxins than ever before; therefore, the quality of living is less secure than it may have been previously. Citing increasing obesity rates, air pollution, and global warming, Finch was decidedly not optimistic about future life extension.

Religious Cohort Remains

While gerontologists debated the relative flexibility of the human life span, there remained another element that continued to oppose the antiaging movement on moral and religious grounds. Leon Kass was a biochemist turned bioethicist at the University of Chicago. In 2001, President George W. Bush announced he would create the President's Council on Bioethics, and he appointed Kass as chair. Kass's primary charge was to monitor stem cell research and to "recommend appropriate guidelines and regulations, and to consider all of the medical and ethical ramifications of biomedical innovation." In that position, Kass led national discussions on other questions beyond stem cell research, including therapeutic cloning, reproductive cloning, and antiaging medicine. Proponents of the antiaging movement generally viewed him quite negatively because Kass usually opposed new research involving the questionable treatment of human life, especially at the embryonic stage.

Kass was raised Jewish, but he described his childhood home as a "moral home" rather than a "Jewish home." He clearly reflected religious principles, but he did not assume any particular denominational position. His ethical philosophy was based on the premise that human life is sacred on its own merit. Quite contrary to the mechanistic view of most evolutionary biologists, Kass believed that all life is defined by its connection to an immaterial reality. He did not reject evolutionary theory, but he adopted a view similar to Christian humanists of the previous century. In short, Kass supported medical innovation and other forms of biotechnology as long as the treatments were used to cure disease, relieve suffering, and restore health. Other uses that would seek to overcome (or enhance) the natural limitations of human nature were viewed as ethically dangerous.

In part, Kass's views rested on the long-standing philosophical traditions of Christian humanists of the past centuries. He also reacted to the historical abuses of scientific theory demonstrated by the Nazi and Communist regimes during the 20th century. In his core philosophy, Kass believed that science and technology require an external moral standard to ensure they are directed toward positive rather than destructive means.

The antiaging community generally reacted with hostility to Leon Kass and those who shared his views, such as Yoshihiro Francis Fukuyama and Daniel Callahan.

Web sites such as fightaging.com called them "mystics" and "modern alchemists" who imposed their religious views on scientific knowledge. At heart, the problem was that the modern antiaging proponents did not accept the reality of a transcendent spiritual realm upon which standards of ethics and morality should be based. In a 2003 article, Kass wrote, "Conquering death is not something that we can try for a while and then decide whether the results are better or worse. . . This is a question in which our very humanity is at stake, not only in the consequences but also in the very meaning of choice. For to argue that human life would be better without death is, I submit, to argue that human life would be better being something other than human." In a later television interview, Kass explained, "The people who think that you can just tinker with the life span and not worry about its implications for the kinds of beings who will live . . . that to simply say life is good and more is therefore better—if that's as far as your thinking goes, then I would say it's shallow."

For religious believers, the prospect of radical life extension involves removing barriers that were set in place intentionally by the forces that created life. It also means never having an opportunity to experience immortality of the soul. For evolutionary biologists who do not believe there is any intention behind the existence of life and that there is no spirit or vitalistic essence beyond the biochemical machinery of the human flesh, there is nothing inherently natural about death, and these sorts of criticisms lose their meaning. To a certain extent, the antiaging movement requires skepticism of an immaterial existence after death.

CONCLUSION

The academic debate within the gerontological community had very little impact on the public demand for antiaging products, treatments, and regimen plans. The fears that Olshansky and Hayflick voiced in 2002 did not become realized a decade later. Certainly, the bourgeoning market for amateur antiaging remained more or less untamed by scientific prerequisites. At the same time, the available funding for geriatric medicine and age-related research likewise increased. In 2016, the NIH funded a study of nearly 800 elderly men with low testosterone levels to determine whether testosterone supplements might restore some of their youthful vitality, including diminished mobility, sexual function, and fatigue. This kind of study would have been extremely unlikely in the 1980s and 1990s, when anabolic steroids were viewed mostly in terms of athletic dishonesty and performance enhancement. It was the sort of study that Robert Goldman and Ronald Klatz promoted in the mid-1990s and the traditional gerontological community strongly criticized. Yet, by 2016, the funds for age-related research had begun to span both the traditional and the antiaging sides of the spectrum.

Sometime near the start of the 2010s, a quiet truce emerged between the traditional gerontologists and the antiaging advocates (both moderate and radical). In part, this arose because the public demand for some sort of scientific action for age-related disorders continued to grow as more and more baby boomers reached retirement age. There was also an understanding that the scientific discovery was not antithetical to business marketing. In 2010, Juergen Bludau wrote a book titled *Aging, but Never Old: The Realities, Myths, and Misrepresentations of the Anti-aging Movement.* Bludau is a geriatrics practitioner in New England and served as the executive medical director of the Elliot Memory & Mobility Center. He is firm believer in fixed life span, and from the start of the book, he quotes João Pedro de Magalhães to explain that aging is a "loss of viability and increase in vulnerability." He adds, "Aging is not a disease or a collection of diseases." It is inevitable and irreversible. Nevertheless, when confronted with the question of whether the anti-aging movement is medicine or business, Bludau responds, "The answer is both."

Bludau flatly rejects all of the five main areas of antiaging treatments: cosmetics; antioxidants and vitamin supplements; hormone replacement therapy (including hGH); dietary restriction and resveratrol (the active agent in red wine); and gene manipulation and stem cell therapy. He said, "None of the anti-aging products can truly treat aging or reverse it." At the same time, public demand has also inspired a great deal of research in traditional geriatric medicine, particularly in Alzheimer's research, mobility issues, and psychological well-being. The sensationalism of Audrey de Grey's predictions helped both the gerontological and the antiaging communities.

In 2014, Google Ventures, which is the investment arm of Google.com, set aside $425 million for investment in firms with potential return. The company regularly sets aside $300 million for such purposes, but in 2014, Google Ventures president Bill Maris announced he was looking to invest the money in antiaging ventures. This was in addition to $700 million that Google's research and development company, Calico (short for California Life Company), received, with promises of up to $1 billion more if needed. The research objectives of Calico are to combat aging and associated diseases. Google's founder, Larry Page, and Apple chairman Arthur Levinson are strong supporters of the antiaging movement. They publicly announced their commitment to "cure" aging and extend the human life span by another 100 years.

As the 21st century entered its second decade, the antiaging movement moved away from its origins in philosophy and theory and entered a new era of practical application. The popularity of eternal youth fueled academic interest, and the prospect of continuous innovation seemed unstoppable. The moral and ethical considerations that defined the start of the movement, and which continue to voice alarms and concerns about its direction, no longer play a dominant role in public decision making.

SECTION TWO

Modern Paths to the Fountain of Youth: A Topical Approach to the Practice of Antiaging

The fountain of youth may owe its origins to ancient dreams, but in the 21st century, it is viewed by many as a potential reality. We no longer search for mythical fountains, but instead plan on practical scientific discoveries to show the way to extended life, perhaps even to the extreme of scientifically engineered negligible senescence (SENS). The modern antiaging movement includes a broad spectrum of people who range from radical enthusiasts to moderate supporters. For each group, the fountain of youth takes on a slightly different meaning and is made accessible through a variety of methods. For some, the fountain of youth represents a watershed moment in the history of evolution, when humanity finally overcomes the boundaries of old age and death. For others, the prospect of prolongated life spans is viewed as a positive outcome of gradual and consistent scientific breakthroughs. Just as the expression of the modern fountain of youth changes with the different supporters, so too do the means and methods for attaining it.

In this section, we examine each alternate approach to the modern fountain of youth. We begin with the more subtle approaches for living healthier and potentially longer lives and end with the more radical approaches that seek to reverse aging or delay the onset of aging indefinitely. Each chapter begins with a summary of the current state of scientific knowledge on the given approach, including a list of specific research studies to support the claims. They end with a balanced overview of the costs and benefits of the approach in terms of quality of life and its antiaging objective. The information is not intended to serve as prescriptions for activity, but rather to provide a survey of current scientific theories and guesses. There is considerable disagreement inside and outside the circles of science, and these chapters are not intended to provide definitive answers. Instead, they present alternatives and let the reader form his or her own conclusions.

The chapters are organized topically according to key questions that help define the various approaches to antiaging. And they may be read independently, which means they may be read in any order without losing continuity. Chapters 6 and

7 begin by defining the terms of the discussion. What is life, that we may extend it? And what is death, that we might delay it? Even at these primary levels, there is debate, and the final picture of eternal youth looks different according to each answer. Chapters 8 and 9 examine what can be done without involving internal medical treatments. These include cosmetic enhancements that disguise the appearance of aging and general recommendations about health and fitness to disguise the feeling of being old. These treatments do not pretend to reverse or even slow down aging, but they may extend the quality of life within the parameters of the natural life span.

The next three chapters consider antiaging options that involve some level of medical treatment. Chapter 10 presents an overview of the most common age-related diseases and examines the current treatments available as well as theories for preventing their onset. Chapter 11 outlines the various supplements and diet regimens that are legally accessible without a prescription—their effectiveness most likely depends on individual expectations at the outset. Chapter 12 discusses potential treatments that require a doctor's oversight. These may include hormone therapies or other pharmaceutical remedies to address metabolic changes. The costs and benefits of these approaches may be speculative or based on presumptions that have not been demonstrated. The section ends with a consideration of the most intrusive and speculative treatments conceivable, including genetic manipulation, selective stem cell cloning, and intelligent prosthetics. Some advocates may call these the cutting edge of antiaging science, while others may view them as dangerous trends.

Throughout the section, religious conviction is set alongside scientific positivism, and they are examined according to their respective influences on successful treatment options. In many cases, the mind plays an important role in influencing health and the perception of aging. One of the defining characteristics of the modern antiaging movement is the degree to which supporters sincerely believe that science might someday find a solution to the problem of age-related diseases and possibly death itself.

Chapter 6

What Is Life, That We May Extend It?

The definition of life is complex. It is relatively easy to visually distinguish living things from dead things, but it is difficult to explain precisely what it is that separates the two. A body may be living in one moment and then be dead in the next. What happened to cause that life to extinguish? What was it that was removed or that ended to cause the living cells or other organic materials to cease functioning on their own? Life is not visible or measurable. We can only identify it by its effects. A living thing moves, changes on its own, reproduces, takes in nourishment, and grows. Perhaps, most importantly, a living thing can die. It is that absence of life that most distinguishes living from nonliving matter. Yet, that is a circular definition and does not really define what life is.

The question is important for the antiaging movement, because if we seek to protect life and prevent it from weakening or dying, we need to understand what it is that needs protection or what it is that is being extended. Natural scientists in biology and chemistry have a working definition of life, as described above: living things move or respond to stimuli, reproduce, take nourishment, grow, and die. But that is mostly a theory of negation. Science can really only measure when life is over. It measures the effects of life, and it can identify when those effects have ended—therefore determining when life has ended. Yet, material science alone has yet to provide a definition that extends beyond measuring life's impact on other physical characteristics. Life always begins with life, and scientists have not been able to find the cause, the substance, the chemical combination, or any other physical characteristic that will transform nonliving materials into living materials. The best that natural science can do is identify when those living materials have lost their life.

There are other definitions of life that do not rely on material explanations. Since ancient times, life has almost always been defined in religious and philosophical terms. Mostly, life is defined as a sort of divine or immaterial spark that animates organisms. Different varieties of life are still identified by their characteristics, and there is a hierarchy of plants, animals, and humans. Though life takes on many forms, from a religious perspective, the essence of life stems from some immaterial source of energy that enlivens the inanimate matter to transform it into living matter. These sorts of immaterial or spiritual-based definitions of life pose a problem for modern antiaging advocates because they limit their opportunities for action. Scientists can identify and at least try to manipulate those phenomena that are based exclusively in the material world. There is, however, no scientific solution for problems that are based in the immaterial world. As such, most antiaging scientists prefer to rely on the working definition of life used by biologists and chemists, even if it is only a descriptive one.

At its most fundamental level, the definition of life will always depend on certain metaphysical presumptions. Antiaging scientists usually rely on definitions that presume there is nothing outside the material world. Religious believers use definitions that presuppose both a material and an immaterial world. There is no quantifiable proof for either option, so both options reflect a certain kind of faith. Antiaging scientists have faith that there is nothing outside this world, while the religious believers have faith in just the opposite. In this way, life is unavoidably defined by our type of faith. The approach, expectations, and hope for the antiaging movement reflects these presumptions.

TRADITIONAL VIEW: RELIGIOUS SPIRIT

Skeptical atheism is a belief system that rejects anything outside the material world. Agnosticism is a similar system that allows for the possibility of an immaterial realm but believes that it is completely removed from the material realm and therefore unknowable. Combined, both beliefs are held by a relatively small minority of people, estimated at about 14 percent of the world's population in 2002. This means that the vast majority of the world believes there is something beyond the material realm and that immaterial world influences us.

There is often considerable disagreement between various religious traditions as to what exists in the immaterial realm, but the fact that it exists is very commonly accepted. In the polytheistic and animistic cultures of the Far East, the immaterial world is dominated by a host of spirits, deities, and other beings that live immortal lives beyond the physical realm. They exist outside the physical world and as such are rarely seen or felt by those people who live inside the material world. Life of any sort is animated by these spirits, and it is their presence that distinguishes between living things and dead things. When the spirit has left a body, the body is dead. The essence of life has moved on.

In each of the various forms of Buddhism, Hinduism, Jainism, Manichaeism, and animism found throughout Asia, the personhood of each individual is defined by his or her soul. For those who believe in reincarnation, they believe that the soul passes from one body into another over successive generations. There may be a host of other spirits in and around each material body, but the single soul that defines personhood is unique for each individual. Life, then, is more than what we see in our physical bodies. It is defined by that immortal spirit that lives forever and never dies. If that immaterial spirit were to die, that personhood would also die and never again inhabit a physical body.

Polytheism and animism have largely disappeared in the West, having been replaced by Judeo-Christian and Islamic religious views. Yet, the West shares with the East the same basic presumptions about the immortality of the human soul. All three Western faiths, like their counterparts in the East, believe that individual personhood is defined by a unique soul, and human life in particular is defined by the presence of that spirit. The West differs from the East in its belief of how life is manifested in other forms. Not all life-forms have souls. Very few of the various sects of Jewish, Christian, and Islamic believers would accept that plants have souls, or even that animals have souls. Yet, plants and animals are alive. Western monotheistic philosophy generally distinguishes between a "life force" that inhabits all living things and a "soul," which only certain creatures (such as humans) possess. Both the life force and the soul exist mostly in the immaterial realm, and they both owe their origin to a divine source (God). Yet, the life force of plants and animals is generic and not tied to individual identity. A soul is unique to each individual and exists in addition to and beyond the basic life force.

Mind-Body Problem

This contrast between life force and the soul is a simplistic version of what René Descartes described as the "mind-body" problem. He firmly believed in the reality of a soul that exists in the immaterial realm, yet he also believed in the reality of a life force that exists independently in the material realm. He argued that the two realms are distinct, and though he could not understand how they interact, he believed that they do somehow. Humans have bodies that are living as a result of the life force. Yet, they also have souls that carry the burdens of our sins and our virtues because the soul enables free will. The mind-body problem was useful for Descartes in explaining why we should treat science, the natural world, and even the biological mechanics of the human body as completely distinct from the moral burdens of the soul. Biology, chemistry, and physics describe the physical world, and theology and philosophy help to explain the immaterial world. We can use the natural sciences to understand the operations of the generic life force, and we can use the metaphysical sciences (theology and philosophy) to understand the human soul. The two realms are separate. And though he did not know how the soul is tied to the body, Descartes did not believe that mystery needed to be solved for scientific knowledge to be understood.

In the 20th and 21st centuries, most Judeo-Christian philosophies share this same mind-body distinction that Descartes proposed. Human life is characterized by a unique personhood defined by the soul and is deliberately created by God with intention and purpose. When human life ends, the soul departs from the body but does not die. When the life force of the body is extinguished, the soul departs. This explanation helps to distinguish between plants and animals and humans. The basic functions of life that animate a human body may be the same sort that also animate animals and plants, but only humans have souls. There may be some disagreement over whether higher animals may have a different type of soul, but there is very little disagreement that the human soul is unique and particularly ordained by God as a special creation.

This distinction between life force and soul allows some churches to believe in the possibility of biological evolution through intelligent design. As long as God is recognized as the source of individual personhood (the soul), it is less important to identify how God chose to create and spread the life force that enlivens all organisms. The Judeo-Christian perspective believes that God must have deliberately transcended the immaterial realm to create the first spark that triggered the spread of a life force. In this way, belief in the evolutionary process does not necessarily negate the belief in an active God. Human life comes from God, animal life comes from God, and so too does plant life; yet, religious believers are able to distinguish a hierarchy between the different forms of life. The soul makes human life sacred because it reflects characteristics shared by God (free will, often described as "the image of God"). Higher animals may (or may not) have souls, but they do not have souls that are created in God's image (no free will and no reason). Lower animals may have different kinds of souls or none at all. Plants are usually never described as having any souls at all.

Vitalism

The mind-body problem posed a difficulty for early humanist scientists trying to explain life in purely material terms. The human soul was entirely immaterial, so it was recognized as residing under the domain of faith and metaphysical sciences. The mind somehow connected the immaterial soul with the physical body, but it was unclear how—so that was left for philosophers to discuss. Yet, the biological mechanisms of the human body (and other plant and animal life forms) existed in the material realm. As such, the life force was necessarily a material property. The problems were how to describe it and how to identify it?

Francis Bacon used the term *spirit* to identify this life force, but he did not invent the concept. It is possible that Bacon was borrowing from ideas taken from Chinese Taoism and adapting it to Western Christianity. Even before Bacon, though, the concept of an enervating, nonsoul-like spirit that bestowed life on inanimate objects had circulated among Christian scholars for several hundred years. In the late 300s, St. Augustine wrote that the plants and animals were created from the life force that God impregnated in the water and soils at the time of creation. Augustine did not believe it was necessary to assume that the creation of particular animals was limited to six days alone. He believed God created all plant and animal life (the life force) and that, over time, some of these species arose from the living elements. In all cases, though, he believed life came from life. Thomas Aquinas echoed this same explanation in the late 1200s, when he explained that some sorts of life-forms arise through the decomposition of other dead organic materials. Aquinas rejected the alchemist ideas posed by the Arabic physician Avicenna, who suggested that life could be generated from certain combinations of inanimate materials.

This medieval tradition eventually evolved into a theory of spontaneous regeneration. Jean-Baptiste Lamarck used this theory to explain biological evolution over a very long period of time. He argued that life emerges as single-celled forms from the rotting organic materials of both plants and animals. These single-celled forms then evolve into multicellular organisms, and over a very long period of time, these eventually evolve into diverse species of plants and animals. Lamarck believed that God created this system and was the first to bestow life that triggered the process, but he accepted Descartes's argument that the processes of the material world operated independent of the immaterial world. Lamarck would have described that life force as a "vital essence," and his belief that life continually spawns additional life is often called "vitalism."

The Lamarckian concept of vitalism is a later derivation of Bacon's *spirit*, which was itself a later derivation of Aquinas and Augustine and a host of other early philosophers. The difference between Lamarck's vitalism and Augustine's concept of impregnated soils and water is that Lamarck argued the process was continual and ongoing every spring. Lamarck pointed to the ponds that had frozen over the winter (and where all life had seemingly been killed), which were reawakened each spring with microorganisms swimming along the top layers of water. Similarly, he pointed to the appearance of maggots in rotting flesh and concluded they were created from the meat itself. Augustine believed the creation of particular sorts of animals occurred very near the start of creation, and they were uniquely ordained by God to arise at the appropriate times later in history. He did not see it as a natural nor continual phenomenon that could occur with any collection of decomposing materials.

The modern Lamarckian definition of vitalism suffered a blow from biologists in the mid-1800s when they discovered that microorganisms come from other microorganisms and do not spontaneously regenerate from any sort of rotting materials. As early as 1688, the Italian Francesco Redi hypothesized that maggots formed in rotting meat because flies had lain eggs too small to see. When he covered the meat and let it set for many days, he found the meat never grew maggots. Yet, it was not until the mid-1800s that Louis Pasteur set up several experiments to show that protected meat will never develop organisms. When a broth is pasteurized (cleansed of any microorganisms) and then covered completely, the broth remains free of organisms indefinitely. If, however, the broth is left in an open vessel, organisms and maggots will develop. Pasteur proved that single-cellular life does not arise spontaneously from rotting organic materials but only from preexisting microorganisms already present.

As vitalism was so strongly tied to spontaneous regeneration, Pasteur's discovery caused many natural scientists to dismiss the concept altogether. The problem is that the two concepts are not synonymous. When Francis Bacon referred to spirits that provide nourishment to living tissues, he was not referring to spontaneous regeneration. He was referring to some material life force that exists in the physical world that is responsible for maintaining life in organic materials. Ironically, Pasteur's experiments actually reaffirmed Bacon's sense of spirit or vitalism, even as they refuted Lamarck's ideas of spontaneous regeneration. Pasteur proved that dead materials, even if they are organic, cannot bring about life. Life must come from some existing life source. It cannot be spontaneously regenerated from inanimate materials. From the perspective of Judeo-Christian traditions, the narrowly defined sense of vitalism (as a life force) would remain affirmed even in the 20th and 21st centuries. Nevertheless, because of its ties to spontaneous regeneration, modern secular scientists usually dismiss vitalism out of hand as an archaic theory of life.

MODERN EVOLUTIONARY BIOLOGY VIEW

Charles Darwin fervently rejected the vitalist theory of life—not necessarily because of vitalism's association with the theory of spontaneous generation, but because of its presumption of immaterial properties. Darwin rejected any life-force theory that relied on the existence of an intangible substance or essence to animate life. He explicitly rejected the possibility that God, or any spiritual agent, could have any role in the creation or development of life. Lamarck had already introduced the theory of biological evolution, and Darwin's primary thesis in *The Origin of the Species* argues that biological evolution occurred randomly and without God, through the unavoidable competition of the natural environment. Modern evolutionary biologists have largely followed his lead in this respect.

Part of the problem of the life-force definition is that science has yet to develop a tool that can measure (or in any way quantify) immaterial phenomena. Any theory that relies on some agent outside the material realm is automatically suspect because it cannot be proven or disproven by physical evidence. One implication of Descartes's mind-body problem was that any explanation for a phenomenon in the natural world must rely on material, demonstrable, and replicable evidence. That insistence is what most characterized the scientific revolution. It was also partially why Francis Bacon asserted the existence of spirits to explain how living tissues retain their life (and eventually lose it). Bacon assumed the spirits were materially based substances that therefore might become measurable if the right tools were invented. There was more room for mystery in Bacon's era, even within the physical realm. In our 21st century of biochemistry and quantum physics, such mysteries are no longer tolerated. Modern evolutionary biologists reject the theory of a life force because they are incapable of measuring or interacting with such an immaterial force.

The theory of evolutionary biology does not require someone to be an atheist or agnostic, yet the two often go together. If you reject anything that cannot be measured as irrelevant to scientific theory, it is a small step to reject the very existence of any immaterial reality. If there is no life force, it is just as possible that there is no soul, no spiritual realm, and no God. Scientific materialism may lead to atheism. At the same time, if you begin with atheism or agnosticism, then vitalism must be rejected because it presupposes a source of life outside of this material realm. In this way, atheism always requires scientific materialism.

What then is life for an evolutionary biologist? The official definition of life used by the National Aeronautics and Space Administration (NASA) in determining whether life exists on other planets does not refer to "life" outside of measurable effects. For NASA, life is defined by movement, reaction, growth, reproduction, and death. Life is only those effects, and nothing more. This definition is sometimes referred to as a mechanistic view of life because it looks at the human body as a biological machine. When the parts are in the right order, the machine works. When they go out of the order, the machine begins to break down and eventually dies.

The difficulty with the strict machine analogy is that life must come from life—even evolutionary biologists recognize that. Louis Pasteur concluded that new life only grew when it was seeded by old life. Yet, in the context of a machine, the parts are assembled and then the machine can be turned on and off at will. There is no "life" of the machine because it depends on a human to turn it on or turn it off. The analogy does not exactly fit with biological machines because organic matter has never yet been "turned on." In terms of organic biochemistry, the characteristics of life are only ever displayed by organisms that have inherited that condition of life from a previous generation. Scientists cannot assemble the parts of an organic compound and then turn the material on and make it come alive. The fact of this impossibility is the stuff of fictional stories, such as *Frankenstein* or *Re-animator*. It is also a basic premise behind the bulk of zombie movies in the 21st century: dead things somehow come back to life, not as humans but as living forms. The general theme behind these stories is that the reanimation is unnatural and always dangerous.

Spontaneous Generation in Evolution

If life must always come from preexisting life, and if evolutionary biology presumes that all life originated from a single source, then where did that single source begin? How then do evolutionary biologists explain the origin of life? Many evolutionary biologists have attempted to provide an answer, and they all follow the same basic pattern. As Richard Dawkins explained in *Selfish Gene*, the world was formed through some sort of gravity-based attraction (the origin of the universe is usually left to astrophysicists, such as Albert Einstein or Stephen Hawking). In the beginning, the surface of the planet was mostly composed of simple molecules such as water, carbon dioxide, methane, and ammonia. Over time, with some sort of electrical agitation, these simple molecules formed into more complex amino acids. Over a much longer period of time, these amino acids formed together through some sort of accident to create a single "replicator" molecule, which could make copies of itself. When that occurred, the basic foundations of life were set in place, and the rest was simply a process of natural selection and biological evolution as that life-form evolved and developed into multiple expressions.

Ironically, the essence of evolutionary theory relies on the probability of spontaneous generation. Except, unlike Lamarck's concept of spontaneous *regeneration*, the new evolutionary theory does not presuppose any previously existing organic materials. Somehow, over a very long period of time, the nonorganic materials became organic and created the first spark of life. From thence, all other life-forms have arisen. Unlike Lamarck, who asserted the process of regeneration occurs continually (mostly in the spring), evolutionary theory has the advantage of stipulating that it need only have occurred once, after billions of years of not occurring. The extreme length of time seems to make the spontaneous generation more likely for evolutionary biologists. As life obviously exists now, they conclude that it must have happened.

Transhumanism

What does it matter whether life comes from an immaterial source or stems from material characteristics alone? The answer poses serious implications for the anti-aging movement. If life is the by-product of an immaterial life force, there is little that material science can do to alter its natural course. In ancient China, the animistic Taoists believed the material and immaterial worlds were so intertwined that they could use certain substances and techniques from the material world to compel the immaterial world to obey and sustain earthly life indefinitely. Such alternatives do not exist for Western skeptics who do not believe in the immaterial realm or that material actions can hold any effect on it. Antiaging advocates in the West must believe in an entirely mechanistic view of life to hold any hope of significant life extension.

If life is simply a collection of characteristics found within biological machinery, there is hope that the machinery can be adjusted to facilitate longer life spans. Perhaps more promising, if life is only found in the collection of biochemical characteristics, the line between animate and inanimate may be less rigid than previously supposed. Mechanical objects implanted in an organic medium and interfaced with living materials would result in an "enhanced organism." It sounds rather like science fiction at first, but there are already many examples of technological implants that enhance or repair human tissues: pacemakers help regulate heart-beats, artificial joints help to extend the longevity of load-carrying limbs, cochlear implants provide hearing for the deaf, and dialysis machines help to replicate the function of the kidneys. In each case, the inanimate biotechnologies enhance the living tissues without changing the nature of the living organism.

The theory that technology might directly enhance human life by enhancing senses, or adding new ones, or otherwise overcoming natural biological limitations through some sort of implantation was introduced by Julian Huxley in the early 1950s. He called the idea "transhumanism." It was not new to Huxley, and the idea had been played with by numerous science fiction writers (see *Slan* (1946) by A. E. van Vogt and *More Than Human* (1953) by Theodore Sturgeon). As scientific technology increased, science fiction stories followed suit. With the advent of computers came both the threat and the promise that computers might develop an artificial intelligence as well as human emotions. In 1950, Alan Turing wrote an article, "Computer Machinery and Intelligence," in which he predicted that one day a human might interact with a computer over a distance and not be able to tell that it was not human. Writers such as Samuel Butler, Arthur C. Clarke, Isaac

Asimov, and Ray Bradbury speculated about how the meaning of life might change if computers could replicate the characteristics shared by human life—particularly the idea of free will and intelligence. Like *Frankenstein* and the zombie genre, these stories often predicted negative consequences for existing life.

During the early 2000s, the theory of transhumanism merged with the antiaging movement. Rather than fear machines becoming more like humans, the new hope was that humans might become more like machines. As the processing power continued to increase and the available random access memory and other fixed memory drives expanded, the dream of unlimited human potential emerged among certain futurists, such as F. M. Esfandiary (author of *Are You a Transhuman?* (1989)); Max More and Tom Morrow (founders of the Extropy Institute); Nick Bostrum and David Pearce (founders of the World Transhumanist Association); and Zoltan Istvan (2016 presidential candidate for the Transhumanism Party). Technology seemed to exist to enhance human life, perhaps by uploading human consciousness into

Presidential Hopeful Zoltan Istvan

Transhumanism moved from philosophy to politics when Zoltan Istvan formed the Transhumanism Party in 2014. He was elected by other party members to run as the Transhumanist Party presidential nominee for the 2016 election. In an interview, Istvan explained, "I'd say the number one goal of transhumanism is trying to conquer death." The Transhumanist Party platform includes the following priorities:

1. Implement a Transhumanist Bill of Rights mandating government support of longer life spans via science and technology
2. Spread a proscience culture by emphasizing reason and secular values
3. Create stronger government policies to protect against existential risk (including artificial intelligence, plagues, asteroids, climate change, and nuclear warfare and disaster)
4. Provide free education at every level and advocate for mandatory preschool and college education in the age of longer life spans
5. Advocate for morphological freedom (the right to do anything to your body so long as it does not harm others)

Istvan is a self-proclaimed atheist who believes "religion has damaged the species and held back science." He campaigned in a school bus that was refashioned to look like a giant coffin, with the name "Immortality Bus" painted on the side. Explaining his media campaign, Istvan said, "We're just normal people that realize that, without a culture of techno-optimism, nothing gets done. And the reason is that 100 percent of the U.S. Congress, the Supreme Court, and the U.S. president is all religious—they all believe in afterlives. They don't see a reason for wanting to live indefinitely." According to Istvan, transhumanists strive to be "godlike" and are not bound by religious presuppositions.

a computer or by implanting computerized accessories in humans that allow for online storage of memories and experiences directly in mechanical devices inside the body. In essence, transhumanism provided the hope of another option for life extension. If the medical sciences cannot preserve the body indefinitely, then anti-aging advocates looked toward physical technologies to permanently extend the life of individual consciousness, even if the physical organic body fails and dies (see chapter 12).

Transhumanism is only conceivable if human identity is strictly limited to the neuron transmissions and brainwave activity of the biological body. It presumes there is nothing more to each person than the physical biochemical reactions that occur somewhere in the brain and nervous system. If those processes were duplicated and recorded, the human person could be copied and transported into any variety of mechanical devices. On the other hand, if it turns out that life is anything more than these physical interactions, transhumanism loses its potential meaning.

BALANCED OVERVIEW

How we define life determines to a great extent how we choose to protect and preserve it. If life is immaterial by nature, then our definition of preservation is necessarily immaterial, at least in part. If life is entirely physical and material, then our definition of preservation must also be entirely physical. There are benefits and consequences to each belief. Most often, however, an individual's belief will also likely determine whether he or she believes the implications are positive or negative.

Implications of Religious Definitions of Life

The primary advantage to a religious definition of life is that it presumes that life was created with potential and inherent meaning. If life owes its source to a larger immaterial reality outside the physical realm—in other words, if God created each individual soul deliberately and with intention—then the life of each person has some particular meaning and purpose. At the very least, the belief in a life force and a soul allows the possibility for intentional meaning in both. Meaningfulness in life is the fundamental requirement of all religious faith and a primary justification for moral conduct. If life has no inherent meaning, there are no expectations or moral standards that govern life, no hope for reward or punishment for misspent lives, and no reason to act in any other way than as one desires.

Beyond the promise of meaningfulness, a religious definition of life also opens a pathway for eternal life outside of this physical world. It presupposes the existence of an unseen, unmeasured world that parallels, transcends, and yet remains removed from the material world. If life begins in this immaterial realm, and if our individual identity is linked to a soul that exists in that same realm, there is hope that life will continue even after the physical body dies. It is the promise of heaven that makes the spiritual definition of human life so compelling.

The drawback of a supernatural definition of life is that it is not measurable in any physical way. Belief in the soul or in a generalized life force is entirely based on faith in its existence, just as the belief in God is an act of faith that extends beyond physical proofs. That does not mean that there is no indirect evidence, only that the essence of either one cannot be measured by scientific equipment. Indirect evidence is measured in the same way that evolutionary biologists measure life, through its characteristics. It requires faith, however, to believe those characteristics are enlivened by an unseen, immeasurable force. It is worth noting that as life cannot be created from inanimate materials, it also requires an equal amount of faith to believe that there is no unseen, immeasurable force. Both the religious and the atheistic definitions of life require an element of faith.

Perhaps the most critical side effect for antiaging advocates of a religious definition of life is the imposition of unseen limitations. If life is created and made meaningful by some supernatural purpose, there are rules about what types of research should or should not be pursued. If human life is sacred, science must observe moral restraints with regard to human research and experimentation. Embryonic stem cell research, human cloning, and radical life extension need to be examined according to whether these practices devalue life or otherwise violate the religious expectations of morality. During the early 2000s, Leon Kass was harshly criticized for his unwillingness to support these types of research during his tenure as chair of the Presidents' Council on Bioethics. The primary criticism against Kass was that his religious definition of life limited the pace of scientific research. Ironically, what nonreligious believers see as a drawback of moral restraint is often viewed by religious advocates as one of its greatest benefits.

Implications of Evolutionary Biologists' Definition of Life

For antiaging advocates, the primary advantage of a strictly material evolutionary biological definition of life is that life is potentially unbounded. It can be changed, adapted, and possibly made more or less eternal. For natural scientists, then, life is exactly what it appears to be and nothing more. The benefit of this strict materialism is that eventually, given enough time, science can reveal everything there is to know about the machine of human life, its biochemical processes, and all the potential loopholes that might be used to adapt and change the machine to fit particular needs.

Another potential consequence of the mechanistic view is that it holds no hierarchical value to life. As life was not created with any meaning or purpose, there is no reason to assume that one form of life is better or superior to another. In terms of tolerance of human differences (such as race, class, or gender), the mechanistic view holds no favorites. Even limitations that appear to be bound by natural order, such as biological sexuality, are defined only in terms of biochemical interactions. Men can choose to become women, if they make the necessary biochemical adjustments, and women can choose to become men. From this viewpoint, gender and identity is not fixed to any sort of biological or supernatural imperative. For antiaging advocates, that also means that the long-standing limitation of the human life span is equally adjustable, and scientific research should be able to modify its length and extent as each person desires. In short, there is nothing "natural" about nature because nature can become whatever scientific adaptation allows it to be.

One of the most commonly discussed benefits of an entirely mechanistic view of life is that it imposes no artificial limitations on natural science. If there is no transcendent purpose to life, there are no rules as to what can and cannot be researched or studied. Embryonic stem cell research, human cloning, and radical life extension are all permissible fields of study. Of course, this is precisely the source of its greatest criticism from opponents. In its most extreme form, the strict mechanistic definition of life evaluates research only according to whether the research leads to practical results. This was the guiding principle behind the eugenic research conducted by scientists during Nazi Germany. If human life is nothing more than a set of biological characteristics, the value of human life is determined by the perceived success of those characteristics. During Nazi Germany, the supposed Aryan supremacy became the ultimate standard of research success. The horrors of the Holocaust caused even the most skeptical evolutionary biologist to reconsider his or her definition of human life. One reaction was to carry the neutrality of life to its extreme and argue that there are no standards of excellence and that human life was no better, nor worse, than a parasitical tapeworm because each found success in adapting to its environment. From this viewpoint, the arrogance of Aryan supremacy was that it based success on completely arbitrary standards. Another reaction was to move the other direction and argue that human life could be endowed with meaning through a common consensus of humanity. From this viewpoint, the consensus of the world identified the grotesqueness of Nazi human experimentation and genocide as a crime against human civilization. In either extreme, however, human life remained free of any intrinsic meaning.

From a strictly scientific perspective, the mechanistic definition of life suffers from an inadequate explanation of its origins. Where does life come from? Whether human, animal, or plant, one critical presumption of evolutionary biology is that life comes from life. The various plants, animals, and humans were not individually "created," they all evolved from a single source. It is a fundamental premise of evolution that all life-forms are related to a single common source. Yet, the theory also presupposes that the first single source somehow spontaneously generated out of nonliving matter. That is a difficult contradiction to resolve.

Typically, the most common solution is to argue that the probability of inanimate matter producing animate life is extremely small, but not zero. As long as there is some probability at all, then given enough time—perhaps billions of years—even the most improbable options become probable. Religious critics argue that the explanation is unsatisfying because it relies on the same degree of faith that is required for believing in a divine act of creation. There is no evidence that inanimate matter can ever produce living matter. Religious believers would then argue that the probability of inanimate material suddenly becoming animate is zero. Therefore, no amount of time would change the outcome. Strict materialist skeptics nevertheless believe it must be possible because life clearly exists now. As material skeptics do not believe in God, the only other possible explanation for the presence of life is spontaneous generation. It is the lack of faith in the divine that makes the possibility of strict mechanism so compelling.

CONCLUSION

The definition of life will not be resolved through scientific methodology. It is a reflection of individual faith and will always depend on basic metaphysical presumptions. Religious definitions to do not preclude the possibility of extending the average life expectancy or promoting healthier lifestyles. Yet, the ultimate determination of life span is determined (or regulated) by forces outside of human control. Conversely, the antiaging goals of extending the human life span beyond the existing limitations imposed by nature do require mechanist definitions of life. They may share common cause with religious advocates in terms of promoting a longer period of active living, with less disease and disability. Ultimately, though, the goal of ending or reversing the aging process to radically extend the human life span presupposes there is nothing to life except forces of physical biochemistry. As modern society has become more secular, the demand and urgency for antiaging technologies has increased proportionately.

Chapter 7

What Is Death, That We Might Delay It?

Death is somewhat easier to define than life. In its most basic meaning, death is the ending of life. As we identify the physical characteristics of life, we can mark the cessation of those characteristics and know the organism has died. The more difficult task is to identify the processes and stages that lead to death. We sometimes refer to that process as "dying," but it may be more precise to simply say "aging." Most people think of dying as that last period of physical decline when the strength and senses of the body begin to fail, just before death. Yet, as the first-century Roman poet Marcus Manilius wrote, "We are dying from our very birth." It is very difficult to know precisely at what point the body ceases to grow and begins to decline. It is best to consider the process of aging to include all the steps that each organism takes from its beginning to its end.

Life is not a process; it is a condition of being. That means the definition of life necessarily involves some article of faith because we cannot know for certain whether that condition of life is limited to this material world only or also extends into the immaterial realm. By contrast, aging is not a condition but a biological process, and one that occurs to all living beings in the physical world. Faith plays little role in defining aging because natural science can identify certain markers of age and measure its effects on the human body. The physical characteristics of aging are apparent for everyone to see, and since the 2000s, scientists have tried to identify particular genetic markers for aging. These should be measurable and quantifiable. Moreover, there are numerous scientific theories as to why and how we age. This chapter discusses each of these theories in turn.

There is some philosophical debate over the question of aging—not in the sense of questioning how or why we age, but rather in the sense of questioning whether we must age at all. So far, science has not been able to conclusively determine whether the biological process of aging is adjustable. This question concerns the antiaging movement most directly because the movement explicitly seeks to stay, slow, or reverse the aging process. These advocates must believe that the aging process is open to change and can be altered or stopped altogether. There are, however, others who do not believe that aging can be changed. The deciding factor over whether a scientist believes or does not believe in the immutability of the aging process has little to do with faith because aging is entirely a physical process.

Nevertheless, faith does play a small role in understanding the inevitability of aging (and death). Religious believers hold that God created life with a particular purpose and that eternal life is found only in the immaterial world (heaven). They usually presume that aging is inevitable and that death is necessary. On the other extreme, certain radical antiaging advocates argue that human life can be extended permanently and that death may become optional or accidental. They generally do not believe that there is anything outside the material realm. Often, the radical antiaging position views death as a reversion into nothingness, after which life simply ends (no heaven or supernatural existence). The imperative to find a solution to aging and death increases as faith in an immaterial reality decreases.

Atheists may also believe that aging is inevitable and death unavoidable, though for different reasons than their religious counterparts. Many natural scientists, religious or not, argue that aging is a natural by-product of living in a physical universe. As all material substances break down and decay over time, they conclude that no material thing can last forever, especially living tissue. These realists may or may not believe that death is a reversion into nothingness, but they also believe that there is little that science can do about it. The central debate between antiaging advocates and these realists is over the question of whether science is capable of manipulating the environment in such a way as to render the effects of time meaningless. The antiaging advocates believe that it is possible, and the realists do not.

This chapter begins with a brief overview of aging trends over the past century to identify whether there is evidence for claiming that the process of aging has already been altered by modern medical practices. Most theories of aging can be divided between those that assume the process is alterable and those that do not. Each theory is considered in light of both proponents and critics. The chapter concludes with some discussion on the positive and negatives implications of the two perspectives on the inevitability of aging and death.

BASIC DEFINITIONS

Every person experiences the effects of aging, no matter how old they are. In the case of childhood and adolescence, the effects of aging are tied to physical growth and sexual development. In the case of adults at the peak of their maturity, the effects may be tied to sustaining physical conditioning and reproductive health. In the case of older adults, the effects are more frequently tied to the loss of physical abilities and the eventual onset of death. Most biogerontologists distinguish the early effects that lead to growth as "development" and generically identify the later effects that lead to decline in biological functions as "aging." It is this last stage of life that receives the most attention in terms of antiaging treatments.

Biodemographers study the comparative lengths of each stage of aging and are able to trace the aggregate changes over time. The cultural markers of adolescence appear to have changed significantly over the course of the 20th century among developed nations, as teens are provided with longer periods of time to develop the technical and intellectual skills necessary for adulthood. Nevertheless, at a biological level, the spans of childhood and adolescence seem to have remained relatively constant. Some evidence suggests that girls experience the onset of puberty at younger ages than in previous centuries, but the research is mixed. The biological evidence of other markers for age is not consistent. Also, there is very little evidence that boys have been maturing at younger ages. At the other end of the spectrum, however, there seems to be considerable evidence that adults are postponing their late adulthood to increasingly older ages. More people are living more active lives until later ages. The average life expectancy continues to increase, apparently suggesting that onset of death is, on average, also being pushed into later years.

These sets of demographic evidence suggest that the rate of aging has already adapted according to modern industrial living conditions. In theory, if the rate of aging appears to be changing, then the length of the human life span should expand accordingly. There is, however, considerable debate on this last point. The average life expectancy is increasing, but there is little evidence to suggest the maximum life span has changed.

Life Expectancy versus Life Span

Biodemographers rely on very specific vocabulary to describe changing variables of life and death in a given society over a given period of time. Average life expectancy refers to the average length of time between birth and death for a population. This statistic is cited most often as an indicator of lengthening life span, but in fact it does not say very much at all about potential length of life. It merely provides a statistical snapshot of a given population.

The average number of years between birth and death must also include a percentage of people who died at birth or at very young ages as well as those who died from accidents or disease during middle ages. These low numbers are weighted against all those who died at very old ages. The statistic does not indicate what the maximum capacity for any individual might be if there were no diseases or accidents. If infant mortality is high, the average life expectancy will be low. If infant mortality and the number of accidents and diseases affecting adults at middle age are reduced, the average life expectancy will increase. This remains true even if the number of people living to really old ages remains exactly the same. No person in recorded history has lived past the age of 122. Only five women have lived past 115, while only three men have lived past 114. Statistically, current evidence suggests that the human life span is at least 122, but there is not enough evidence to know whether that maximum is unique or fixed.

Statistics cannot determine maximum length of life, but it can identify previous trends. The increase in average life expectancy suggests that people are getting older. In 1850, the average life expectancy in the United States was 40 years. By 1910, it had increased to 50 years. That is a 10-year increase over a 60-year period. By 1930, the life expectancy had increased to 60, which is the same amount of increase in one-third the time (20 years instead of 60). If that rate were to continue,

Mortality Rates

There are other sorts of statistics that attempt to provide more meaningful information about individual life spans. Mortality rates refer to the number of people that die at a given age within a population. In 2009, a little less than 1 percent of infants died before their first birthday. That percentage declines precipitously until children reach the age of 5, in which case their mortality rates hover at just over 1/100th of what it was 4 years prior. Less than 1 out of 10,000 children died (for any reason at all) between the ages of 5 to 9 years. Those rates begin to increase at age 10 and are again significant after age 15. Between the ages of 20 and 30, people die at a rate of just over 1 out of every 1,000. After 35, mortality rates increase at a steady rate, with mortality rates of 1 out of 100 at age 65, 1 out of 10 at age 85, and approach nearly 9 out of 10 at age 100. These statistics suggest that as we approach the end of our natural life span, the likelihood of dying increases.

Yet, mortality rates only give odds of living. At age 65, women face a 50 percent probability that they will live another 20 years, and a man has a 50 percent chance of living 17 more years. At age 80, a man has only a 30 percent change of living 10 more years. At some age point, the probability of living one more year becomes exceedingly low. Yet, even then, the probability only refers to past evidence and does not say much about individual likelihood of survival.

In 2016, 100 percent of the people aged 117 years died (both of them: Andrew Hatch of Oakland, California, and Misao Okawa of Tokyo). That left 116-year-old Susannah Mushatt of Brooklyn, New York, as the oldest living person. What is the likelihood that she will continue to live to reach the oldest recorded age of 122 (a record held by Jeanne Calment of France)? Given the very small number of similar examples, any guess at probability is not very meaningful.

we would expect life expectancy to increase to 70 years in 1940, 80 years in 1945, and 100 years by 1950. These statistics can be misleading. In fact, it took 65 years for the life expectancy to reach 75 (only a 15-year increase.) Since 1995, the average life expectancy has increased less than 4 years during the 20-year period to 2015.

Bruce Carnes and S. Jay Olshansky have published numerous statistical studies on average life expectancies between 1800 and 1900 and concluded that the increasing life expectancy does not indicate extended life spans. The initial jump in the average from 1850 to 1930 was a result of new sanitation methods and antibiotic medicines that had reduced infant mortality and increased survival rates through the ages of young adults. Subsequent increases in life span since the 1950s have been the result of further medical treatments for diseases that affect adults in later age groups. The rate of increase of life expectancy, however, is gradually diminishing, and Carnes and Olshansky predict that for the average life expectancy to reach 85, the mortality rates at every age group would have to be cut by 50 percent.

Olshansky explains that this trend is not pessimistic but rather realistic. He describes it as a matter of physics and uses the analogy of breaking the Olympic records for the one-mile run. The first man to break the four-minute barrier was Roger Bannister in 1954. Since then, the record has been broken 18 times. If we considered statistical rates alone, rather than maximum capacity, we would conclude that the record would continue to be broken until it reached zero (the point when someone managed to complete the mile at the instant the starting pistol was fired). Obviously, physics prevents that sort of speed. Olshansky argues that the same limitations exist for human life.

Other antiaging advocates, such as the biologist Stanley Shostak, argue that statistical models are inappropriate for either side of the argument. The example of trends in breaking the one-mile record is misleading because the context is fixed within specified parameters. It does not include the possibility of athletes jumping on motorcycles or jet engines to break the record. Yet, antiaging proponents seek to accomplish just that sort of feat by using technology to maintain existing life functions into extreme old age. Moreover, there is a natural limit to how fast something goes, but there are no limits to how slow something goes. Therefore, it is physically more probable to slow or stop aging than it is to increase its rate to geometric proportions. In either case, statistics on aging do not provide sufficient evidence to determine the possibility of altering its processes.

CHARACTERISTICS OF ADVANCED AGING

Usually, the most depressing chapter in any book on antiaging is the section that outlines all the characteristics that indicate someone is in their advanced years and approaching death. This is a traditional section that seems to have been included in every text since Aristotle's lecture "On Youth and Old Age" in the fourth century BCE, in Avicenna's *Canon of Medicine* from the 1200s, and in Francis Bacon's *Cure of Old Age* in the 1600s. Over the course of 2,500 years, the description has changed very little.

Physical characteristics of advanced age include changes in physical size, metabolic functions, and sensory acuity. Both men and women tend to shrink in height (due to bone loss) and often lose weight (due to muscle loss), though sometimes weight increases due to excess fatty deposits. Metabolism declines, which causes changes in the elasticity of the skin due to the loss of subcutaneous fat deposits. Wrinkles form, and the skin becomes thinner. Hair becomes gray and sometimes becomes thinner, leading to partial or complete baldness. Fingernails thicken as do the walls of the heart muscle. Rates of cardiovascular disease increase after age 50, but the pumping function of the heart remains relatively constant. Other organs begin to lose function, especially the kidneys, lungs, and pancreas. Women lose their reproductive functions through menopause around age 50, and men begin to lose their testosterone levels around the same time. This results in gradual loss of muscle strength, which can lead to loss of mobility. Vision, hearing, smell, and taste become impaired, and the immune system changes with increasing autoimmunity functions (leading to increased rates of cancer). The brain shrinks due to lost cells that are not replaced, and cognitive functions begin to decline, with slower responses to stimuli, impaired learning functions, and gradual loss of memory. These physical characteristics have been more or less consistently documented, though with varying descriptions, since ancient times (see chapter 11).

Antiaging advocates recognize the universality of these characteristics, but they often argue that it is undetermined whether these traits are an inevitable result of time or a result of environmental factors that may be modified. For example, recent research suggests that the appearance of wrinkles may be more a result of exposure to the sun than a reflection of old age. Graying hair and baldness may be more a result of family history than old age, as it often affects young adults who go on to live very long lives. Similarly, high blood pressure and muscle loss may be more related to genetics and lifestyle choices than to cellular decline.

One solution to this problem is to find epigenetic markers among the nucleotide combinations on the DNA molecule. Researchers at the National Institute on Aging think that these markers are not affected by disease or ethnicity, which means they may reflect molecular maturity alone. They are trying to isolate particular markers for the purpose of research. By comparing differences in these molecular aging markers rather than collecting statistics on mortality rates and average life expectancies, researchers may be able to identify the precise rate of aging for a given individual.

As of 2013, up to 70 markers had been identified as potentially useful, but none had been recognized as consistently useful. Moreover, there is still insufficient evidence to determine whether these rates are unique for each individual or universal for all humans. If they are not universal, the next question is, why do some individuals age faster than others? Is it a genetic issue or an environmental issue? In either case, can these rates be alterable within the individual? At this point, there is no conclusive answer.

THEORIES OF AGING

There are numerous ways of categorizing the theories of aging. Scholars such as Leonard Hayflick organize them according to where the "action" of aging occurs: in the organs, in human physiology, and in the genome. Others, such as Robert Arking, organize the theories according to whether they arose from systemic processes or from single random events. The various theories of aging are not necessarily mutually exclusive; they usually just reflect one aspect of a larger body of knowledge. Though some researchers firmly adhere to one theory more than another, most scientists recognize that there may be multiple causes for aging, and therefore there is not one single universal explanation (yet). This complexity can pose a difficulty for antiaging advocates because it means that there must be multiple solutions for the process of aging to be slowed or reversed. In this book, we organize theories of biological aging into two broad categories: those that imply a fixed life span and the immutability of the aging process and those that imply a flexible life span with an aging process that is open to change.

Fixed Life Theories (Realists)

Belief in a fixed life span does not necessarily mean denying that age might be extended through proper medicine and health care. From very early in the modern era, scientists have recognized that long life is often a reflection of how we live. In the 16th century, Francis Bacon argued that the traditional biblical age limit of "three score and ten" (70 years) was more symbolic than actual, and he believed the antediluvian ages of several hundred years were possible with proper lifestyle choices. Nevertheless, he never doubted the inevitability of both death and old age—he simply disagreed as to when these events were bound to occur. Similarly, most modern researchers recognize that our greater understanding of science and medicine may well push back the length of years as active healthy adults. Yet, they still believe aging is inevitable and death is absolutely unavoidable, and their theories of aging reflect that presumption by emphasizing the natural conditions that all organisms are susceptible to in the physical world.

Entropy

Physics is the study of the forces that affect the natural world, especially matter and energy. A physicist does not often distinguish between forces acting on a living object as opposed to forces acting on an inanimate object. The properties of matter and energy should be the same for both. The entropy theory of aging argues that the biochemical reactions of a living organism are ultimately bound by the laws of thermodynamics, which include the law of conservation of energy, the law of increasing entropy, and the third law stating that entropy declines with temperature. In terms of human biology, the law of entropy means that as energy transfers or is transformed through the metabolic process in the human body, some portion of that energy is lost in the process. Our bodies are able to constantly refill that energy through breathing and eating. Yet, entropy implies gradual disorder, and at the molecular level, objects that are ordered will gradually become more disordered over time. That means that as our cells continually perform their functions and express their genetic codes, they will eventually lose their orderliness. Over time, more and more errors enter into the biochemical process, and the various metabolic functions of an organism begin to break down.

There are numerous versions of this theory, though they all reflect the basic presumption that physical things (whether organic or not) are bound to decay. The primary difference between the various theories is over how and where that decay occurs. Antiaging advocates criticize this view by arguing that living things are different from inanimate objects because they are able to repair themselves. The stone wall that is untended may last a few centuries, but a stone wall that is constantly monitored and repaired might last indefinitely. Antiaging scientists point out that the law of entropy applies to closed systems (that are not influenced by outside forces), and biological organisms are not closed because they constantly take nourishment and respond to their environment. Supporters of entropy theory respond that the increase in disorder also affects the repair mechanisms, resulting in gradual decline. A repaired stone wall may last indefinitely in theory, but the people that repair it are constantly changing. That change inevitably leads to increased disorder over time.

Metabolic Rate

Another version of the entropy theory focuses on the rate of living. Since the Renaissance, scholars have recognized the link between large-sized animals and their average life spans. Until the 18th century, elephants were believed to live for hundreds of years, while common field mice only lived a matter of months. A theory emerged that the life span of an organism is based on the particular metabolic rate (the rate at which food is converted into energy) per gram of body mass. Larger animals with more mass and lower metabolic rates could continue to live for a very long time. Smaller animals with higher metabolic rates live shorter lives. Aging, then, is caused by the gradual usage of metabolic energy that is stored in physical size. Over time, the animal exhausts its stores of energy and simply dies.

This rate of living theory was first articulated by the Comte de Buffon in 1749 and was rearticulated using modern science in 1929 by Raymond Pearl. Both theories were related to ancient heat and moisture arguments made by Galen and Aristotle from Greek and Roman eras. Most modern biologists dislike this theory primarily because it suggests the existence of some sort of invisible source of living energy, which is strikingly similar to vitalist theories of life. The idea that there is a fixed amount of energy per animal suggests that some source of that energy exists outside the material realm, and many natural scientists do not approve of such presumptions.

Other criticisms to metabolic rate theory arose after it became clear that body size does not always indicate life span. Modern science has revealed that most elephants actually have shorter life spans than humans, and some rodents can live quite a long time. The tiny naked mole-rat, for example, has a life span of over 30 years. Also, research in *Drosophila* fruit flies indicates that individual groups within the same species (same size and weight) may share the same metabolic calorie intake per day and yet still demonstrate significantly different life spans, depending on other conditions.

Wear and Tear

Both Francis Bacon and August Weismann (from the late 1890s) argued that aging is a by-product of the accumulated gradual wear and tear that every organism experiences through the natural course of living. The body gets normal cuts and scrapes and bruises and will repair itself, but the healing will not be perfect. Over time, these wounds lead to a gradual breakdown in function. Bacon focused on the assaults that occur to the skin and body, while Weismann focused on viral assaults that occur within the organs and metabolic system. Both men argued that the average life span could be increased if these assaults were limited throughout life.

Modern researchers criticize the traditional version of wear and tear by pointing to the fact that laboratory animals who live in perfect sanitation and are completely removed from the dangers of the natural environment still die after roughly the same life span. Nevertheless, the theory remains strong, though in different forms. The most recent versions focus on the gradual weakening of the body's ability to heal. Sometimes referred to as the "failure to repair" class of theories, these theories emphasize the systemic damage occurring at the molecular level that seem to trigger age-related disorders:

- *Cross-linkage Theory:* Over time, proteins cross-link with other proteins in unexpected ways, creating new chemical properties. For example, the collagen tissues found in joints, tendons, skin, and elsewhere become less flexible as a result of cross-linking proteins, which effects shape, size, and nimbleness of our bodies, making us more susceptible to age-related diseases. This gradual rigidity of tissues renders them less likely to heal themselves.

- *Altered Protein Theory:* Protein processing slows down with age for some as yet unknown reason related to cytoplasmic pathways within the cells, resulting in the creation of altered proteins over time, which inevitably changes their functions. Over time, these altered proteins may interact or otherwise impact a cell's functioning, leading to senescence.

- *DNA Mutation or Damage Theory:* After numerous replications, the order of the nucleotide base pair sequences within the DNA molecule are altered in some way: some are added or deleted, or they are rearranged. This may be preprogrammed by some system within the genome, or it may simply be a matter of random alterations that occur after each replication. Either way, the likelihood of these random mutations increase over time, impacting cell functions and rendering aging inevitable.

- *Error Catastrophe Theory:* Just as errors may occur within the process of DNA replication, so too errors may occur at some other random point of protein synthesis, resulting in imperfect protein molecules. Most minor fluctuations trigger feedback loops to cleanse the body of the imperfect protein (a repair mechanism). At other times, though, the imperfect proteins may trigger other self-destruct mechanisms within a collection of cells. Some researchers have speculated about a "death hormone" that is triggered when multiple protein errors are found; the result is the widespread death of cells in various parts of the body, including the brain and organs. These reactions can lead to the physiological functions of aging. As with the DNA mutation theory, the longer that a system operates, the more likely these sorts of errors will result.

- *Dysdifferentiation Theory:* Related to error catastrophe, dysdifferentiation theory suggests that cells may lose their ability to operate properly over time. The fact that the entire genome is contained in every cell is a great mystery for geneticists because somehow each cell knows how to use only those parts of the genetic code that it needs (liver cells express different genetic sequences than the heart cells or the pancreas cells). Over time, cells may lose their ability to distinguish which genes ought to be expressed and which ought to be suppressed. This confusion could result in cell failure (and cell death).

- *Inflammation (Autoimmunity) Theory:* This is a very broad category of theories that argue the body loses its ability to distinguish between good cells and bad cells, resulting in unnecessary inflammation and, eventually, to cell death. Some of these theories suggest that cells in the thymus, which are responsible for much of the body's immune system, develop a sort of memory over time, causing them to be more prone to attack and resulting in increased (and uncontrollable) autoimmune reactions. The hyper immunity system causes the body to attack itself, which may result in aging and age-related diseases.

Researchers continue to identify different ways in which gene expression is limited, cell replication is halted, or metabolic functions are altered over the natural course of time. All of these, though known by different names, reflect a general presumption that the body suffers from gradual wear and tear over its lifetime, either from larger events outside the body or microscopic events inside the body. In either case, these are unavoidable reactions that are triggered over time that make biological aging inevitable.

Hayflick Limit (Telomere) Theory

This last theory of aging may be classed as either a fixed life span theory or a flexible life span theory. The difference depends on how researchers view the possibility of overcoming it. In 1961, Leonard Hayflick demonstrated that certain cells appear to be limited in the number of times they can replicate themselves. Once that limit is reached, the cell enters into senescence and eventually dies. Two decades later, researchers Elizabeth Blackburn and Jack Szostak connected Hayflick's limit to the existence of telomeres at the end of the DNA molecules. The cells of every organism appear to include a small length of repetitive nucleotide pairing sequences at the end of the DNA molecules. That length of sequences is called the *telomere*. Each time a cell divides, the length of telomere is reduced, and when the length is reduced to a certain point, the cell enters senescence. Hayflick's discovery of limited cell division became a major theory for explaining the aging process: when cells reach their natural limits, they die, and the body gradually begins to fail. Hayflick believed there was no way around this limit.

There was some debate, though, because some cells experienced a clear limit, while others (like those found in cancer) do not. Hayflick argued that those cells that escape senescence eventually turn into cancer cells, and death is triggered through an alternate route. In the 1990s, Carol Greider and Elizabeth Blackburn discovered a new enzyme called *telomerase*, which serves as a template for the DNA to replicate telomeres. They discovered that cells that contain telomerase are able to replicate indefinitely, while those without the enzyme are subject to the Hayflick limit and subject to senescence.

The Hayflick theory of aging is on the cusp between fixed and flexible life spans because there is some question as to whether or not telomerase holds the key to avoiding senescence (and curing cancer). If a telomerase supplement could enable continued regeneration of good cells, and if an antitelomerase supplement could

Telomere Length and Reproduction

Since the discovery of a connection between telomere length and cellular senescence, scientists have been struggling to better understand the reasons why some cells naturally maintain longer telomeres, while others do not. In the process, some unexpected correlations arose. In 2016, Simon Frazier University published a study that found a correlation between an increased number of childbirths and the increased length of telomeres. The research team examined 75 Mayan women from Guatemala and measured the length of their telomeres after a 13-year interval. They found that women who gave birth to more children had longer telomere lengths than women who had fewer or no children. Researchers theorized that the estrogen may play some role in contributing to telomere length. Estrogen levels increase significantly during pregnancy.

Men also experience increasing telomere lengths over time, though it is not connected to successful reproduction. A 2012 study published by the National Academy of Sciences found that older adult males produce children with consistently longer telomere lengths. Males maintain strong concentrations of telomerase, the enzyme that repairs telomeres, in the testicles. Researchers believe that, over time, the telomerase concentrations increase in older males, resulting in sperm with longer telomere lengths. These sperm produce children with longer than average telomere lengths. Subsequent correlational data suggests these long telomeres may persist for two generations.

turn off the regeneration of cancer cells, then death might be avoided indefinitely. There is a great deal of debate on this subject, and most researchers tend to hold with the side of Hayflick arguing that senescence and death are unavoidable.

Very recent research suggests telomere length is only partially responsible for cell death. Some types of cells, such as those found in the brain and the heart, never divide, and yet they will eventually die for reasons unrelated to telomere length. Current theories speculate that there is another undiscovered mechanism that triggers cell death. The connection between telomerase and the eventual formation of cancer cells is so strong that many scientists argue that cell senescence is actually a natural defense mechanism against cancerous tumor growth.

Flexible Life Theories (Antiaging)

Other theories of aging place less emphasis on physics or wear and tear and more emphasis on the biological purpose of death. Why do organisms die? Theology and philosophy were removed as methodologies for answering this question, so biologists turned to evolutionary theory. The field of gerontology tied itself to evolutionary biology early on, but Michael Rose's 1990 text, *Evolutionary Biology of Aging* (1990), provides a useful construct and vocabulary for explaining the need for aging and death outside of a religious context.

The central premise behind the evolutionary theory of aging is that life evolved to survive the natural environment up to the point of reproduction. Diseases that kill an organism before it can reproduce are not passed down to other generations. They are self-selected out of the gene pool. Yet, diseases that harm an organism after the age of reproduction are unaffected by natural selection, and they will likely remain. The evolutionary theory of aging assumes that because there is no incentive to continue to fight for life after the age of reproduction, organisms eventually succumb to whatever diseases arise, resulting in old age and death. As Robert Arking wrote in his textbook *Biology of Aging* (1998), "Aging has evolved not because it is adaptive but because the force of natural selection declines with age (we age because there is no reason not to age)."

Antiaging advocates depend on evolutionary theory to explain aging because it provides an element of flexibility in the process of aging. If death evolved, it is not necessarily inevitable, and it might be changed if scientists can cure the ailments that natural selection ignored. Most of the evolutionary-based theories of aging include some hope that the cause of biological aging can be addressed and possibly altered or even reversed.

Multiple Hormone Deficiency Theory

The primary purpose of natural selection is to preserve the organism long enough to reproduce; therefore, the bulk of the metabolic energy is directed to producing sex-related hormones up to the point of successful reproduction. After the period of reproduction has passed, the organism no longer devotes energy to making sex-related hormones. The result is that the development, peak, and decline of hormones correlate to youth, adulthood, and old age. In humans, hormones such as testosterone, estrogen, and human growth hormone (hGH) follow a life cycle arc of low levels produced during childhood, high levels produced in early adulthood, and increasingly lower levels in later adulthood.

Even before hormones were fully understood in the late 1800s, such scientists as Charles Édouard Brown-Séquard believed that sexuality was somehow linked to age. After testosterone was isolated and identified in the 1930s, there were some who believed it held the key to the fountain of youth. Modern biochemists recognize that there are a host of interrelated hormones working in the endocrine system that influence the physical vitality of youth. Nevertheless, it remains an active scientific question whether the onset of aging triggers the loss of hormones or whether the loss of hormones causes the onset of aging. There are many antiaging advocates who believe hormone replacement therapy may hold the answer to combating aging.

Oxidative-Damage (Free-Radical) Theory

Oxygen is an essential source of energy for cellular activity. Inside each cell, hundreds of mitochondria produce energy by combining the carbon molecules taken from digesting food with the oxygen molecules taken in by breathing to create molecules that bind with the bulk of all organic molecules in the body. Oxygen is critical to human life, and if it is cut off, we die almost immediately. At the same time, too much oxygen is also harmful because it creates too many highly reactive molecules, called *free radicals*. Mitochondria produce free radicals as a normal part of their operation because they carry a strong negative charge that draws them to other molecules in the vicinity. The problem is that too many radicals may create unintended bonds. Over time, these free radicals can create damage both to the mitochondria and to the cell itself. Free radicals are suspected in causing heart disease, cancer, and a host of other age-related diseases.

The body carries several natural defenses, called *antioxidants*, to protect against free radicals, but over time, the increasing ratio of free radicals may overwhelm the defense mechanisms, resulting in age-related disorders. Waste accumulation theory is a related hypothesis that suggests that free radicals and other damaged enzymes and proteins caused through cross-linkages lead to an excess of waste products in each cell. These toxins not only crowd the cell but may damage the various organelles and the DNA itself. The usual mechanisms for cleaning the waste become ineffective, and basic cell functions become impeded, leading to senescence.

The free-radical theory is very popular among antiaging researchers because it provides a potential pathway for solving the problem. If scientists can devise natural and synthetic antioxidant chemicals to remove the unneeded free radicals (and retain the necessary ones), then cells may avoid senescence. Similarly, other biochemicals might be found to clean out the waste toxins that accumulate in each cell, thereby refreshing and renewing cellular life. This suggests a potential for genuine biological rejuvenation.

Part of the problem, though, is that the very act of creating free radicals within the inner membrane of the mitochondria creates added stress as new molecules repeatedly pass through the membrane walls. Healthy functioning of the mitochondria appears to create stress in the cell over time, which is essentially another version of the wear-and-tear hypothesis. Nevertheless, researchers hope that other repair functions may be found to heal the damage caused by the stress and thereby extend the life of each cell.

BALANCED OVERVIEW

How we define aging and death greatly influences our confidence in the potential effectiveness of antiaging solutions. If scientists are convinced that the human life span is fixed and that aging is an evitable process of physics, their research will primarily focus on extending healthy living. The result may extend the years of active adulthood and compress the years of morbidity (the time just before death), but it will not likely impact the aging process nor delay death.

On the other hand, if scientists are convinced that the human life span is an arbitrary limit imposed by the forces of evolution, their research will focus on processes that seem to have a direct impact on aging and age-related diseases. From this evolutionary perspective, age is itself a disease or the aggregate by-product of a collection of diseases. Their research goals are to extend healthy life indefinitely by avoiding the onset of aging. Along the way, they also hope to extend the period of active adulthood to increasingly later years.

The scientific debate between these two interpretations is far from settled. As of yet, no medicines or treatments have been introduced that conclusively slows or eliminates aging as a biological process. At the same time, gerontologists seem to be continually uncovering new details about the process of cellular senescence, which provides constant hope for future breakthroughs. For the foreseeable future, the antiaging movement will continue to follow the same path as traditional gerontology in so far as they both target the causes of age-related diseases.

Aging and the Meaning of Life

Biology does not seek to define the meaning of life, nor does it require a particular religious faith. Yet, the definition of death (and the inevitability of aging) does often reflect certain religious beliefs. If we believe life is limited to this material world only, then death means an end to that life with nothing more to come. If we believe that life continues in the immaterial realm (heaven), then death is merely a passageway from this material world to the next. Also, the belief in a potential spiritual death can influence behavior and decision making related to physical actions. The urgency with which we want to defer physical death or to find a solution to aging will often reflect these religious beliefs.

As a rule, biologists are loath to apply moral or religious considerations into their theories. Yet, there are some difficult philosophical questions related to human motivation and free will that arise depending on whether the human life span is fixed or flexible (indeterminate). Religious opponents of antiaging research, such as Leon Kass, argue that the inevitability of death motivates individuals to plan for a life that is limited in scope. Death tends to compel people to search for meaning—either existentially, for life in general, or personally, for their life in particular. Have I done what I could have or should have in the limited years that are available to me? Both theologians and psychologists recognize the power that death holds over individual motivation. What would happen if death were no longer mandatory?

On the opposite side, antiaging advocates such as Aubrey de Grey respond by saying that death is only influential because it is so strongly associated with fear. Most people do not want to die, and they often make poor decisions because they hope to avoid it (or, in their despair, potentially embrace it). If, however, death were recognized as a personal decision rather than an imposed condition, people might spend more of their lives extensively planning and developing long-term goals. They also might be more prone to taking fewer risks, knowing that a near indefinite future life span may be at stake. Finally, antiaging advocates often argue that most of the pains and discomforts of life are related to diseases that come with the onset of aging and as precursors to death. From this perspective, they say it is unethical not to try to cure those diseases (including death), if it were possible.

There are other moral implications regarding the decision-making process involved in choosing to accept or to avoid death. In Judeo-Christian traditions, life is bestowed as a gift of God alone and should only be taken away by God alone. This is the fundamental reason behind the immorality of murder at any point in the human life span. Death by natural means (old age, disease, or accident) removes responsibility for any particular individual. Death by intentional means is viewed as murder, or homicide, and this viewpoint usually applies to all life at any age. Religious opposition to abortion is based on a belief that life begins at conception, and its deliberate termination is an act of homicide, even though the child is still in the mother's womb. Similarly, euthanasia and suicide are often contrary to religious beliefs because they are viewed as an act of self-murder. The successful creation of antiaging treatments would shift the cause of most deaths away from disease to either accident or personal decision. If death becomes largely voluntary, then the decision to extend life through medical means creates an unavoidable voluntary decision to end life later on. The decision to stop taking medicines and die might be viewed as the moral equivalent of suicide. As such, the decisions to begin taking the medicines might hold the same degree of moral scrutiny.

Clearly, these sorts of decisions are only dilemmas if the person making them believes that life and death are left to God alone. Antiaging advocates rarely believe there is an immaterial eternity after death. As such, they also often reject the view that an immaterial realm holds any influence on human decisions. For these believers, the decision to extend life holds no moral implications. As they do not believe in heaven, there is no threat of its loss by choosing the length of their life on earth.

CONCLUSION

The field of biogerontology is constantly improving its understanding of the process of biological aging. At this point, however, the various theories of aging remain just theories. There are no absolute or conclusive explanations. As such, though, moral questions about the meaning of life and death should be considered even now; as a practical matter, they may not become imperative until scientists have actually been successful at altering or changing the rate of aging. If the human life span is, in fact, fixed, these discussions lose their meaning.

Most theologians and philosophers would agree that healthy living is always a good thing in and of itself. Whether medical advances lead to life extension or just to an extended period of active adulthood, the short-term result of healthier living applies to all. In the short-term, it does not matter whether aging is inevitable. Any effort to extend the average human life expectancy will improve quality of life and be applauded by both sides. Antiaging and traditional gerontologists both support the maxim of "pro-health" (as do religious advocates), and the field of gerontology benefits from both perspectives.

Chapter 8

What Makes Us Look Younger?

During the thousands of years that preceded this century, eternal youth has been only a dream, and, most often, it was not even a positive dream. It might be more accurate to say that the historic quest for youth has rarely been so much a pursuit of long life as a desire to reclaim the experiences of being young. When we are children, we want to look older, like the ideal model of young adulthood. When we reach that age, and older, we want to look young again to reclaim that ideal youth that we did not fully appreciate at the time. The dream of the fountain of youth has been to look and feel young as long as we live. The promise of delaying or evading death is often a side effect of that first priority.

The cosmetics industry experienced a transformation when it joined causes with the antiaging movement. A new term, *cosmeceutical*, was invented in 1984 to advertise the lotions and creams that were also marketed for their antiaging properties. Albert Klingman coined the term to describe a line of retinoid-based skin-care products that served as "a topical preparation that is sold as a cosmetic but has performance characteristics that suggest pharmaceutical action." Since then, the industry has embraced the argument that makeup is about more than just beauty; it is also about healthy skin and reducing the appearance and effects of age. Global sales of cosmeceutical products reached $35 billion by 2012, and it represents the fastest-growing market segment of the personal care industry. Consumers are taught that cosmetic enhancement not only adds beauty but is also part of healthy living. As a practical matter, though, the Food and Drug Administration (FDA) does not make any distinction between cosmetics intended to beautify and those that are intended to be therapeutic. There are no regulatory standards that companies must follow to describe their product, and claims of "age-defying" technology are not tested by scientific evidence.

The desire to look young affects both men and women. But women tend to link their self-worth to their perceived body image, whereas men tend to connect their self-worth to money and influence. These gender differences explain why women make up nearly 90 percent of the cosmetic antiaging market. Most women retain similar ideals of a perfect body image over the course of their lifetime, even though their age makes attaining that image more and more difficult. For many women, the appearance of youth is the primary objective of antiaging products (external youth), while for men it is usually the extension of life (internal youth). The field of radical antiaging advocates is almost exclusively dominated by men. Evidence suggests, though, that both men and women tend to believe that looking younger generally indicates more youthful vitality. In the 21st century, the proportion of men seeking surgical and nonsurgical antiaging treatments has increased slowly but steadily.

The antiaging movement enjoys a mutually reinforcing relationship with the cosmetics industry, media, and other cultural standards of youth and beauty. The constant desire to match the popular image of the perfect body type provides added incentive to discover scientific solutions to aging and age-related disorders. At the same time, the growing academic interest in antiaging provides popular culture with a sort of scientific legitimacy to what might otherwise be viewed as vanity. The most common results for a Google search of "antiaging" are all cosmetics related. Yet to date, none of these cosmetic remedies or procedures have been shown to have any impact on aging. In some cases, these remedies may actually increase the risk of cancer or other terminal diseases; yet, the market for cosmeceuticals grows stronger with each passing year. In this case, it is the appearance of youth and not the actual retention of youth that seems most important.

THE MARKET FOR YOUTH

The human desire to find cosmetics to make us more beautiful dates back to ancient times. Some of the earliest archeological finds in ancient Egypt include palettes for holding makeup. Rouge and other powders are mentioned in the Old Testament, and the Greek philosopher Xenophon observed the practice was so common that he warned of its innate deception. The cultural demand for the tools to improve face and figure is hardly new to the recent centuries. Yet, the standards by which we define beauty have gained a more consistent definition as modern telecommunication technologies transmit the same common images of youthful beauty throughout the world.

Entertainment media, especially, has spread images of beauty to the far corners of the globe, limiting the degree of cultural differentiation that used to exist. In a 1999 study, researchers found that the ideal body image among young girls of the Pacific island of Fiji changed dramatically just a few years after television was introduced to the community. Previous standards of beauty had promoted larger body types for both men and women, and eating disorders were completely unknown. After the introduction of television with Western programming, surveys given to high school girls indicated that most were newly concerned about their weight: nearly 30 percent showed signs of potential eating disorders, and 15 percent reported they had engaged in bulimic behaviors (inducing vomiting to control weight). Studies of other nations in Africa and Asia and among Western states confirmed the power of visual media to promote more rigid standards of beauty. The ideal body type is now thinner and younger than in previous eras.

The quest for obtaining the perfect body changes as we age. The fear of being overweight is most common among preteens, teens, and young adults, resulting in a general increase in eating disorders. This has become a popular subject on college campuses, especially among undergraduates attempting to change the cultural norms of their communities. In 2008, the Tri Delta Sorority launched a "Fat Talk Free" week through a series of YouTube videos that emphasized the use of positive conversations about personal appearances to combat negative body self-image. The video called on viewers to stop lamenting about how they look and how fat they feel, as if being fat were a fate worse than death. Citing research from the Body Image Project conducted at Trinity College in San Antonio, Texas, the video claimed that 54 percent of women would rather be struck by a truck than be fat. The Tri Delta video went viral and was seen by 140,000 people; it was released in different forms over the next three years.

The purpose behind both the video and the sorority's initiative was to build awareness of the prevalence of a thin body image that confronts men and women through media on a daily basis. The new definition of beauty is to be very thin and eternally young, and that is not a possible goal for the vast majority of people at any age. The socialization process begins at very young ages. Some research

The Male Market

Women may be more susceptible to advertisements that cater to improving their physical appearance, but men are often more concerned about their perceived strength and vitality. Changes to the Pure Food and Drug Act in 1994 opened the way for direct-to-consumer advertising of pharmaceuticals and herbal supplements on television and other print media. Pfizer was the first pharmaceutical company to advertise treatments for erectile dysfunction (Viagra) directly on the television in 1999. At first, the phrase "erectile dysfunction" was never mentioned in the ads, but the context of the narrative made it clear to consumers what the product was for. By 2003, competitors like Cialis had launched similar advertising campaigns that were more explicit.

Also, beginning in 2001, a host of other related ads for herbal supplements began appearing on television, including the famous ad with "smiling Bob," the spokesperson for Enzyte—a product purported to increase penis size. The ad said nothing explicit, but instead relied on obvious *double entendres* that made it clear that "Bob" and his television wife were smiling because he had increased the size of his penis through herbal supplements. The campy humor was extremely successful, and Enzyte's manufacturer, Steven Warshek, earned half a billion dollars in a matter of a few years. Growing from 15 employees in 2001, his company, Berkeley Nutraceuticals, increased to 1,500 employees with $250 million in annual sales by 2004.

The market for legal medications to treat erectile dysfunction was $3.2 billion in 2015. The market for herbal supplements for "male enhancement" is undocumented, but estimates place it at multiple billions of dollars per year.

indicates girls as young as 5 and 6 years old worry about their weight, and girls aged 10 and 11 years diet to avoid the 20- to 30-pound weight gain that comes with natural maturation. On the other end of the spectrum, women who experience natural weight gain following childbirth and as they approach menopause are continually guided by a standard that was formed in their minds decades earlier. The shock of the Tri Delta information video is that more than half of the women surveyed seemingly would prefer death to a life of fatness. The same statistic might be applied to the antiaging movement; people would often rather appear young and thin than to actually live a long life otherwise.

Younger people want to look like the Hollywood actors in their late teens and early twenties, so they focus on weight loss and sculpted muscle development. As men and women get older, though, their objectives become less particularized on a certain look and more focused on simply reclaiming the sort of beauty that comes with youthfulness. Those who felt beautiful in their youth tend to have a more difficult time adjusting to the natural changes that accompany aging, but research suggests most women and many men feel unsatisfied by their body image as they get older. These trends are fully recognized by the personal care industry, which built its fortune on marketing strategies that encourage or exploit each individual sense of inadequacy, while simultaneously offering convenient remedies to solve the problem.

The Beauty Bias and Body Image

In 2010, Deborah Rhode's *The Beauty Bias* discussed the often unrecognized discrimination that follows the loss or absence of beauty. The ancient proverb may claim that beauty is in the eye of the beholder, but recent studies suggest beauty is often correlated with facial symmetry, unblemished skin, and particular body types: hour-glass figures for women and muscular height for men. Rhode summarized research collected by the Social Issues Research Center (SIRC) during the 1990s, which indicated that attractive children tend to receive more attention and higher evaluations at school and have greater expectations placed on them, which improves their performance. Attractive applicants are more likely to find a job with higher pay, even with the same qualifications as their less attractive competitors. Attractive people are less likely to be convicted of a crime and less likely to be given as severe a sentence if found guilty. In most social interactions, studies indicate that attractive people are generally treated more favorably than those deemed less attractive.

This cultural bias may result in subtle discrimination in the workplace and may impact personal relationships, yet that does not mean that beauty always leads to happiness. Other studies collected by SIRC indicate that attractive people often feel less secure in their abilities because they tend to question the praise of peers and coworkers. Perhaps more relevant, attractive people are less able to constructively deal with the loss of age-related beauty. The problem is compounded by the fact that most adult women (8 out of 10) are dissatisfied with their appearance no matter how attractive others may find them. In part, this is due to the changing standards of ideal beauty. Around the time of the World War I, the most celebrated female model body type was 5 foot 4 inches and 140 pounds. At the start of the 21st century, the modern ideal model was 5 foot 10 inches and 120 pounds. These ideals are mostly impossible. Only about 5 percent of woman are capable of matching that weight and size without some significant surgical enhancement. Even attractive men and women fall short of the social expectations. The industry of cosmetic surgery largely relies on this constant dissatisfaction.

Advertising may take advantage of natural insecurities, but the media-driven culture is so heavily dominated by images of beauty that there is no need for any coordinated pressure toward physical conformity. Research conducted at the start of the age of cable television, beginning in the 1980s and into the early 2000s, indicates that people become more dissatisfied with their physical appearance after watching programming featuring beautiful actors with thin builds or when they have read fashion magazines filled with pictures of thin models in luxurious surroundings. Women especially can experience depression, shame, guilt, insecurity, and an increase in generalized stress. These cultural pressures were compounded in the 2010s by the rise of social media, which has largely intensified insecurity about body image. Web sites such as Facebook, Twitter, Instagram, and others provide youth and adults with forums for posting and commenting on pictures that generate constant feedback on their personal appearance. The pressure is more intense than previous Hollywood stereotypes because the photos are of seemingly average people who live nearby and who all seem to be attractive and carefree.

A 2016 study conducted by Common Sense Media indicates that the basic problem of social media is that the images are highly selective; they reflect only the most positive features and are often digitally enhanced to create impressions of beauty that are simply impossible to achieve. More importantly, though the posts appear to be interactive, they are usually shallow reactions to unrealistic images. Not only do participants objectify their friends, but they often objectify themselves by binding their sense of self-worth to their external appearance. Several research studies indicate higher rates of depression and personal insecurity following increased hours spent on social media forums. It is difficult to see thousands of pictures of beautiful (often digitally enhanced) images and not compare them to yourself. Rates of negative body image among teens and young adults have increased significantly since the popularity of social media. Not surprisingly, the rates of cosmetic surgery also increased (by 20 percent) following the rise in popularity of Facebook in 2008 and doubled over the next decade.

Gender Differences

Appearance is more important to women than men, but this is rarely related to vanity or self-indulgence. Women are more likely to be judged by their appearance by members of both sexes, and their self-worth is often strongly connected to how they look—or how they feel like they look (which is often not the same thing).

Women tend to feel larger than they are, and if they are obese, they feel less capable than average-sized women. Deborah Rhode cited numerous studies in *Beauty Bias* indicating that obese women are more likely to be in lower-paying jobs and are 20 percent less likely to marry than women of normal weight. Though women tend to judge their own attractiveness severely, they are less likely to consider attractiveness in their potential spouses than men. As women age, they often feel less influential, less noticed, and less empowered. By contrast, men tend to gain a greater sense of authority with age, and their self-worth is often not tied to their physical appearance. These trends have changed over the past two decades as the baby-boomer generation began to reach late adulthood.

All cosmetic procedures increased significantly between 1997 and 2015, by as much as 300 percent for women and nearly 150 percent for men. In the single decade from 2005 to 2015, the total number of procedures for both sexes increased from 10 million to 15 million. These numbers may be a little misleading, as 40 percent of those undergoing cosmetic procedures were repeat patients and a little more than a third of the clients underwent multiple procedures at the same time. Men are significantly less likely to undergo the most invasive reconstructive surgical procedures. In the 1990s, they accounted for less than 5 percent of all procedures. Over the next decade, though, those rates doubled, and by 2012, men claimed nearly 10 percent of the surgical procedures.

Gender differences in rates of plastic surgery do not necessarily indicate differences in their pursuit of retaining their youthful appearances. During the 2010s, the most common surgical procedures performed on men were liposuction (extracting fatty tissues from around the waist), hair transplants, and rhinoplasty (surgical reconstruction, particularly for pectoral enhancement or male breast reduction). During the same period, women typically underwent 12 times as many plastic surgery procedures. These mostly included breast enhancements, liposuction, and tummy tucks (removing excess skin from the waist). For noninvasive procedures, however, the gender differences tend to disappear. For adults aged 50 and above, similar numbers of both genders underwent procedures for removing wrinkles, including injections of neurotoxins to achieve microparalysis of facial muscles (Botox, Dysport, and Xeomin) as well as skin-resurfacing techniques using lasers and microdermabrasions (removing wrinkles by buffing away dead skin). Moreover, both men and women spent roughly the same amount of money on facial creams and lotions.

Women may feel more social pressure to look younger, and they may be more attentive to appearance than men during all ages. Yet, beginning in the 2010s, men were increasingly willing to spend money for antiaging cosmetics that did not require significant effort or recovery time.

The Makeup Marketplace

The marriage between the natural demand for cosmetic enhancement among the aging baby-boomer population and the rising popularity for antiaging treatments transformed the personal care industry by lending a sense of medical legitimacy to their products. As long as the packaging and marketing materials do not claim to cure, treat, or lessen the symptoms of particular diseases, the product is not subject to FDA regulations. Marketing techniques avoided these restrictions by focusing on scientific-sounding solutions that have no actual practical medical meaning. Skin care products "reduce the appearance" of wrinkles and "promote" healthy skin. Some cosmetic companies claim to repair DNA and promote particular gene expression to rejuvenate skin, but their descriptions are not medically tenable. In 2010, the FDA and the Federal Trade Commission (FTC) sent out letters to 10 major cosmetic manufacturers, warning them that their advertisements included drug-like statements that required scientific evidence to substantiate and that they risked regulatory oversight if they were not corrected. No penalties were levied.

There are, however, numerous other antiaging cosmetic treatments that do require a prescription and are subject to FDA regulation. These include hormone-replacement therapies and all dermatological office visits and surgical operations. There are strong marketing campaigns for all types of treatments, but most development money is spent on cosmeceuticals. The world's largest cosmetic company, L'Oréal, spends $1 billion annually on research and development and $8 billion on marketing and promotions for all of its makeup products. Its nearest competitor, Olay, spends $216 million on advertising its "antiaging" skin care products alone. The global sales for cosmeceuticals was just under $40 billion in 2014 and was expected to reach nearly $60 billion in 2019. Cosmetic procedures conducted by dermatologists and plastic surgeons only accounted for a little less than $13 billion in 2014.

TYPES OF ANTIAGING COSMETIC PROCEDURES

There are three categories of antiaging cosmetic products and procedures. The first includes the broad range of cosmeceutical lotions, creams, and related skin care products that can be purchased over-the-counter. The second includes prescription medications and other minor procedures that must be performed at a dermatologist's office. The last category includes the wide variety of plastic surgery procedures that must be conducted by a physician.

Over-the-Counter Treatments (Cosmeceuticals)

The outward appearance of age is most noticeable through visible changes in the skin and hair. People look older when they develop wrinkles and when their hair begins to gray or become white. Hair coloring has been available for centuries, but it does not pretend to provide any medical benefits. By contrast, cosmeceutical skin care products all advertise themselves as nourishing, replenishing, and rejuvenating skin to combat the effects of getting older. The primary objectives for most antiaging skin care products is to remove the signs of wrinkles, to lighten age spots, and to enhance elasticity, color, and smoothness of skin. Despite the optimistic marketing campaigns, no cosmeceutical has been shown to be effective beyond the usual masking of skin blemishes.

The American Academy of Dermatology states annually that the most effective way to protect skin against premature aging is to stay out of the sun, apply sunscreen when outdoors, and apply moisturizer daily. Despite these minimal expectations, there are dozens of products that claim to do more. Unfortunately, repeated consumer product testing suggests that the added benefits are not demonstrable. American Consumer Reports investigations, beginning in 2006, and a German *Stiftung Warentest* (Foundation for Product Testing) investigation in 2015 tested more than 30 antiaging products and discovered no noticeable differences in skin damage. Using high-definition dermatological photography, photos were taken of each test subject before applying the creams, immediately after applying the creams, then one day after, and again six weeks after applying the creams. Though some individuals experienced short-term benefits, the photos did not indicate any noticeable healing or repairing of skin for any of the test subjects. And price did not seem to matter either. There were no noticeable differences in the effectiveness between expensive creams (ranging from $300–$400) and the less inexpensive products (around $15–$20). The primary difference was in packaging and marketing.

Daily moisturizing and frequent application of sunscreen to prevent damage caused by ultraviolet (UV) rays are the only demonstrably effective means of reducing the probability of wrinkles, but these measures are intended for long-term goals only. They are most effective when applied to skin that is already young and hydrated. These preventative measures usually do not become important to consumers until later in life. Only about 20 percent of women aged 18 to 35 believe that skin care products are important to them. For women 35 years and older, more than 45 percent believe proper skin care is important. By that time, though, much of the sun damage to the skin has already been done, and the evidence suggests that the antiaging skin care products have no appreciable impact on healing or reversing that damage. The best that can be hoped for is to maintain the same level of skin health.

Cosmeceuticals are distinguished from ordinary skin care products by their active ingredients, which include a variety of vitamins and amino acid agents. Ordinary moisturizers use emulsions to trap moisture in the uppermost layers of the skin, which is prone to loss of hydration through exposure to the sun's rays. Antiaging moisturizers and sunscreens include nanotechnology (very small particles sometimes only a hundred times larger than the width of an atom) to convey vitamins and to provide more penetrating UV protection without leaving greasy or chalky residues on the skin. Some of these nanotechnologies include liposomes, nanoemulsions, solid liquid nanoparticles (SLNs), and zinc oxide or titanium dioxide compounds. The primary benefit of these added chemicals is that they can preserve the active ingredients and make them last longer on the skin.

Most other antiaging cosmeceuticals seek to rejuvenate skin by increasing the collagen levels, which improve flexibility and smoothness. Collagen decreases with age and often breaks down with the exposure of UV rays and other environmental pollutants that can affect the skin. Some of the most popular active ingredients are

Pro-retinol A and nanoencapsulated Triceramide, both of which seek to preserve existing collagen levels and to weaken or destroy the factors that lead to the break-down of collagen. Most of these compounds are variants of particular vitamins. Retinol belongs to the vitamin A family, but it is diluted in strength to avoid the need for a prescription. Vitamin C is added to soften fine lines, and vitamin B_3 is used to lighten dark spots. Copper peptides are used to enhance healing. Other facial cleansers include alpha hydroxy acids (AHA), which help to remove dead skin. They also leave the skin more vulnerable to harmful UVA and UVB rays and are usually followed by a coenzyme Q_{10} supplement, which is taken in a pill form and used as an antioxidant to promote the skin's ability to resist sun damage. Some cosmeceuticals made outside the United States contain mercury, which has been linked to skin cancer and other neurological disorders (and has been banned by the FDA).

Other technological developments include the use of nanotechnology in almost all antiaging cosmetics. Dior was the first to use this technology in 1986 with liposome formulations, which are biodegradable, flexible vesicles used to hold active ingredients and to preserve their potency against degradation caused by exposure to oxygen and light. These are especially useful in delivering vitamins A, E, and K as well as other antioxidants. A decade later, L'Oréal introduced the use of nanocapsules for deeper penetration into the skin. By 2000, most cosmetic companies were utilizing some form of nanotechnology, including nanopigments, niosomes, nanocrystals, SLNs, carbon nanotubes, fullerines, dendrimers, and cubosomes. Each of these help to preserve the effectiveness of the active ingredients, ensure deeper penetration into the upper layers of skin, and provide greater UV-blocking protection.

The active ingredients in antiaging creams and lotions may not always be compatible with all skin types and may sometimes irritate the skin, resulting in rashes. The use of nanotechnology, however, carries its own hazards. In addition to the environmental dangers involved in production (which may subject workers to increased risk of inhalation, ingestion, or dermal exposure), the very nature of the nanotechnology is to improve the penetration of topical creams and lotions. Due to their extremely small size, nanoparticles may potentially pass to the lower layers of the skin and reach the bloodstream. Most nanoparticles easily pass out of the body, but some may be absorbed through the bloodstream into various organs. Some nanoparticles are soluble (liposomes and nanoemulsions), but some are insoluble (titanium dioxide and fullerenes). Dermal absorption is minimal on normally healthy skin, but the risk of absorption increases when applied to unhealthy skin (which is a common purpose for cosmeceuticals). Research on the subject is mixed, with some studies suggesting that most nanoparticles cannot penetrate the skin and others finding zinc oxide particles in blood and urine samples. In in vitro experiments, titanium oxide has shown to lead to brain damage in mice and may increase the number of free radicals in the body, leading to cellular senescence, which is often cited as contributing to the aging process.

As a result of these concerns, the FDA sent out a general alert on antiaging skin care products, warning manufacturers to be careful in how they describe the medical benefits of their products. With the exception of daily moisturizing treatments, the majority of over-the-counter antiaging treatments are intended to provide immediate short-term benefits that mask or hide skin blemishes. The long-term side effects are undetermined at best and, in the worst cases, may be harmful.

Prescription Treatments

Dermatologists and other health care physicians can prescribe tretinoin, which is a more potent version of retinol, from the vitamin A family. It is a cream used to kill off the old and dead skin at the upper layers so that new cells can form. Side effects often include itching and patches of redness and rashes for the first few weeks, until the new skin cells develop. The goal is to tighten the skin, provide more even tones, and thicken skin by preserving collagen levels. Most patients do not see beneficial effects for at least three to six months of daily use. Patients need to be extra careful of further sun damage because the skin is left more exposed while the treatment is underway.

The most common form of prescriptive treatment is conducted at the dermatologist's office. These treatments include chemical peels and microdermabrasion, which serve the same function as tretinoin. In microdermabrasion, the dermatologist uses a power buffing wand with diamond particles to scrape off the top layer of skin to facilitate new cell growth below. The process is faster than the prescription cream, but it still may require multiple procedures over the course of several months. A slightly more expensive approach is to use chemical peels, which provide the same results and require a similar number of treatments. Results might last anywhere from one month to several years, depending on the depth of the treatment. Another approach dermatologists use is to substitute the buffing wand with a laser that can remove variable layers of skin at once in a process called skin resurfacing. The procedure can be 10 to 20 times more expensive than microdermabrasion, but the results are expected to last two to five years.

The most popular antiwrinkle procedure involves neurotoxin injections applied directly into the areas of the face that show the most wrinkles. Botox was the first FDA-approved injection, in 2009; other competing brands include Dysport and Xeomin. Each uses the same active ingredient of botulinum type A to paralyze specific facial muscles by blocking the nerve impulses to smooth out the appearance of wrinkles. Results typically take from three to seven days to become manifest, and the paralysis lasts between three and six months. Effects can last longer after multiple procedures, but this also reflects potential negative side effects, including the possibility of long-term paralysis.

Another common, though often illegal, cosmetic antiaging therapy is a hormone replacement regimen involving anabolic steroids or human growth hormone (hGH). Testosterone and its analog variants have been used discreetly by bodybuilders and athletes to enhance performance since the late 1950s. By the

1980s, the general public had become aware of its widespread use after the Olympic Games ejected dozens of athletes who had tested positive for performance-enhancing drugs. Massively muscular bodybuilders and professional wrestling stars had achieved near superhuman proportions using the drugs. During the 1997 and 1998 seasons, Major League Baseball drew national attention as Mark McGuire and Sammy Sosa repeatedly broke home run records. Several years later, news broke that both players had used anabolic steroid variants to achieve their victories. To the public, steroids were largely viewed as a form of cheating. News reports of unpredictable emotional outbursts and excessive competitive behaviors served to tarnish the drugs as harmful and toxic.

Yet, steroids and other performance-enhancing drugs continue to be used for cosmetic purposes. In 2004, television actress Suzanne Somers launched a series of books on her personal experiences with weight loss and fighting the effect of menopause through hormone replacement therapies, including the use of hGH. Like anabolic steroids, hGH stimulates cascading sequences in the endocrine system that promote muscle development. Unlike steroids, hGH appears to have fewer immediate side effects (violent mood swings and hair loss). In 2012, a *Vanity Fair* article disclosed the prevalence of hGH use not only among actors and actresses striving to look perfectly toned and fit but also among producers and directors wanting to maintain higher levels of energy. As one talent agent explained, "Any actor over 50 you're still seeing with a ripped stomach and veins in his forearms is probably taking H.G.H." The article claimed that Hollywood icons had previously used steroids but switched to hGH to avoid the unpredictable emotional outbursts that often disrupted their professional careers.

When used in moderate doses and combined with an aggressive exercise regimen, both anabolic steroids and hGH can provide immediate results in lowering body fat, tightening muscles, and increasing physical endurance. They are also only approved for cases of hormone deficiency, typically related to wasting diseases (such as HIV) or hypogonadism (such as dwarfism). Nevertheless, some doctors who specialize in antiaging practices can be creative in how they diagnose hormone deficiency (see chapter 12). Both testosterone and hGH levels decline as men get older, and a doctor could argue that the declining levels represent a deficiency. This potentially opens the way for prescribing the drugs to anyone in their late fifties and older.

The potential long-term side effects of anabolic steroids include increased risk of heart disease, joint stress, and mood disorders. Long-term side effects of hGH include increased risks of heart disease, cancer, and diabetes. There is little question that these drugs are used for their short-term benefits at the potential cost of serious long-term consequences.

Surgical Procedures

Plastic surgery as a treatment for aging is rarely described as anything more than a cosmetic enhancement. There is no pretense of slowing or reversing the effects of aging on the human body. The most common procedures include liposuction, eyelid surgery, facelifts and tummy tucks, and male breast reduction. Every surgical procedure involves some level of risk, especially those involving general anesthesia. Typical risks include lung infection, stroke, and heart attacks—any of which could prove fatal. The most common risks associated with plastic surgery include nerve damage, infection, scarring, and blood clots (known as deep vein thrombosis). Blood clots are especially dangerous because they can travel to the lungs to create a pulmonary embolism and may be fatal. Liposuction may damage internal organs and could potentially puncture organs and other membranes, leading to internal blood loss, which also may become fatal.

CONCLUSION

Cosmetic approaches to antiaging will not solve, halt, or reverse the effects of growing older. Though some procedures may involve potent medicines and surgery, they can only disguise the visible effects of aging and are not much different in nature than the use of ordinary makeup. Nevertheless, public demand for cosmetic enhancement increases every year. In part, the pressure to match some ideal of the perfect human body is a reflection of cultural norms that some critics find destructive. By contrast, advocates argue that the quality of life is improved significantly by a more attractive physical appearance. History reveals consistent demands for cosmetic enhancement in every society during every age. Only recently, though, have they found common cause with the growing antiaging movement.

The general rule for evaluating medical treatments is to weigh the potential short-term benefits against the probable long-term risks associated with implementation. Potential short-term benefits of cosmetic antiaging treatments are mostly psychological in nature. People may feel better about themselves and their self-worth when they look younger. At the same time, there is a risk that the underlying insecurities of a negative self-image have little to do with appearance and more to do with internal dissatisfaction. Evidence from social media and other passive visual media sources suggest that an increased emphasis on external comparisons to other people may actually undermine an individual's sense of self-worth.

In all accounts, the potential long-term risks for cosmetic enhancements are not negligible. In some case, the risks may even be life-threatening over the long-term and may increase the likelihood of shortening the expected life span rather than prolonging it. Nevertheless, cosmetic antiaging treatments are really mostly intended to address a short-term pursuit of youth. They cannot make any promises of long-term youthfulness.

Chapter 9

What Makes Us Feel Younger?

Traditionally, the search for the fountain of youth is shrouded in a promise of looking and acting in the prime of health forever. The perfect dream would be to enjoy the wisdom of 85 years and yet look as if we were 25, with the expectation of continued vibrant health for the foreseeable future. Antiaging researchers work tirelessly to find the medical answer for curing "aging," as if it were a disease, and the cosmetics industry responds with practical solutions for continually looking younger than our years. At heart, the antiaging movement strives to somehow turn back the hands of time because old age is perceived as an evil to be avoided.

Yet, there is a third strain of the antiaging movement that seems to defy both these approaches and their presumptions. This strain has no convenient name, but it is characterized by an emphasis on feeling young without worry or concern about age or its negative connotations. Sometimes described as the "successful aging" movement, its goals emphasize growing old gracefully by accepting age as it comes, with an emphasis on living youthfully throughout all stages of life. Those who advocate successful aging or feeling younger do not necessarily worry about the appearance of age or adding years to their life span. They seek to find enjoyment and satisfaction at every age. In some cases, the methods for feeling younger are similar to those science suggests may help extend our life spans. In other cases, these methods may actually undermine our ability to disguise age or look younger. This approach does not necessarily reject the antiaging movement, but its objectives focus on the more immediate concerns of life at the moment.

There is a substrain within the successful aging movement that is more controversial. The modern antiageism movement emphasizes the need to change cultural values so that aging is treated as a normal condition of living, without negative associations. Ageism is defined as a cultural prejudice that discriminates and stereotypes people on the basis of their age. Whereas the successful aging movement strives to find ways that individuals can continue to feel vibrant and active as they get older, the antiageism movement seeks to change social constructs and to remove the barriers and stigmas associated with getting older. The first concentrates on internal perceptions of the individual, while the second addresses the external expectations of society.

Antiageism often comes in conflict with programs that promote successful aging and feeling younger because they reject the presumption that aging can be unsuccessful and that feeling older is undesirable. Antiageism advocates argue that old age is no different than young age and that society ought to change to accommodate natural differences rather than marginalize one end of the spectrum over another. Presumptions that portray age as a less desirable condition are seen as forms of cultural discrimination.

The greater conflict is between *antiageism* and the goals of the *antiaging* movement. The long-standing antiaging movement presumes that age is a disease that must be fought and defeated if society is to progress. By contrast, the antiageism movement argues that the effort to "cure" aging is similar to an effort to "cure" blackness or to "cure" femaleness—as if they were handicaps that needed to be corrected. Antiageism advocates view the antiaging movement as a form of implicit cultural discrimination that needs to be fought if society is to progress.

The irony is that all three of these strains, antiaging, successful aging, and the antiageism movements, arise from a common desire to extend the time of middle age between adulthood and death. Whether through compressed morbidity (shortening the time between declining health and death) or an expansion of the years before declining health, both cases prolong the period of time when individuals live active and engaging lives.

SUCCESSFUL AGING

The United Nations (UN) defines *youth* as that period between "the dependence of childhood to adulthood's independence," which for statistical purposes is defined as persons aged between 15 and 24 years. Few advocates seek to halt the biological process of aging to 24 years, and far fewer are hopeful that such a goal is attainable. The UN definition defines the label in economic and sociopsychological terms. For the most part, *youth* refers to those people who have not yet gained their economic independence and to those people who have not yet asserted themselves as masters of their own time and decisions.

Not all aspects of youth are desirable. All three strains of the antiaging movement (antiaging, successful aging, and antiageism) consider youth in strictly biological terms related to health and vigor. There is no movement to turn back the time of experience and wisdom that only age provides. Common objectives of maintaining youthfulness seek to preserve only those characteristics that made life exciting at young ages into older ages, without the immaturity that often made life scary. The proponents of successful aging contend that most of the characteristics of youth are associated with an active lifestyle and personal mobility and are not necessarily dependent on biological limitations. They do not seek to deny the physical passage of time, but they do seek to maintain the feeling of youthful energy for as long as possible.

Youthful Identity

Most people feel youthful by default. According to a research study conducted in 1986 by S. R. Kaufman, people may experience considerable changes in physiology and social interactions as they get older, but their inner sense of identity does not change nearly as quickly. Kaufman describes it as an "ageless self": no matter how old we get on the outside, we tend to feel the same age on the inside. Numerous other studies conducted during the 1990s and 2000s seem to affirm this conclusion. One study on Midlife Development in the United States (MIDUS) found that, as far as internal age identity, people in the 25- to 29-year-old age group tend to experience hardly any difference between how old they feel they are and how many chronological years they actually are. Every other age group tends to stay nearer to that 25- to 29-year-old optimum. People do feel older, but they tend to do so at a much slower rate than their actual years.

There were some important exceptions to these trends. About 75 percent of Americans feel younger than their actual age. Yet, people who experience health issues tend to feel the same or older than their chronological age. These correlations suggest that there is a connection between how old you *feel* and how old you may *become*.

Several factors influence individual age identity. Typically, the ideal age that people would like to be mirrors the age they feel like they are. The oldest age cohort (70–74 year olds) generally want to be about half their current age (around 35–40). Their age identity, then, usually remains close to that ideal age they hold in mind. Similarly, the ages that people typically think of as when midlife begins or ends can also influence age identity. Most people view midlife as somewhere between 44 and 59, and their age identity usually stays close to the age of either entering or leaving that midlife period. Other factors include personal perception. Those who believe they have remained essentially the same person over time (self-continuity) will likely view themselves as younger, as will people who only emphasize their positive characteristics and often fail to see the negative (self-enhancement). As antiageism advocates would point out, cultural pressures also play a role in the sense of age identity. When a society places greater value on youth than on old age, people tend to want to be younger than their actual age.

The sense of a younger age identity is not merely a matter of self-deception. A series of studies conducted between the 1980s and the early 2000s found that younger age identity is linked to successful aging. People who feel younger than they are tend to maintain positive mental health and a healthier sense of well-being. One study in the *Journal of the American Medical Association* in 2015, by researchers at Seattle University, found a correlation between feeling younger and living longer. After studying 6,500 test subjects with an average age of 65 years, they found that the mortality rates over the next 8 years was 18.5 percent for those who felt 3 or more years younger than their actual age and nearly 25 percent for those who felt more than a year older than their actual age.

To a large extent, good physical health plays a major role in developing youthful age identities. People tend to feel younger when they are healthy. Perhaps more importantly, though, the correlations appear to remain true both ways. Other studies suggest that the more youthful a person's age identity, the more likely he or she is to maintain better health over time. The advocates of successful aging contend that feeling young may actually lead to longer middle-age vitality.

Characteristics of Youth

When teenagers speak of youth, they often speak from immaturity and emphasize the drawbacks of their dependent condition. Teens are unable to make their own choices, they are unable to pay for the things that they are most interested in, and they do not have the security of a known future—in short, they often do not get to do what they most want to do. Yet, when an older adult speaks of youth, those sorts of dependencies are largely forgotten. Instead, they tend to emphasize the positive characteristics that teens usually take for granted: youthful strength, endurance, and the ability to more quickly heal and bounce back from physical and emotional wounds. In short, it is the abundance of energy in all its forms that seems to define youthfulness.

Mobility

Many symptoms of declining strength and endurance are not evident until after age 60, and they are often not noticeable until they affect an individual's ability to move around. Yet, impaired mobility is not exclusive to older adults. A Harvard Medical School study (2001) found that problems of mobility are common to all age groups and become most pronounced after age 60. Using a cross-sectional survey of 19 million adult males, the study defined loss of mobility as any difficulty in standing, walking, or stair climbing. The average age of people who had experienced mobility issues was between 59 and 67 years, yet nearly a third of those people indicated that they had begun experiencing major symptoms before age 50. In many cases, the impaired mobility was not necessarily a result of age; it was often a result of an accident, disease, or problems associated with obesity.

A strong correlation exists between how healthy you feel, how old you feel, and how able you are to move around. Nearly 40 percent of people reporting limited mobility perceived themselves to be in poor health. There is another strong correlation between obesity and impaired mobility at every age, though researchers could not determine whether obesity caused the impairment or vice versa. There were, however, significant connections between people with limited mobility and significantly greater risks of osteoarthritis and other signs of declining cardiovascular and respiratory fitness.

The problem for defining youthfulness by strength and energy is that the characteristics of average youth have changed significantly over the past four decades because of increasingly sedentary lifestyles. Since the 1970s, children have become less active in their daily routines, and the average height-to-weight ratios have increased proportionally. Surveys conducted in 2015 indicate that nearly one-third of children are clinically obese. Around 70 percent of obese children have at least one cardiovascular risk factor, and nearly 40 percent have two or more risk factors. Characteristics of impaired mobility and compromised health profiles may begin at very young ages and are not necessarily limited to older adults.

Active Lifestyles

The definition of *youthfulness* may not necessarily include high energy and increased strength and endurance. Many youth lack motivation, are overweight, and live sedentary lifestyles that can compromise their health. It is popular to blame television, video games, and smartphones for this lifestyle, but the causes are less important than the trends. These trends suggest it is possible to feel younger at any age. A sedentary lifestyle can deprive an individual of strength and energy at any age. Conversely, more active lifestyles contribute to a greater sense of vitality at any age. Often, the decision to pursue certain lifestyle choices will have a greater immediate impact on strength, endurance, and energy than the declining biological factors of aging. Feeling old may have less to do with age and more to do with inactivity.

The source of youthful energy may be less biological and more a by-product of mental outlook and resulting lifestyle choices. Young adults who have the greatest biological advantage in avoiding obesity are often less inclined to make necessary lifestyle choices or pursue the discipline of an active lifestyle. At the same time, adults who experienced bouts of obesity in their youth are often more committed to pursuing and maintaining active lifestyles because they had firsthand experiences with the problems that arise from inactivity. Chemical supplements (such as hormone therapies) may produce the increase in energy that is expected from youthfulness, but if they are not also accompanied with continued physical activity, the results are ineffective. Biochemistry only plays a partial role in feeling young again.

Many adults in their forties with declining levels of naturally occurring anabolic steroids claim to feel stronger than they ever did in their twenties, and this is often a result of specific lifestyle changes. A mature adult is often still capable of developing strength and endurance. A 2009 study at the University of Oklahoma reported that two cohorts of men (young college-aged 18 to 25 and another of ages 35 to 50)

Age at the Olympics

The Olympics represent the best and most elite athletes in the world, and often the competitors are in their late teens or early twenties—but not always. During the 2016 Olympic Games in Rio de Janeiro, Oksana Chusovitina (for Uzbekistan) became the oldest gymnast at 41. The average age of most Olympic gymnasts is 16, with a range usually between 15 and 18. Chusovitina first competed in 1992 and has attended seven Olympic Games. In addition, Mebrahtom Keflezighi, also at 41, became the oldest American Olympic marathon runner in 2016. He joined 39-year-old Jo Pavey (United Kingdom) and 40-year-old Scott Westcott in the same games. The average age for distance runners is 25, though older athletes are more common in non-Olympic marathons. Fauja Singh became the oldest distance runner when he completed the Hong Kong Marathon at the age of 102.

In other Olympic events, age has much less meaning. Shooting and equestrian sports often include older competitors. The oldest Olympian man was Oscar Swahn (Sweden), who was 72 when he competed in shooting during the 1920 games. Arthur von Pongracz (Austria) was also 72 when he competed in dressage events during the 1936 games. Hiroshi Hoketsu (Japan) was 71 when he competed in the same event during the 2012 Olympic Games. At the age of 70, Lorna Johnstone became the oldest women to compete during the 1972 Olympic Games (also in an equestrian event).

underwent the same exercise regimens, and the older men gained more muscle mass and lost more weight than the younger set. Despite declining hormone levels, the older adults still managed to retain their strength through active exercise routines.

The decision to live a more youthful lifestyle can have a significant impact on whether you feel youthful. The irony is that young adults often take their biological youth for granted, focusing instead on those characteristics of age that they do not yet have (freedom of decision making and economic stability). The old adage, "Youth is wasted on the young," seems to apply. Similarly, adults often make the same mistake and ignore their advantages of wisdom and maturity by focusing more on their desire for the youthful energy they believe they must be missing. In many cases, the youthful energy is not yet gone.

Active Lifestyle: Diet, Exercise, and Sleep

Weight Control

For those adults who seek a more active lifestyle, the Centers for Disease Control (CDC) recommends losing weight. This can come from reducing caloric intake through a moderate diet, but diet alone will not necessarily result in weight loss. There are hundreds of different diets available, and some promise results without significant lifestyle changes (outside of eating habits). Diet plans can range from low-sugar or low-carbohydrates, to eating only in small portions or only during certain times of the day, to any number of other clever systems. Yet, most of these diets are intended to take advantage of our existing psychological habits and do not necessarily effect weight loss from a strictly biological perspective. Individual metabolism varies, but, ultimately, weight loss occurs when the body burns more calories than it takes in. Weight is maintained, gained, or lost depending on whether the individual consumes more or fewer calories than he or she burns. Diets without an accompanying exercise plan usually fail. Exercise increases the number of calories burned per day, which is more likely to result in the caloric deficit necessary to maintain proper weight.

Weight control is only part of maintaining an active lifestyle. People who are overweight tend to be less active, which affects mobility and impacts their perceived sense of health as well as their mental age. It is the active lifestyle, and not the weight, that is most significant in determining a youthful feeling. Physical activity involves movement, and the very act of exercise—even if it is light, such as walking or cycling—involves some form of movement. It is the feeling of active mobility that plays the greatest role in determining the sense of healthiness.

In addition, weight loss through dieting alone may actually have a negative effect on how young we feel, even if dieting might increase the final number of our years. Evidence suggests that very low caloric intake ratios may extend the natural life span. Antiaging research indicates that dietary restriction (eating about 25 percent less than the daily recommended allowance) leads to as much as a 50 percent increase in life span among lower rodents. Unfortunately, the psychological side effects of constantly hovering at or near starvation include listlessness, an inability to concentrate, and lack of energy. These symptoms run counter to the goals of an active lifestyle and for sustaining the energy required to feel younger. Maintaining a healthy weight through a combination of diet and constant activity may contribute to a more positive outlook, encourage greater mobility, and promote a greater sense of youthfulness.

For the purposes of successful aging, weight control is intended for youthful feeling and not necessarily for aesthetic purposes. Not all people will lose weight in the same way, and an active lifestyle will not necessarily lead to the figure or physique of a 25-year-old model. The goal is to achieve a healthy weight, not necessarily a socially popular weight. Moderately excessive weight only leads to physical symptoms when it results in critical risk factors that include high cholesterol, high blood pressure, or increased insulin resistance leading to high blood sugar. Research suggests that many people gravitate toward a healthy weight that is somewhat heavier than average. In 2012, a 25-year longitudinal study of nearly 44,000 individuals found that some metabolic rates may lead to obesity despite active lifestyles. The study describes this condition as "medically healthy obesity." As long as cholesterol, blood pressure, and insulin resistance remain at normal levels, the excess weight has little impact on health and longevity.

More importantly, other evidence suggests that the psychological benefits of being satisfied with a healthy weight are greater than maintaining a socially attractive weight. The ideal figure promoted in consumer advertising is only realistically obtainable by about 5 percent of the population, which means that most people will fail to achieve that goal without some sort of cosmetic surgery. Constantly dieting to achieve a difficult (or impossible) ideal weight can be highly stressful. Moreover, actuarial studies affirm that people who are either a little overweight or are underweight tend to have the longest life spans. Both conditions may lead to longer life spans, but they are not equal in terms of happiness. Researchers at McMasters University in 2012 found that individuals who are genetically predisposed to being overweight are often happier and enjoy a greater sense of healthiness than people with the same genetic markers at normal weights.

Sleep

Perhaps more important than weight control is access to ample sleep. Many of the symptoms of obesity can be triggered by a lack of sleep, including high blood pressure, insulin resistance, and obesity itself. The body needs sleep to restore many of the hormones associated with youthful energy (including hGH). In addition, sleep helps promote psychological restfulness. Sleep researchers have linked dreams to increased emotional health, based on the theory that the subconscious unravels many of the mental obstacles that occur during the waking day. Several decades of research conducted by Rosalind Cartwright from the National Sleep Foundation found that dreams help us to work through emotional tensions and lead to reduced stress and greater patience overall.

Sleep requirements are age-related. The need for sleep is very high for infants (18 to 22 hours a day), gradually declines for young children (10 to 12 hours a day) and teens (8 to 10 hours), and then plateaus for adults (7 to 9 hours). The amount of sleep needed for adults aged 65 and older is only slightly less (7 to 8 hours). Unfortunately, adults of all ages often lose their ability to sleep as they get older because of emotional tensions that accompany increased family and professional obligations. Age-related fluctuations in levels of the hormone melatonin may also affect an individual's ability to fall asleep. In addition to physical symptoms, lack of sleep may also effect mood, memory, and concentration—all of which are often attributed to advanced aging (see chapter 12).

Sunlight

Strong evidence suggests that a daily habit of routine exercise, healthy eating, and ample sleep greatly contributes to a sense of well-being and promotes a greater feeling of youthfulness. Physical exercise during the day, especially extended walks outside in the fresh air, may help to reduce stress and alleviate problems with falling asleep. Mood and emotional health is strongly related to vitamin D, which is best obtained through exposure to the UV rays found in sunlight, out in the open air.

Walks outside improve mood and emotional well-being. A lack of sunlight can result in a drop in vitamin D and the hormone serotonin, which impacts mood. In climates where it is difficult to walk outside due to extreme temperatures or where there are long periods of darkness (such as the northern regions), residents often suffer from a lack of sunlight that results in seasonal affective disorder (SAD), which is strongly linked to depression. The cure requires both vitamin D supplements and greater exposure to natural sunlight. According to a study conducted by the National Institute of Environmental Health Sciences, exposure of the hands, arms, and face to as little as 5 to 30 minutes of outside sunlight three times a week is sufficient to improve physical and emotional well-being.

Unfortunately, one of the two known preventative measures for reducing the appearance of wrinkles and other physical signs of aging in the skin is to avoid exposure to sunlight. This is a situation where individuals need to weigh the benefits of appearing younger against the benefits of feeling younger. Feeling younger may require a sacrifice of increased wrinkles and increased risk of skin cancer. Fortunately, the other preventative measure for reducing wrinkles is frequent use of a moisturizer. As long as they do not contain UV protection, moisturizers generally do not block vitamin D. Individuals must balance their priorities of feeling younger with the priorities of other physical and cosmetic antiaging techniques.

Cosmetics

At first glance, cosmetic enhancement may seem at odds with the ideal of successful aging because it attempts to disguise or deny the reality of a person's real age. For most plastic surgery enhancements that may be true, but not for all. Reconstructive surgery following mastectomies (for cancer-related reasons) are rarely undertaken to disguise the effects of aging; the motivation is often based on a need for emotional healing rather than cosmetic enhancement. By definition, cosmetic surgery differs from reconstructive surgery because it seeks to enhance tissues from their natural state. Most cosmetic surgery seeks to disguise the effects of aging, but not all cosmetics are used for that purpose. Like reconstructive surgery, some cosmetics are used simply to provide emotional healing. Most of the less intrusive forms of cosmetic enhancement do not involve any surgery at all (hair color, makeup, etc.) and may not necessarily involve a desire to hide or disguise age.

Some common beautification practices such as daily makeup, hair color, and fashionable accessories for women are often motivated by internal rather than external reasons. As discussed in chapter 8, women often use cosmetics to bolster their sense of empowerment and to enhance (rather than disguise) their own sense of beauty. Does the use of cosmetics help women to age gracefully? Research suggests it depends on why women use it. If the primary goal is to look younger, then clearly this does not fit into the model of successful aging. Yet, if the primary goal is to feel confident with the physical characteristics that the individual woman already possesses, then the use of cosmetics does not necessarily imply a desire to defy aging or to escape the physical effects of time.

Advocates of the antiageism movement are more explicit on this point. Women of all ages use makeup, and various beautification techniques are often a matter of artistic self-expression. Young girls in high school may choose bold hair colors as a form of expression, and older women in their later middle ages may choose do the same thing for similar reasons. The freedom to dress, or act, or wear makeup for any reason should be the same for women of older ages as it is for women of younger ages. It can be argued that the cultural expectations that encourage older

The Ugly Truth of Young Centenarians

It is commonly assumed that people who reach very old ages of 100 years or more must have developed healthy habits when they were young. Evidence gathered from centenarians does not reflect that assumption. In 2011, the Institute of Aging Research at the Albert Einstein College of Medicine at Yeshiva University conducted a longitudinal study of 477 adults aged 95 to 112 and surveyed their lifestyle habits when they were younger. This data was compared against surveys taken among the similar age cohort during the 1970s. Those centenarians who survived into the 21st century did not diet more than the rest of their cohort, nor did they smoke less, drink less, or exercise more. In fact, in some cases, the centenarians had less regular exercise and were just as likely to be overweight, though there was less frequency of obesity among the centenarians.

Nir Barzilai, the lead author of the project, theorized that centenarians must have had some other (unaccounted for) longevity gene to result in the longer lives. He explained, "Although this study demonstrates that centenarians can be obese, smoke and avoid exercise, those lifestyle habits are not a good choice for most of us who do not have a family history of longevity."

women not to wear makeup are just as discriminatory as those social pressures placed on middle-aged women to wear makeup to disguise their age. In either case, if age is the reason for the social pressure, it can be viewed as a form of ageism.

THINKING AND ACTING YOUNGER

A sensible diet, frequent exercise, and ample sleep may help us to feel younger than our actual years, but physical strength and energy play only a part of successful aging. Another characteristic of youth is a curious mind and a willingness to learn new things. Again, these traits are often overlooked among teens and young adults who may see education as a burden or an obstacle that needs to be overcome to begin living as an adult. Yet, evidence suggests that for older adults, the continual quest for new knowledge can play a major role in maintaining a sense of youthfulness and an agile mind.

Myths of Mental Aging

Much of geriatric research is dedicated to finding cures for common age-related diseases, including cardiovascular disease, cancer, and Alzheimer's disease. Most funding for this research comes from public sources, which means that numerous national associations exist both to raise funds for research as well as to raise awareness of particular diseases. As a result, the public consumer can be overwhelmed by the frequent fund-raising activities dedicated to specific diseases (walk-a-thons, rides for a cure, and special colored ribbons, to name just a few). These efforts may inadvertently create an impression that old age is marked by constant suffering from one disease or another.

As early as the 1990s, sociologists Meredith Minker and Carroll Estes coined the phrase "biomedicalization of aging" to describe the phenomenon of equating old age with disease and pathology. They attributed this trend to private industries (such as nursing homes and pharmaceutical companies) as well as fund-raising and awareness-building organizations. They also coined the phrase "apocalyptic demography" to describe theories that predict the future economic bankruptcy of public resources if people continue to live longer lives. Many organizations promote dire predictions of social problems associated with aging to attract government research money. Minker and Estes were joined by other spokespersons in the 2010s, such as antiageism journalist Ashton Applewhite and AARP CEO Jo Ann Jenkins, both of whom argue that the realities of old age are not nearly as painful as the images found in popular cultural media suggest.

The Alzheimer's Association's Web page includes headlines that state, "1 in 3 seniors die with Alzheimer's or another dementia" and "Every 66 seconds someone in the United States develops the disease." These and other headlines are accompanied with financial predictions: "In 2016, Alzheimer's and other dementias will cost the nation $236 billion" and "Family caregivers spend more than $5,000 a year caring for someone with Alzheimer's." The statistics are impressive, but they are not always reflective of the total population. The same statistics reveal that nearly 90 percent of adults aged 65 or older do not have Alzheimer's or dementia. As of 2015, only 4 percent of adults aged 65 or older lived in nursing homes, which is down from 5 percent in 2006. Only 10 percent of adults aged 85 years or older live in nursing homes. Despite the fearful predictions of dementia, a more typical generalization is that most people will die at home and not from Alzheimer's or other dementia.

Mental Acuity in Older Ages

Mental acuity for older adults is stronger than popular culture suggests. A longitudinal study conducted at the University of Washington in Seattle indicated that many of the presumptions of declining mental functions are false. After collecting data for more than 50 years, the researchers affirmed that memory and processing speed seem to decline with age, but that abstract reasoning and simple math functions seem to improve with age. The study found that adult brains (between 40 and 70) remain adept at learning and are better at combining previous experiences into new situations, resulting in generally calmer dispositions and a stronger ability to navigate social situations. Other research conducted at the University of Southern California in Los Angeles found that adults tend to focus more on positive information than on negative information, and they tend to be more emotionally stable. This often translates in better ability to judge other people's true intentions than their younger (or significantly older) peers. Additionally, researchers from the University of Toronto found that older adults tend to use more of their brains for similar tasks, including the use of both sides of their brains from various tasks, while younger people tend to favor one side or the other.

It is not inevitable that older adults will lose their mental abilities. Indeed, it would seem that wisdom really does increase with age. Evidence suggests that there are many things that older individuals can do to augment their wisdom while still feeling and thinking younger. Recommendations mostly involve engaging in the kind of mental activity that youth engage in, including being constantly curious, continually learning, and maintaining some hope for the future.

Acting Old—Daily Routines

The Seattle research study suggests that part of the reason why older adults may feel like they are less able to learn new things is because they often spend years, and even decades, developing specialized knowledge of matters related to their professions. Adults continue to learn but often only within narrowly defined knowledge bases. Research from a team of psychologists at Princeton University in 2000 indicates that many of our presumptions of mental limitations are self-imposed based on our own expectations. Older adults may tell themselves that they cannot learn new technologies or new skills, but evidence suggests quite the opposite. Older adults are more adept at combining the new knowledge with the old knowledge, and that translates into greater wisdom.

Evidence suggests adults do well at adapting to new experiences; nevertheless, some older adults are afraid of these new experiences. This may be less a by-product of age and more a result of habituated experiences—daily routines (which is a form of specialized learning). People develop daily routines because they have figured out the best way of managing a particular set of circumstances, and they maintain those routines rather than experiment with new or creative problem-solving techniques.

For some, routines can be very positive because they provide an intellectual structure from which to deal with the other random events in life. People who work with very young children often stress the need for routines to help the children create mental patterns that they can use to better assimilate new information, which for young children is a constant occurrence. Yet, for older adults, those routines could potentially limit new learning. In the early 1980s, the psychologist Robert Kastenbaum coined the term "habituation" to refer to the tendency for adults to depend on daily routines and limited expectations as an energy conservation measure. He argued that mental aging was more an effect of people choosing to classify new events in the same way that they understand old events. This encourages a sense of comfort but may also encourage mental stagnation.

In its extreme form, hyperhabituation may result when individuals are deliberately resistant to new experiences and new challenges. Kastenbaum used the concepts of habituation to explain why older adults appear as if they are less able to learn. He argued, however, that habituation is not biologically determined. It reflects a pattern of psychological choices. Most often, both habituation and hyperhabituation reflect specific lifestyle choices. Choosing to "think younger" means being more open to experiencing new forms of mental stimulation that force the mind to use creative problem solving. If there are fewer random events in life, the routine does not stimulate the mind to assimilate new information.

Anecdotal evidence from centenarians often cite long-standing daily routines to explain why they have lived so long. They wake up at the same hour, go to bed at the same hour, and often eat the same kinds of food, with very similar daily exercise routines. The biodemographer Jay Olshansky explains that these sorts of routines are helpful in that they can protect older adults from unexpected accidents that might impair their biological functions. They do not, however, necessarily impact their degree of mental stimulation. As Lawrence Katz, a neurobiologist at Duke University, argues in *Keep Your Brain Alive* (1999), physical routines are not the same as mental routines, which should be avoided. He recommends older adults, "Do something that challenges and engages your mind, . . . not because it's difficult, but because it's different from what you normally do."

Acting Young—New Learning

There are many ways for older adults to avoid the pitfalls of daily routines that promote mental stagnancy. Some routines may be modified to incorporate new information on a daily basis: watch the morning news to keep abreast of current events, read new books every day, or go out and make new acquaintances. The process of incorporating new experiences into daily routines may preserve both the comfort of established patterns as well as the stimulation of new information. Unlike most youth, older adults often have access to the means and opportunities to develop new experiences. In this way, their age is an advantage over youth.

Travel

One of the most effective methods for breaking daily routines is to travel to a foreign country. The culture shock that follows the new environment forces people to develop new strategies to solve new situations. Everyday habits require new solutions: different currencies, different languages, different social customs, and new foods, art, and architecture all stimulate different areas of the brain. Solutions often require the use of older tools, such as mathematics, language development, and flexible interpersonal relationship skills, as well as adjustments to fine and gross motor skills to the new customs.

In addition, traveling to foreign countries exposes people to new histories, new points of visual references, and often new friendships. Interacting with people from completely different backgrounds forces us to reconsider what we say or what we assume during our interactions. Often, the wisdom and experience of age better prepares older adults to solve these problems than younger adults. Discernment, patience, and adaptation are improved with age as long as physical impairments do not compound the challenges of culture shock.

New and Deeper Relationships

Travel is very effective for encouraging new problem-solving skills, but it is not always an available opportunity for those who do not have the funds or who suffer from impaired mobility. Nevertheless, many of the same benefits may be found without leaving home. There are new situations, cultures, and experiences right at home. Older adults who make new friends with members from a younger generation or from a different cultural or socioeconomic background may gain many of the same experiences as traveling abroad.

The greatest risk from habituation comes from following patterns of behavior that do not require new solutions. Changing daily routines to include new experiences, such as joining a new club or a new organization, requires learning new customs or traditions. Similarly, sharing new experiences with old friends may achieve the same results. Eating different foods, listening to different music, or reading different kinds of books and then sharing those experiences can create new pathways for mental stimulation without necessarily disturbing the comfort of a daily routine.

Forging deeper relationships with old friends (as well as with new ones) also involves problem-solving skills, though in a different way. In a 2010 meta-analysis of almost 150 research articles, psychologists at Brigham Young University found a 50 percent increase in longevity among those men and women who formed strong personal relationships. The sense of being well connected can provide the same sort of comfort found in a daily routine, which results in less stress and allows individuals more opportunities to develop mental stimulation in other ways.

Married couples generally live longer than individuals who never married, yet such demographic trends do not have obvious causal explanations. Stanford Medical School professor and past president of the American Geriatrics Society Walter Bortz wrote three books on successful aging. He explains, "It's a matter of survival. People that have sex live longer. Married people live longer. People need people. The more intimate the connection, the more powerful the effects." Biological changes have only a modest impact on the ability to engage in sexual activity, and a majority of people aged 50 to 80 continue to be sexually active. Though divorce rates were very high in the 1970s and 1980s, modern statistics indicate that nearly 75 percent of married couples living in the 2000s will remain so until death.

There is a risk of habituation within a strong marital relationship, as each partner becomes accustomed to the other's habits to form strong daily routines. This risk of isolated relationships that depend heavily on the spouse stems from the dramatic sense of loss that occurs when the relationship ends through death (or some other reason). Negative effects of hyperhabituation may become magnified, as the surviving spouse seems to lose his or her will to live rather than continue in a world without his or her loved one. To offset that risk of habituation, a broad network of friendships with many people can help to break the isolation that may occur when the emotional bond of friendship is limited to only one person. Evidence from research conducted at the Department of Human Development and Family Studies at Texas Tech University suggests that a strong intimate bond with your spouse generally decreases daily stress while also providing opportunities for developing broad friendships and other platonic relationships with a variety of other people. The combination of a marital bond with a broad circle of friends and hobbies helps to promote more durable relationships and to avoid habituation.

Education Never Ends

In addition to forming broad relationships, the feeling of youthful inquiry is easily stimulated through continual education. This may include something informal, such as learning a new hobby, arts and crafts, or a new recreational skill or activity. The impact is enhanced when the hobby is shared by new friends and acquaintances, especially with younger adults. As the Seattle longitudinal research study indicates, there is very little evidence to support the adage that "you can't teach an old dog new tricks" (even for dogs).

Formal forms of education are also an excellent source of mental stimulation. Teens and young adults may lament the challenges of high school and college, but for older adults, these venues provide an opportunity to learn completely new fields of knowledge. The 2010 U.S. Census indicates that more than 170,000 adults aged 65 and older are enrolled in undergraduate and graduate programs. About 15 percent of college students are 35 years or older, and the number of adults returning to the classroom, for economic or other reasons, has steadily increased since 2000. Nearly 40 percent of the students in graduate school are 35 or older.

Work and Vocation

A critical aspect of thinking younger involves hope for the future. For a teen or young adult, the future may pose some frightening challenges as they discern what career path they may be most suitable for. This anxiety may continue even after youth, but, generally speaking, mature adults tend to settle on a particular occupation or vocation that occupies their time, provides income for sustaining themselves and their families, and promotes continual planning for short-term and long-term projects that stimulate mental activity through creative problem solving.

Retirement creates challenges for older adults who have become habituated to a routine that involves daily work or an identity that is tied to a professional occupation. In a 2009 study conducted by the RAND Corporation, researchers found that people who retired without developing a suitable vocational activity quickly lost cognitive abilities, including the speed of mental processing and abstract reasoning. Early retirement, before age 65, appears to compound these effects. The study suggests that people may become mentally stagnant after retirement because they have removed themselves from an environment that required frequent problem solving and because they lost incentives for engaging in the world around them.

Both problems, loss of a mentally stimulating environment and loss of engagement, may be remedied by deliberately pursuing a second vocation. The term *vocation* is broad enough to include any activity that involves dedicated work and effort and provides personal satisfaction. It does not necessarily involve earning money, and older adults living on the retirement of a prior career are often in the unique position of being able to pursue a vocation that is low paying or even voluntary. This opens up a broad array of opportunities that younger adults may not be able to enjoy. In addition, if the new vocation requires additional learning with new relationships, the benefits are multiplied.

Acting Older and Wiser

The antiaging movement often associates age with debility and decline. By contrast, youth is usually associated with energy, strength, endurance, and curiosity. It is easy to forget the negative associations with youth. Due to their lack of experience, young adults are often impulsive, unrestrained, and may be unmotivated because of fear of failure or an inability to appreciate the importance of long-term planning. Young adults may be impulsive or overly cautious because they lack the experience to trust their instincts or to believe that they can recover from a failure.

In part, youthful immaturity may be largely due to biological reasons. Child psychologist Alison Gopnik at the University of California at Berkley argues that youth that are caught between midteens and midtwenties are still developing physical pathways within the brain. Up until age 13, children have hyperdeveloped language skills, but as they enter their teen years, those parts of the brain become less active. Yet, the frontal lobes that contribute to decision making and abstract reasoning do not become fully developed until the midtwenties. The result is that high school and college-aged youth often make decisions based on emotion rather than on rational consideration. Students may experience severe mood swings and may not be able to explain why they feel the way they do, which continues to foster the sense of frustration and fear or impulsiveness and lack of restraint.

Mature adults have the benefit of complete biological development. Mature adults are no longer growing; as a result, their physical bodies begin to stabilize (before eventually declining). This process of aging is precisely what the antiaging movement seeks to remedy. Yet, this maturation process is also the primary reason why adults tend to have calmer dispositions, are more emotionally stable, and are better able to discern other people's true intentions, as reported by researchers at the University of Southern California in Los Angeles. It is precisely that sort of wisdom and experience that best explains the justification behind the successful aging movement.

CONCLUSION

In part, the antiageism movement is based on a conviction that cultural stereotypes about aging and its inevitable debilities and decline play a significant role in undermining widespread hope among older adults. If you are convinced that your elder years will result in disease, dementia, and death, it makes sense that you would do everything you can to avoid it. The antiaging movement is based on the attempt to remain young and youthful and to avoid all those negative consequences of aging. The antiageism movement, by contrast, seeks to destroy the negative associations by creating new cultural norms that accept the physical and emotional changes associated with aging in the same way we might accept similar changes among those who are young and maturing. Aging is a part of life and no worse than the alternative.

The antiageism movement strives to make political policy changes to encourage new cultural norms about aging. This effort is challenged by the inescapable reality that human bodies do not live forever and that age does in fact begin to limit physical abilities. The scientific arm of the antiaging movement is working diligently to prove that generalization wrong. They hope to find a biochemical solution to physical aging that would allow bodies to continue to heal themselves indefinitely. In the meantime, however, our bodies get old, and at one point we will no longer be able to be physically active.

The successful aging movement recognizes that human bodies get old, but they take a little from both the antiageism and the antiaging movements to argue that the effects of aging are not as inevitable as it is commonly assumed—particularly in terms of how we feel—and that some aspect of aging can be avoided with a proper mental outlook. The goal of feeling younger is to maximize the physical potential of an active lifestyle for as long as the biological capacity of the human body allows.

Religious Conviction

One aspect of successful aging that seems to defy the label is a gradual recognition and acceptance of the inevitability of death. It is the firm conviction that life is limited that drives the desire to live a more complete life. In this way, religious belief can play perhaps the most critical role in successful aging and in feeling young late into old age.

Scientific research into the role that spiritual and religious faith plays in successful aging is a relatively recent development. The White House Conference on Aging in 1971 helped to set the foundation for the formation of National Institute on Aging three years later. It featured a discussion on the value of religion for older adults; yet, the roundtable forum was limited, and most researchers preferred to avoid the subject. It did not become popular among geriatric researchers until the late 1990s. Nevertheless, among older adults, religion is one of their most dominant concerns. Multiple surveys in 2008 indicate that though religion plays an increasingly less important role in the daily lives of all adults (18 and over), it remains a consistent priority for adults 65 and older (between 80 and 90 percent). A large percentage (34 to 36 percent) of young adults aged 30 and younger describe themselves as atheistic or agnostic, yet the evidence from decades of demographic research suggests that the number of people who profess no faith declines significantly as they get older.

Scientific evidence suggests religious belief plays a major role in successful aging. Beginning in the 1990s, with the McArthur Research Network on Successful Aging, and continuing into the 2010s, research indicates that spirituality and religious participation encourages social connectedness and promotes hopefulness in the future. A 2001 study conducted at the University of Alabama reports that religious belief plays as important a role in successful aging as diet, exercise, mental stimulation, and self-efficacy. In part, this may be because religious faith has the potential of encouraging a sense of meaning to life that creates its own incentive for more active living. Other studies conducted that same year suggest that religious belief provides a critical social function in promoting positive attitudes, encouraging self-enhancing behaviors, and providing a mechanism for dealing with the inevitability of death and loss.

The successful aging movement finds its greatest support among those who hold religious convictions. Yet, the same demographic studies that show the importance of religion among older adults also show a gradual decline of religious conviction over the past 20 years in the population as a whole. There is little evidence to suggest that the culture will lose its majority religious identity, but there is significant evidence to expect that the percentage of nonreligious identification will continue to grow, especially among the younger age groups. It is from this subset that the antiaging movement finds its greatest support. As the society becomes increasingly secular, the sense of urgency within the antiaging movement will likely increase.

Chapter 10

What Kills Us (and How Can We Escape)?

Traditional gerontologists often argue that the antiaging movement sets up unrealistic goals when it strives to "cure" aging and death, as if they were diseases. In his defense of the growing antiaging movement of the 21st century, the English bioethicist John Harris countered this sentiment by arguing that all doctors must support antiaging. He explained that the physician's goal is to save lives, and therefore every treatment that helps save a life is "simply postponing death to another point." He added that all medical knowledge is more or less a practical application of the antiaging movement. To oppose the goals of the antiaging movement, one would have to oppose all routine therapeutic interventions for life-threatening illnesses. Doctors would have to let people die when they got sick—a sort of indifference that contradicts the basic creed of medical practice. As such, Harris reasoned, all medicine must necessarily promote antiaging. Science is constantly improving, and, ultimately, medical technology should seek to improve indefinitely. Once doctors find cures for all diseases, life spans should have no logical limit with medical care.

Critics among traditional gerontologists may debate the overgeneralized meaning of "antiaging" research, which could also include other medical innovations, such as genetic manipulation and cybernetic implants. In practice, however, John Harris's basic argument remains untested because science has yet to find cures for even a strong minority of the age-related diseases that lead to death. In this pursuit, traditional researchers in geriatric medicine happily join forces with the more recent antiaging advocates to find cures for cancer, Alzheimer's and dementia, cardiovascular disease, and a host of other ailments that impair the quality of life as we get older. There is no disagreement that medical science should do all it can to understand and solve these life-threatening diseases and thereby improve the quality of life for people of all ages.

There is, however, a risk of overgeneralization when we automatically associate aging with death and disease. The antiageism movement (as discussed in chapter 9) portrays the conditions associated with older ages as just another stage of development in the human life cycle. The uncomfortable truth remains that those age-related conditions often involve diminished biological functions and capacities. People typically begin to lose their hearing, sight, strength, mobility, and often

The Myth of Tithonus

In Homer's "Hymn to Aphrodite," the Greek poet told the story of Eos, an immortal daughter of two Titans, who is the personification of the morning dawn. She is said to have fallen in love with the Trojan warrior Tithonus, who was mortal and therefore doomed to die. In an effort to protect their love forever, Eos asks Zeus to grant Tithonus eternal life, which he does. However, she forgets to ask also for his eternal youth. In the legend, Tithonus grows older and increasingly infirm, and yet he never dies. Eos is forced to watch her lover become so incapacitated that he is no longer able to move, communicate, or even remember her love—yet, he still lives. In this way, his extended life is a curse and not a blessing. For the Greeks, there was a distinction between the conditions of age and the ailments that led to death.

their memory as they enter into older ages. In addition, these diminished functions increase our risks of contracting certain diseases, such as cancer, diabetes, and cardiovascular and respiratory diseases.

Antiageism advocates do not deny these facts, but they argue that the automatic association between age and disease is a form of social discrimination. In this, antiageism finds support among antiaging advocates, who argue that science has yet to determine whether age causes these conditions and diseases or the conditions and diseases cause the signs of aging. If scientists can find cures for the age-related problems, the negative associations will fade away automatically because chronological age will then have no connection with diminished biological functioning and capacity.

Part of the difficulty for gerontologists is in distinguishing between the "conditions" of diminished biological function that change with age and the "diseases" that are most often associated with age. This is illustrated by the myth of Tithonus, who gained eternal life but not eternal youth. For some traditional gerontologists, extending life indefinitely by curing the diseases that cause death will not likely benefit society if science does not also solve the debilitating conditions that follow aging. Maintaining life for its own sake is not as important as ensuring the quality of life. Antiaging researchers contend that the conditions of aging and the diseases of aging are inseparable. If they treat the conditions as a form of disease, they can solve both sorts of problems at once. As a rule, antiaging advocates argue that Tithonus is a myth both for the Greeks and for modern medical science; they do not believe life extension will happen that way. Avoiding natural death and prolonging the natural life span will necessarily involve finding cures for all age-related ailments. If the cures are not found, the life span will not be extended.

For this chapter, we consider first the most common age-related conditions that lead to diminished biological function and capacities. As of yet, there are no cures for these conditions, but we will examine what science offers as potential remedies. Then, we consider the most common age-related diseases and discuss the extent science has found cures or therapeutic treatments for them. There is no successful treatment for aging, and though science can cure specific instances of disease, it has yet to discover a way of reversing the age-related conditions that lead to these diseases. Nevertheless, there is great excitement among medical researchers that significant breakthroughs are possible, and perhaps even imminent, in both areas.

AGE-RELATED CONDITIONS

It is difficult to distinguish precisely which conditions are due to age-related deterioration of biological function and capacity and which are due to some other ailment independent of age. If we call them "diseases," we assume these conditions are disorders that impair normal biological function and were not the result of an accident or physical injury. In fact, the term *disease* is itself difficult to define because it presupposes a specific set of characteristics of normal health. The World Health Organization defines health as "a state of complete physical, mental and social well-being, not merely the absence of disease or infirmity." That definition is certainly inclusive, and the antiageism movement supports the implied conclusion that older adults can be healthy even if they have lost some of the biological functions and capacities that they may have enjoyed at younger ages. At the same time, the definition suffers from being so broad that it does not recognize that some age-related conditions can be debilitating, even under normally healthy conditions. Old age may not be classified as a disease, but these conditions can significantly impact the quality of life nevertheless.

In practice, gerontologists often use the terms "age-related conditions" and "chronic diseases" interchangeably. As adults grow older, they are more susceptible to conditions that impair their existing abilities. These conditions are not limited only to older adults, but they are common enough to be identified with age alone. In fact, by age 65, more than 88 percent of Americans will suffer from at least one chronic condition that cannot be cured by a vaccine or medication. Though there is no single uniform definition of chronic disease, a 2013 study overseen by the Centers for Disease Control (CDC) identified three basic characteristics: (1) chronic diseases do not cure themselves (they are not "self-limiting" and do not just disappear); (2) they are associated with persistent and recurring health problems that cannot be cured by vaccines or medications; and (3) their duration is measured in months or years, not in days or weeks. Chronic conditions are not necessarily deadly, but they do affect the quality of life and often make patients more vulnerable to other diseases.

Chronic diseases and other age-related conditions are not inevitable. In a very few cases, older adults may escape their effects entirely. Also, these conditions are not exclusive to older adults and may be found in youth as well, depending on their particular lifestyle choices; those who smoke or use drugs, engage in poor eating habits, and live sedentary lifestyles may develop many, if not all, of these conditions. The exceptions seem to support the claims of antiaging advocates, who argue that these conditions are not unavoidable by-products of aging but specific

diseases that should be treatable. They contend that older adults are more susceptible to chronic diseases because they have more years of experience and have an
increasing likelihood to suffer the cumulative effects of unhealthy behaviors. More
traditional gerontologists would disagree. They argue that the aging body develops
these conditions as a consequence of normal wear and tear of the biological system
and that they are unavoidable. The debate remains unresolved.

The Brain

For many people, one of the most frightening aspects of getting older is the prospect that they might lose their memory or their sense of identity. As discussed in
chapter 9 there is significant pressure from public awareness campaigns to remind
all Americans of the dangers and hardships associated with Alzheimer's disease
(AD) and other forms of dementia. As a result, it is not uncommon for people
to assume that forgetfulness and temporary confusion arising from interrupted
routines are both early warning signs of aging and dementia. Fortunately, recent
research indicates that the vast majority of older adults will not contract AD. It is
a growing pathology, and the medical community is devoting an increasingly large
percentage of research into better understanding its causes. They are continually
searching for potential treatment options. Nevertheless, it is not a natural condition of growing older. Most people can live to very old ages without ever developing the condition.

Mild Cognitive Impairment

Most recent research has distinguished between the more obvious symptoms
of fully developed dementia and the less obvious characteristics of mild cognitive impairment (MCI). Patients specifically suffering from AD not only experience memory issues but also encounter difficulties with attention, language, and
a generalized sense of confusion. Cognitive impairment may be expressed as a
broad spectrum of conditions that include trouble remembering or learning new
things and difficulty concentrating or making decisions. Severe cases manifest as
AD or some other form of dementia and usually result in an inability to live independently. Mild cases often go unnoticed by the patient or his or her family and
friends and do not necessarily progress into advanced stages. The symptoms of
MCI and early-onset AD are the same. The difference is that, over time, the cognitive abilities of patients with AD will gradually decline, while patients with MCI
may remain stable or perhaps improve over time.

Physicians may be able to diagnose MCI to determine whether it represents
early-onset AD or is an unrelated condition. Certain biomarker tests of the cere-
brospinal fluids and brain-imaging techniques (including magnetic resonance
imaging (MRI) and positron emission tomography (PET)) as well as basic examinations of reflexes, balance, and mood can identify early-onset AD. If AD is not indicated, then MCI may simply be a result of some other biomedical or environmental
conditions, such as depression or anxiety. A Mayo Clinic College of Medicine study

in 2011 examined 1,600 people aged 70 to 89 with no memory problems and found that about 7 percent developed MCI per year. Of those who developed the symptoms, only about 10 percent (or less than 1 percent of the total) developed AD over the course of the next four years. But there is evidence to suggest that over 10 years a large number of patients diagnosed with MCI would eventually develop AD, though at least 20 percent would not.

Generally speaking, statistics still suggest that most people will never develop dementia or MCI, and as such, it should not be considered a necessary condition of aging. There are differences in cognitive abilities between older adults and younger adults (as discussed in chapter 9), but these are often due to more specialized learning experiences or habituated routines and may be avoidable with the adoption of certain lifestyle choices.

Depression

Some conditions of old age reflect common lifestyle choices rather than biological impairment. Older retired adults often share similar sociological conditions, and public perception often ascribes common characteristics to age rather than to the other social conditions that they share. After leaving the workplace, retired adults typically experience a decline in social interaction. Research indicates that adults over 65 spend on average 8–10 percent of their free time with friends and family. It is not uncommon for them to also experience symptoms of depression. Surveys indicate that 15–20 percent of adults over 65 suffer from depression. It is probably not coincidental (though the evidence does not indicate a causal connection) that the CDC also indicates that 20 percent of adults aged 65 and older deal with some form of substance abuse, which includes a dependency on alcohol, tobacco, opiates, or other prescription painkillers.

Loneliness and depression are not necessary conditions of getting older. Rather, it is more accurate to say that adults who are less active and who no longer share their homes with dependent children tend to be at greater risk of suffering from depression. The solution to this condition is to increase their activity and to develop greater networks for social interaction. The loss of a sense of purpose and self-worth is often a reflection of changing vocational conditions. Most older adults retire from their lifelong professions, and therefore most adults will be forced to confront the common situation of having to determine how to devote their retirement years. This is not a disease, but it is a common psychological dilemma and can often became a source of stress. Statistics also suggest that the majority of older adults eventually settle on satisfying choices and avoid depression.

Bones, Joints, and Muscles

After age 50, adults often begin to lose their mobility due to inflammation of their joints and the gradual reduction of tissue mass in their bones. Osteoporosis and osteoarthritis share similar sounding names, but they are diagnosed differently, treated differently, and often stem from entirely different conditions. The CDC estimates that 54 million people aged 50 and over suffer from osteoporosis, the loss of bone mass, which increases the risk of fractures and breaks. Similarly, almost 50 percent of adults aged 65 and older suffer from osteoarthritis, a degenerative joint disease that affects any place where two bones come together (such as knees, wrists, fingers, toes, spine, and hips).

Osteoporosis

The loss of bone density is frequently undiagnosed until the problem becomes severe enough to cause injury (a fracture or a break). It is easily detected with a bone mineral density test, but it usually goes untested until some other symptom appears. In some cases, the disease can cause older adults to lose height (the bones shrink, and the overall skeleton becomes slightly shorter).

There are a variety of potential causes for developing osteoporosis, including diets low in calcium, smoking, and excessive alcohol use. The toxins in tobacco can generate free radicals that undermine basic cellular health throughout the body, including the bones. Specifically, these toxins can impede the hormone calcitonin, which is used to build bone mass, and may also increase the level of cortisol hormones, which lead to the breakdown of bone tissues. Women are especially susceptible because nicotine and free radicals may produce other enzymes that harm estrogen levels, which also affect bone development. Whether they smoke or not, women are more susceptible than men to osteoporosis as they age because their estrogen levels are significantly reduced following menopause. Estrogen helps the body process calcium, which is a primary building block for bone health.

Other factors may include family history and the lack of weight-bearing exercises. The body naturally adjusts its needs according to physical habits. The more weight applied to the bones, the more the bones will respond with increased density. Although obesity may contribute to osteoarthritis, it has very limited impact on osteoporosis, as the added weight on the skeletal frame tends to increase bone density.

There is no cure for osteoporosis. The best treatment option is to avoid developing the condition through healthy lifestyles choices that include avoiding tobacco use, regular weight-bearing exercises, and a balanced diet that includes calcium and vitamin D. Numerous medications have been approved to treat symptoms of osteoporosis, but most involve painkillers to deal with the aftereffects of breaks and fractures.

Osteoporosis is a chronic condition, but it is does not lead to death. It may, however, contribute to a gradual loss of mobility, including permanent disability, which in turn may lead to more life-threatening conditions related to heart and respiratory health. Younger adults may develop the disease as a side effect of certain medications and other ailments, but typically the risk of developing osteoporosis is tied strongly with age.

Arthritis

Almost any condition that impairs the proper functioning of joints may be generically labeled as arthritis. In fact, there are two main types of arthritis, and only one is associated with age-related conditions. Rheumatoid arthritis (RA) is an autoimmune condition, which results in the inflammation of tissues surrounding the joints. The body essentially attacks itself because it misidentifies healthy tissues as diseased tissues, resulting in inflammation that renders the joints difficult to move. Patients with RA can be of any age, and treatment options include a variety of prescription medicines that target the body's immunity responses. Patients with RA often develop osteoporosis as a side effect of their medication.

The more common age-related arthritis is called osteoarthritis (OA), and it is a degenerative joint disease that often develops as a result of overuse. Patients suffering from OA tend to be older because they have had many more years of using their joints in repeated motions that tend to wear away the cartilage between the two connected bones. Even normal activity may result in OA over the course of many years as the joints slowly wear down. Yet, younger patients who engage in excessive sports may also develop OA if they abuse their joints and harm their cartilage through unusual and repeated activities that cause undue stress.

Both forms of arthritis can lead to impaired mobility, which in turn increases the likelihood of obesity, which can lead to a host of other diseases. Similar to osteoporosis, there is no cure for OA as of yet. Once the cartilage between the joints begins to wear away, there are few treatment options for repairing the damage. Treatment options include several pain-relieving medications, such as nonsteroidal anti-inflammatory drugs (NSAIDs), physical therapy, and other analgesic remedies to dull the pain (including topical creams, hot and cold packs, massage therapy, and acupuncture). Some surgical options include joint replacement, but these are not permanent and often require additional replacement after a limited number of years. Most physicians require patients to be above a certain age before they recommend joint replacement.

There is some hope, however, because arthritis is a major area of research and new innovations in biotechnology are continually being pursued. In 2016, researchers at Washington University working with the biotech firm Cytex developed genetically engineered cartilage made from a patient's own stem cells. Using a biodegradable scaffolding form and 3-D bioprinters, the stem cells are arranged according to the precise measurements of the patient, and as the cells originate from the patient, there is no fear of rejection. This breakthrough provides some hope for curing the most common symptoms of OA. As of 2016, the technology was still in the experimental stages.

Loss of Muscle Strength

As a result of naturally high levels of anabolic hormones (testosterone, estrogen, and human growth hormone (hGH)), young adults develop increasing muscle strength and endurance until they reach their late thirties. After that point, the levels of anabolic steroids naturally produced in the endocrine system begin to taper off, and unless they are deliberately engaged in strenuous activity, muscle mass and function begin to decline (about 3–5 percent per decade). Inactive lifestyles will accelerate the rate of muscle loss. This condition is not a disease but a natural reaction to the declining levels of hormones that are responsible for muscular tissue growth, and it is entirely age-related. In medical terms, it is called age-related sarcopenia (ARS), and even with deliberate exercise programs, the muscle loss is very difficult to avoid. The rate of ARS increases after age 75, though adults may experience this acceleration at any time between ages 65 and 80. It is the leading cause of frailty among older adults.

Though not life-threatening, ARS is a significant factor in the increasing rate of falls and fractures among older adults, which is a leading cause of mortality. The CDC reports that 30–40 percent of adults aged 65 and older fall at least once per year, resulting in 2.5 million visits to the emergency room. Of those, 20 percent result in serious injuries, including broken bones, hip fractures, or head injuries. Nearly 95 percent of all hip fractures are caused by falling. Though there are a variety of factors that lead to falls, including declining vision, loss of balance, cognitive impairment leading to confusion, and physical obstructions in the home, ARS is usually cited as a leading cause.

ARS is not curable as a condition, but it is treatable. Hormone replacement therapy (HRT) with testosterone and hGH can help to offset declining levels of anabolic steroids, but the side effects to mood and the stress on joints are unpredictable. Anabolic steroids have no effect on degenerative joints, and the added muscle mass may actually increase the pain and discomfort of osteoarthritis. In addition, there is some evidence that HRT may increase the likelihood of certain cancers. For these reasons, the most prescribed treatment for ARS is exercise and resistance training to increase muscle strength and endurance naturally. Such training may also increase the natural levels of anabolic hormones within the body in ways that supplemental HRT may not achieve.

Eyes and Ears

More than 90 percent of the information entering the brain is perceived through the ocular and auditory senses. Gradual loss of vision and hearing can seriously impair an individual's ability to interact with the world around them. These conditions may not be life-threatening, but they can have a significant impact on the quality of daily life.

Eyes

Eyesight begins to decline between the ages of 40 and 45, resulting in a condition called *presbyopia*, which affects 100 percent of the population after age 45. Presbyopia refers to the loss of ability to focus on distant and near objects, and its most common manifestation is when older adults lose their ability to read small print. Reading glasses with bifocals may correct the condition.

More serious conditions, such as cataracts and age-related macular degeneration (AMD), become more common as patients reach age 65 and older. Cataracts occur when the crystalline lens of the eye becomes cloudy or opaque. Early stages do not present obvious symptoms to the patient, but they can quickly increase in density, resulting in a rapid loss of vision. By age 80, nearly 50 percent of adults will have cataracts. Cataract surgery replaces the crystalline lens of the eye (called an intraocular lens implant), often with corrective refraction to restore vision to the level experienced in youth. More than 3 million cataract surgeries are performed each year, making it one of the most common surgical procedures in the United States.

By contrast, AMD is less common and more difficult to treat. AMD destroys the part of the eye that provides sharp central vision, often resulting in a large central blind spot in the field of vision. About 2.5 percent of white adults aged 50 and older suffer from the condition, though the rates jumps to 14 percent among white adults aged 80 and older. For some reason, race plays a factor. Rates of AMD for black, Hispanic, and other nonwhite races remain steady at just under 2 percent for all ages 70 and above. There are no effective treatments for AMD, but there are some medicines that help to slow the rate of vision loss. There are also some miniature prostheses (such as the implantable miniature telescope) that may help to magnify images to improve relative vision.

Glaucoma is another ocular disease that becomes more common after age 40. It is a condition that damages the optic nerve and is the leading cause of blindness in the United States, affecting 3 million people, 90 percent of whom are over the age of 40. There is no cure for glaucoma, but there are some therapeutic and surgical treatments that can reduce the rate of nerve damage. Race also plays a role in glaucoma rates, with African Americans developing blindness six to eight times more often than white and Hispanic races. Glaucoma often shows no early symptoms and causes no pain. Early detection is only possible by having annual eye examinations.

Ears

Unlike eyesight, hearing loss is not guaranteed, but it usually begins to affect people after age 40. Just over 10 percent of the population aged 44 to 54 suffers from presbycusis, which is age-related hearing loss. Rates increase with age, affecting a quarter of the population between ages 55 and 65, with more than half affected by age 75. Presbycusis is a complex condition that involves a gradual reduction of the ear's ability to hear certain high frequencies over a long period of time, often many years. Gender plays a role, with more men suffering from hearing loss than women.

Though hearing loss is directly linked to aging, other environmental factors can also play a significant role, including exposure to loud noises, smoking, and other diseases. Family history may also be a factor. Presbycusis is not curable, but treatment usually involves amplification devices such as hearing aids. Some patients may also benefit from cochlear implants, but not all. Research for various chemical therapies is ongoing but as of yet unsuccessful.

Digestion and Urogenital

As we age, our bodies begin to lose the ability to process foods and control waste flow with the same efficiency as our youth. In the stomach, the opening of the lower esophagus loses its ability to close tightly, which allows the acids of the stomach to leak back into the esophagus, resulting in gastroesophageal reflux disease (GERD), more commonly known as *heartburn*. A wide variety of over-the-counter antacids exist to treat GERD, but stronger prescription-strength medications called *H-2-receptor blockers* may be prescribed. GERD can affect people of all ages, from infants to adults, but it can become a chronic condition after age 40, with instances occurring once or twice a day. Half of those diagnosed with GERD serious enough to warrant prescription-strength medications are between the ages of 45 and 64.

On the other end of the alimentary canal, older adults often experience loss of bladder control, or *urinary incontinence*. Nearly 10 percent of adults aged 65 and older suffer from this problem. Women tend to be more likely to have bladder control problems than men, but men are more likely to have more difficulty with urinary constriction. As men age, their prostate tends to grow larger, often constricting the urethra and resulting in decreased or halted urine flow.

These conditions are not life-threatening, and there are many treatment options that include a variety of medications to treat overactive bladder (frequent need to urinate), urge incontinence (sudden urge to urinate), and stress incontinence (leaking urine when laughing, coughing, or sneezing). Other behavioral remedies include avoiding certain foods, limiting the amount you drink, and certain pelvic (Kegel) exercises. Surgical and nonsurgical devices can be used for both men and women to help support the bladder and the urethra. Most commonly, these conditions affect the quality of life by making social situations more awkward.

Teeth, Hair, and Skin

Dental care is a lifelong concern, and it affects young children as often as it affects adults. The difference is that, over time, the repeated instances of cavities, gum disease, and other tooth decay may have a cumulative effect of total tooth loss. Approximately a quarter of adults aged 60 and older have no natural teeth at all. The rates of gum disease and tooth decay among older adults are higher than with children, and the severity of the gum disease is also higher. Modern treatments include use of dentures and artificial implants.

One of the most obvious signs of aging is the loss of hair color. Hair follicles produce a pigment called *melanin*, and as adults age, that pigment begins to decline. Gray hair often appears at age 30, and for most adults, their hair eventually turns completely white. The rate of hair color change often depends on family history. At the same time, the thickness and quantity of hair may also decrease over time. Men are more likely to show significant hair loss than women, but some loss of density is common to both sexes. Treatment options are mostly cosmetic and include hair coloring and surgical transplants.

The skin also shows signs of aging through wrinkles and sagging. Over time, as a result of exposure to the sun and increased dryness, skin becomes thinner and loses its fat. Older adults often suffer from dry skin and an inability to quickly heal from common scrapes and scratches. Rashes and cracked and scaly skin also

The Gender Gap in Okinawan Longevity

Okinawa is a collection of 44 islands located about 800 miles south of the Japanese mainland. They are culturally and ethnically different from Japanese traditions and have been influenced by China, the United States, and other civilizations in Southeast Asia and the Pacific Rim. There are a little more than a million people among the islands, and they tend to be among the least economically developed regions in Japan. Yet, in the 1960s, they were also found to have the longest life expectancies in the world, with a significant proportion of centenarians, though those numbers mainly apply to Okinawan women, rather than men. Typical life expectancy among women is more than 86 years and nearly 78 years for men.

Though the diet and lifestyle of Okinawa is noticeably different from that of mainland Japan, the life expectancies are relatively similar. In fact, Japanese men tend to live a year longer than Okinawan men, though Japanese women expect a year less. Nor are Okinawan men unique in the world. Italian men tend to live almost six months longer than Okinawan men, though Italian women expect to live two and a half years less than Okinawan women. In both countries, though, the women will outlive their men by five and nine years, respectively. It is the exceptionally long life expectancy of Okinawan women that so greatly influences their longevity statistics. This is also true elsewhere in the world. On average, men in Sweden and Switzerland tend to live as long as the Japanese and at least a year longer than Okinawans. Again, women in those two countries generally outlive their men by anywhere between four and six years, though not as long as Okinawan woman.

In terms of the relative proportion of centenarians, Greek men aged 100 and above are more common than Okinawan men, with French men only slightly as common. But the prevalence of centenarians among Okinawan women is twice as abundant as in France and three times as abundant as in Greece. There are more than seven women aged 100 years or over for every one Okinawan man. Among the top dozen countries with the highest life expectancies in the world, five times as many women tend to reach 100 years than men. Only in Greece is the ratio close to 2 to 1. Okinawa earned its reputation for exceptionally long lives primarily because of the longevity of their women.

become more common. The cosmetics industry offers a plethora of treatment options, including moisturizers, concealers, and cosmetic surgery (see chapter 8). Ultimately, though, there is no cure for aging skin.

Few of these conditions of old age are life-threatening, and most are not curable. They are chronic conditions that affect daily life and manifest as symptoms of age. At the same time, however, medical researchers strive to find biochemical or technological solutions for some of the most cumbersome ailments that affect the aging body. As of yet, the solutions are mostly temporary and cannot halt or reverse the ultimate causes of these age-related conditions. There is no successful treatment for aging.

AGE-RELATED DISEASES

The natural conditions of growing older are unavoidable and, so far, incurable. They affect the quality of life but do not necessarily change the natural duration of life. Older adults may suffer from several chronic conditions and yet still be regarded as normally "healthy" individuals. Age-related diseases belong to a different class because most of these pathologies can lead to death if left untreated. They not only affect the quality of life in so far as they diminish mobility and biological functions and capacity, but they also require significant therapeutic interventions. Some patients may find cures for these diseases within their lifetime and eventually die from some other ailment. Others may find successful treatment strategies that allow them to live relatively normal lives despite these conditions. For many others, these conditions often result in the patient's death.

In this section, the age-related diseases are categorized according to general type and are ordered to reflect their ranking as a leading cause of death in the United States. These lists are not comprehensive, but they are intended to show the range of pathologies that affect the aging body. Though older adults tend to be most at risk for developing these diseases, they may afflict anyone at any age.

Cardiovascular Disease

The heart is perhaps the most essential organ in the body because it is responsible for dispersing the flow of oxygenated blood to all the various organs and tissues. Without oxygen, the cells are unable to burn the sugars and fatty acids necessary to produce energy, and they die. Different tissues are able to sustain themselves for varying lengths of time without constant blood flow: bone and skin tissues may survive up to 8 to 12 hours, while muscular tissues can sometimes last for 6 hours. However, death usually follows within two minutes after the heart stops because nerve cells require constant blood flow. If brain tissues die, the entire body is dead. The heart and its cardiovascular system is critical for maintaining a constant supply of oxygen throughout the body to all tissues, especially the brain.

Though the heart is the primary organ responsible for pumping the blood, the entire network of arteries and vessels work in conjunction to ensure the proper transmission of oxygen. If a blood vessel is constricted or blocked, the tissues that are fed by those vessels will likely die. Blocked blood vessels can be dangerous in any location in the body, but they are often fatal when they are located near the brain or the heart.

The single greatest risk factor for cardiovascular disease is age. As we age, the arteries and blood vessels become less elastic and more constricted, and the heart begins to lose its efficiency with irregular rhythms. Heart tissues become thicker, and heart valves may thicken or leak. The heart's tolerance for increased workloads decreases. Obesity and inactivity may compound these problems at any age, but older adults become more susceptible to cardiovascular disease even without these added risk factors.

Heart disease is the leading cause of death of adults aged 65 and older, affecting more than a third of men and more than a quarter of women. One in four deaths can be linked directly to cardiovascular disease, which is more than all the deaths caused by respiratory disease, stroke, Alzheimer's disease, diabetes, influenza, and pneumonia combined. Only cancer ranks as a close second as a cause of death, yet heart disease kills more people than all forms of cancer combined.

Coronary Artery Disease

The most common source of coronary artery disease comes from the hardening and narrowing of the arteries, known as *atherosclerosis*. It is responsible for most heart attacks, strokes, and other peripheral vascular diseases (poor circulation in the legs). The interior lining of blood vessels (endothelium) is smooth at young ages. As we grow older, and especially if we expose our arteries to excessive stress (from high blood pressure, smoking, or low-density lipoprotein (LDL) cholesterol), the endothelium cells may become damaged, resulting in a sort of reactive scar tissue known as *plaque*. Over time, the buildup of plaque in the arteries restricts blood flow. If the flow is blocked, patients may experience pain when they exert themselves, called *angina*, which is due to the pressure of increasing blood flow against the constricted arteries. When the plaque completely blocks the artery or ruptures, the blood will clot inside the artery. If this occurs in the heart, it results in a heart attack (also called a *myocardial infarction*), and the heart muscle may die. If this occurs in the brain, it is called a *stroke* (also known as a *cerebrovascular disease*), and brain tissues may die. Both conditions are more often lethal than not.

Most treatment options for coronary artery disease require significant lifestyle changes. Research conducted at Harvard Medical School in 2012 suggests that reducing caloric intake and increasing exercise might trigger a genetic defense response that encourages rejuvenation of endothelial cells and may help reduce atherosclerosis and arterial stiffness. Unfortunately, these conclusions are based on research conducted on insects and lower rodents and have not been demonstrated in human physiology. Nevertheless, the CDC strongly recommends exercise combined with a healthy diet low in saturated fats and high in fiber. Low sodium and cholesterol will also help reduce blood pressure, lessening the stress on the arteries, as will avoiding other risk factors, such as smoking, heavy drinking, use of stimulants, and obesity.

Prescription medications can help treat the risk factors associated with coronary artery disease, especially treatments that can lower blood pressure and prevent blood clots from forming. Blood pressure and heart rate are often managed using angiotensin-converting enzyme (ACE) inhibitors, angiotensin II receptor blockers (ARBs), beta blockers, calcium channel blockers, and diuretics. The levels of LDL cholesterol in the blood may be controlled with statins, niacin, fibrates, or bile acid sequestrants. Aspirin is most commonly prescribed as an antiplatelet tool for reducing the risk of blood clots. Other remedies for chest pain (angina) include nitrates, such as nitroglycerin. These treatments, though, do not resolve the primary cause of atherosclerosis.

Other surgical procedures may include tools to clear out some of the plaque buildup inside the arteries (angioplasty) or tools to reinforce the walls of the arteries to prevent rupture (stents). Surgeons may also graft blood vessels from another part of the body to create new pathways for avoiding the diseased areas, called coronary artery bypass surgery. More than 700,000 angioplasty procedures are performed each year, and more than 250,000 bypass procedures. Survival rates are very high, with nearly 90 percent of patients surviving more than five years after surgery.

Heart Disease

In addition to diseases that affect the various pathways and highways of the blood, the heart itself can become more susceptible to disease over time. Any disease that affects the heart muscle is referred to collectively as *cardiomyopathy*. Some of these pathologies result in a thickening of one or more heart walls (hypertrophic cardiomyopathy) and the enlargement of the heart (cardiomegaly). These conditions are often caused by the cumulative stress of high blood pressure. The most serious consequence of heart disease is congestive heart failure, which refers to the inability of the heart to pump blood through the organ. If the blood is unable to move, the flow of oxygen is halted, and the heart may simply stop, resulting in sudden cardiac death.

Other forms of heart disease affect the electrical impulses that control the pacing and rhythm of the heartbeat. Irregular heartbeats (arrhythmia) can create asynchronized contractions between the upper and lower chambers of the heart. If these irregularities persist, either the upper or the lower chambers may "quiver" (fibrillation). If this occurs in the upper chamber (atrial), the patient may suffer from the feeling of heart palpitations, dizziness, and shortness of breath. The disruptions may come and go with no problems, or it may cause a pool of blood to collect in the chamber, increasing the risk of clotting and stroke. If the fibrillation occurs in the lower (ventricular) chamber, the flow of blood may become disrupted and lead to immediate congestive heart failure. The patient usually succumbs or faints. Unless CPR and an automated external defibrillator (AED) are used immediately to resuscitate the heart, the patient will suffer sudden cardiac death.

If the arrhythmia is detected early enough, patients may be equipped with a pacemaker, which is a small prosthetic device that sends out electrical signals to keep the heart beating regularly. More than 600,000 pacemakers are implanted each year, and they often take less than an hour to insert. Pacemakers rarely interfere with a patient's lifestyle. For more extreme cases, surgeons may use other surgical solutions that involve lasers or applying surgical cuts directly to the tissues that are sending out the irregular electrical signals.

Recent research out of Harvard Medical School suggests that some causes of heart disease may be due to the cardiac cells' inability to properly replace themselves. Over time, the genetic material in the heart cells may become damaged through oxidation, free radicals, and other biochemical disruptions that occur at molecular levels. These cells simply stop functioning in the way they used to, and healthy cells are unable to replace the damaged cells quickly enough to ensure continued heart health. The same research study indicated that reduced caloric intake and increased exercise triggers genetic responses that encourage more rapid cellular repair mechanisms. As these processes occur at such microscopic levels, and in vitro, scientists have yet to establish exactly how they operate or how they might be replicated through a synthetic pharmacological solution. In other words, they are looking for a prescription medicine to trick the body into triggering these repair mechanisms but have so far not succeeded in finding one.

Cancer

Nearly 600,000 people a year die from cancer, and cancer is second only to cardio-vascular disease as a leading cause of death. The scientific community has made great strides in understanding the nature and process of cancer since the 1990s, particularly after the advent of tools to better understand DNA transcription and translation. Cancer is now recognized as a genetic disease that affects the way cells develop and replicate. We categorize any disease that divides without stopping and spreads to neighboring tissues as a cancer, and we usually name the cancer according to the region where it began (lung, brain, breast, colon, etc.). There are more than 100 different cancer types, but what most distinguishes cancer from other diseases is the process by which it spreads.

Cancer cells are not necessarily toxic in themselves. Most often, they remain undefined, and when they replicate, they do not become specialized for specific functions as a normal cell would. Each cell contains all the genetic material (DNA) for every organ and process in the body, but only a small portion of the DNA nucleotide sequences are expressed in any given cell. Liver cells specialize in functions necessary for the liver, while cells in skin, muscle tissue, and other organs each specialize for the function of their region in the body. Cancer cells do not specialize; they simply replicate. They become deadly when they take over the resources of particular organs and when they cause other neighboring cells to halt their own specialized functions. Cancer in the liver may slowly grow into a tumorous mass that takes over the normal healthy liver cells and eventually causes the liver to cease functioning entirely. Cancer cells can be deadly precisely because they have no natural replication limit, and they do not easily die on their own.

The single greatest risk factor for developing cancer is age. Cancer affects younger people, but the likelihood of developing malignant tumors increases significantly as you get older. For example, the average age of patients suffering from lung cancer is about 70, with less than 3 percent of the 228,190 lung cancer patients in 2013 under the age of 40. Scientists have identified a number of potential carcinogens that increase the likelihood of developing cancer, including tobacco use, radon, radiation, and other pollutants. The fact remains, though, that medical researchers have been unable to find direct causal connections between specific risk factors and the development of cancer.

Many risk factors are identified primarily because they are generally toxic to the body and not because they are specifically identified with a particular disease. Tobacco use greatly magnifies the chance of developing lung cancer, but it also significantly increases the risks of developing heart disease and blood diseases, interferes with fertility, and generally increases the risk of disease in almost every other organ of the body. The carbon monoxide and other chemicals from tobacco smoke interfere with the transmission of oxygenated blood through the circulatory system, and they weaken the immune system in almost every organ. Tobacco use is strongly correlated to lung cancer: when tobacco use declined in the 1980s and 1990s, lung cancer rates also declined. Nevertheless, the linkage is not absolute. A 2006 study found that 85–90 percent of smokers never contract cancer, including more than 75 percent of heavy smokers (five or more cigarettes a day). Perhaps more significantly, about 20 percent of lung cancer patients never used tobacco (16,000 to 24,000 people each year). The one common variable among all cancers is that aging cells are more likely to become cancerous than younger cells.

Tumor Suppression and Oncogenes

Cancer is a genetic disorder, and gene mutations can occur through environmental causes (called *acquired mutations*) or may be passed down through family inheritance (called *germline mutations*). Recent statistical studies of the human genome have uncovered several genetic markers that seem to link germline mutations to certain cancers types. Lung cancer is associated with the EGFR gene among young patients, and the ALK and ROS1 genes are linked to lung cancer in nonsmokers. Breast cancer (BRCA) gene 1 and 2 and the p53 gene have been linked to breast and ovarian cancers. These genes seem to be responsible for tumor suppression, and those individuals who do not have these genes become more vulnerable to developing the associated cancers. They are, however, still not guaranteed to ever develop the disease.

In addition, there are other genes called *proto-oncogenes* that are responsible for normal cellular replication. If these genes are damaged through acquired mutations, they may be responsible for transforming normal healthy cells into immortal cancerous cells. Two common oncogenes are HER2 (which promote cellular growth) and RAS genes (which help to program necessary cellular death). Most cancers are not linked to any particular genes, and many cancers develop without any of these markers being present. Cancer is a genetic disorder, but medical researchers are as of yet unable to identify precisely how any particular disorder can be prevented or reversed.

Telomeres and Telomerase

Several theories developed to explain why cancer is so strongly linked to old age. In the 19th century, physicians believed cancers grew as a result of the body depositing excess wastes (lymphs, blastema, or some other unidentified fluid), which gradually accumulated over time to develop into tumors. The discovery of microbiology and the endocrine system largely deflated these theories, and for the bulk of the 20th century, cancer remained a mystery. Genetic research in the 1970s led to the discovery of tumor suppressor genes and oncogenes, which greatly transformed the understanding of cancer development and growth.

One of the earliest of the modern theories used to explain the correlation between cancer and old age suggested that, over time, cells in older adults develop genetic damage and become more susceptible to mutations that lead to cancerous growth. This new theory resulted in greater research and attention toward discovering potential environmental carcinogens and in understanding how those cells became damaged, thereby allowing health care officials to devise preventative measures. A more recent theory from the 21st century places less attention on carcinogens and more emphasis on the prevalence of tumor-suppression genes that seem to thrive within younger cells. As they replicate over time, it seems that these suppression mechanisms begin to fade, and tumors begin to arise naturally as a result of age.

The goal of modern research is to determine how to maintain those suppression mechanisms within the cells of older adults. In 2014, researchers at the National Institute of Environmental Health Sciences pointed to DNA methylation, which is the process by which specific biochemical compounds (methyl groups) operate to activate or silence certain gene sequences. The research team led by Zongli Xu and Jack Taylor theorized that these methyl groups become less active as we age and no longer function properly to turn on the necessary tumor-suppression genes.

The discovery of the link between telomeres, telomerase, and cellular senescence caused a great deal of excitement among antiaging researchers in the 1990s (see chapter 5). Researchers found that the telomere tails connected to the ends of DNA strands—which serve as a natural "clock" that limits the number of times a cell can replicate—could be influenced by the presence or absence of the telomerase enzyme. The potential for unlocking the natural genetic timecode for cellular death seemed a potential solution for radical life extension and possibly the key for curing death itself. In the decades that followed, however, genetics research has been unable to break the link between excessive telomerase and inevitable cancerous tumor growth. By the 2010s, numerous studies had appeared that seem to conclude that telomeres are a necessary tumor-suppression mechanism. If cells do not die naturally, they will inevitably become cancerous.

Despite the potential that immortal cells may lead to cancerous growth, researchers at the University of Utah continue to place great hope in telomeres as a key to solving both cancer and premature cellular death. One of the functions of telomeres is to provide the DNA strands with "extra" nucleotide base pairs so that the transcription of the DNA can begin at the very start of the strand rather than somewhere near the end. As the telomeres become shorter, there is greater likelihood that the DNA will be copied incompletely. The research team led by Richard Cawthon discovered that people with shorter telomeres tend to die younger. They also discovered that cancer cells tend to replicate with very short telomeres—it is only the presence of the telomerase enzyme that enables the corrupted DNA strands of the cancer cells to continue to replicate. Their research is looking for a way to increase telomere length to avoid cancerous cells and then to more precisely regulate telomerase to ensure longer-living lines among healthy cells.

Since the turn of the 21st century, antiaging researchers have devoted a great deal of energy toward understanding the causes and development of cancer. An old adage among doctors in the 20th century says, "If you live long enough, and you do not die of anything else, then you will eventually die of cancer." The very strong association between aging and cancer risk prompted many researchers to believe that understanding cancer is the key to significantly extending human life. If researchers can discover a cure for cancer as a class of diseases, what would remain to cause untimely deaths?

Respiratory Diseases

Many respiratory diseases are not age-related. Asthma is the most common chronic condition, and almost a quarter of asthma sufferers are children. Asthma is also often tied to allergies, and allergic reactions comprise a significant portion of respiratory problems and are not linked to advancing age. There are also some very serious lung diseases, such as cystic fibrosis, that are usually genetically determined and also not tied to age. Nevertheless, the most commonly lethal forms of respiratory diseases are chronic lower respiratory diseases, specifically those known as chronic obstructive pulmonary disease (COPD), which directly interfere with airflow. Nearly 80 percent of respiratory deaths (130,000 per year) are a result of COPD, making it the third leading cause of death in the United States and in the world. Two of the most common forms of COPD are bronchitis and emphysema, both of which are strongly linked to age.

Breathing may be affected by general age-related conditions related to osteoporosis and sarcopenia. Bones often become thinner as a result of osteoporosis, and age-related sarcopenia may weaken the muscles that support the diaphragm. Both conditions may contribute to difficulty in breathing. Similarly, the lungs may begin to lose their shape, causing the air sacs to become baggy and more difficult to expand. These conditions may lead to diminished levels of oxygen reaching the bloodstream and insufficient removal of carbon dioxide. The lack of fuel and waste removal often undermines the immune system, making the older patient more susceptible to infections and diseases. As with many age-related conditions, the most effective treatment for these sorts of ailments is to increase physical exercise and regain muscle strength.

Advancing age may generally weaken the body's defenses against illness, but the most common forms of COPD seem to be more associated with environmental irritations than with cellular breakdown. Bronchitis refers to the inflammation of the air tubes in the lungs (bronchi) and is characterized by chronic coughing, shortness of breath, mucus, and general discomfort in the chest. Over 70 percent of patients suffering from bronchitis are aged 45 years or older. Emphysema refers to damage done to the lung's air sacs (alveoli), which makes it difficult to blow air out or suck air in. Emphysema is a progressive disease, and there is no known cure. More so than bronchitis, the risk of emphysema increases with age, as 90 percent of patients with emphysema are 45 years or older.

Some researchers suggest COPD may be linked to specific genes (alpha-1 antitrypsin, or AAT) that make certain individuals more likely to develop respiratory problems. Other evidence, however, suggests that COPD develops as a result of long-term exposure to certain toxins in the air that irritate the lungs. Over time, the cumulative effects of those irritations lead to obstructions that impair breathing. Smoking is an obvious risk factor, as it causes inflammation and destroys bronchioles within the lungs. Yet, like lung cancer, about 20 percent of patients who develop COPD have never smoked, which suggests that other equally toxic airborne irritants are responsible or that the aging lung tissues simply become more vulnerable to airborne irritants.

Pneumonia

Pneumonia is an acute lower respiratory tract infection that results in about 50,000 deaths per year. It is dangerous at any age, but it is more lethal for infants and older adults. Most youth and adults are able to recover in as little as one to three weeks. Young children under the age of 5 are vulnerable because their lungs have not yet fully developed. About 15 percent of childhood deaths are due to pneumonia, though those rates are declining in the United States. At the other end of the spectrum, adults aged 65 and older are also more likely to die from the disease. Traditionally, medical researchers tended to blame the increased vulnerability of older adults to their compromised immune systems caused by other concurrent diseases or chronic conditions. Recently, though, research in 2010 studied pneumonia patients admitted to intensive care units in Canada and found that the likelihood of dying increased proportionately to age, regardless of other conditions. For every 10-year age group (65–74, 75–84, etc.), there was a 25 percent increase in the likelihood of dying. The study suggests that older adults are simply less equipped to fight pneumonia. It may not be an age-dependent disease, but it becomes more lethal with age.

Endocrine and Nervous System Diseases

The endocrine system is that informal network of glands, organs, and chemical communication systems that tell the body which biochemicals to produce, how much, and when. Every organ produces a variety of hormones that travel through the bloodstream to enter the cells of target tissues and tell them to turn on or turn off various functions. A complex assortment of feedback loops control all of the processes of the human body: the kidneys, liver, heart, thyroid, pancreas, and other organs function because of the presence or absence of certain hormones that trigger other chemical reactions. These reactions control digestion, blood sugar levels, muscle development, sexual development and reproduction, and a million other biological operations that occur simultaneously each moment. In a perfectly healthy body, the intercommunication of all the organs together achieves a sort of balance called *homeostasis*, which ensures that every part is working as it should. In an unhealthy body, these functions break down at one or more points, and the communication is lost somewhere. Doctors often prescribe medication in an attempt to help offset the disruption. Sometimes they are successful, and other times not.

The nervous system is very similar to the endocrine system, except that instead of communicating through biochemical hormones, it sends electrical pulses through a network of neural transmitters. Instead of communicating through the natural highways of the blood and circulatory system, the neurons communicate through the highway of nerves that often follow parallel paths. The endocrine system is often regulated locally at the site of organs and tissues, while the nervous system is regulated by the central nervous system (the brain). Most of these communications operate involuntarily, which means we have no control over them. Both systems serve as the underlying infrastructure of the body. Diseases in either of these systems can affect digestion, reproduction, mobility, cognition, and even mood. The most common diseases of diabetes, Alzheimer's disease, and Parkinson's disease kill nearly 200,000 people per year, making them (collectively) the fourth leading cause of death.

Diabetes

Diabetes is the most common disease that afflicts the endocrine system. It is a disease that affects the pancreas, causing it to produce either too much or too little insulin, which is a hormone used to trigger the absorption of blood sugars (glucose) into cellular tissues to produce energy. Type 1 diabetes occurs when the pancreas makes too little insulin or no insulin at all. This is most common among children and is commonly developed by older adults. Type 2 diabetes occurs when the pancreas produces insulin, but somehow the feedback loops have been disrupted in such a way that the body does not effectively use the insulin to regulate glucose levels. People of all ages may develop type 2 diabetes, but it is traditionally associated with older adults who are less active and overweight or obese.

Recently, the predominance of electronic forms of communication and entertainment have contributed to a more sedentary culture, and the rates of childhood obesity have significantly increased the number of new cases of type 2 diabetes among youth. These statistics defy historical trends, which most often link diabetes with old age. Yet, these counterexamples help to demonstrate that the disease is not necessarily age-related. It is the loss of mobility, the increasing likelihood of obesity, and the sedentary conditions that most often trigger type 2 diabetes. Nevertheless, age does seem to magnify the risk.

More importantly, type 2 diabetes tends to have more damaging effects for older adults. If left untreated, the unregulated glucose often intensifies the effects of atherosclerosis, which magnifies the risks of heart disease, stroke, and poor circulation to the legs and extremities. As the electrical impulses used by the nervous system and the brain require considerable energy, unregulated levels of glucose may also lead to nerve damage, including damage to the optical nerve, leading to blindness. For patients with already compromised systems due to the natural conditions of older age, type 2 diabetes can be particularly dangerous.

Diabetic disruptions may also have an impact on kidney function, which is necessary for filtering and cleaning toxins from the blood. Unregulated glucose levels may damage small blood vessels. As the primary blood filter, the kidney is filled with a multitude of tiny blood vessels, so they are often affected. The most common side effects of kidney disease (known as *renal failure*) are malnutrition, weight loss, and sarcopenia, which older adults are already partially susceptible to. These symptoms may trigger a cascading effect that leads to multiple physical and cognitive disabilities.

Diabetes may also harm the gall bladder, which is used to collect and store the bile necessary to break down fat in the bloodstream. Excessive glucose may overwhelm the gall bladder, resulting in gall stones or infections requiring the removal of the gall bladder altogether. These are not lethal consequences, but the undigested fat may intensify problems related to atherosclerosis.

Treatment options for diabetes include a variety of prescription medicines to help artificially regulate glucose. Most of these must be used in conjunction with frequent monitoring of glucose levels. Modern technology has rendered both tasks relatively painless, yet these treatments mostly address the symptoms of diabetes and not the underlying causes. The most commonly prescribed treatment options require lifestyle changes of proper diet to control weight and frequent exercise.

Dementia

Alzheimer's disease (AD) leads to nearly 84,000 deaths a year and affects almost 10 percent of the population aged 65 and older. Diagnosis is difficult because early symptoms share many of the same characteristics of mild cognitive impairment (MCI). Moreover, because it carries such fears, people are often prone to jump to the amateur diagnosis whenever they become forgetful or temporarily confused. Nevertheless, it is a very real and progressive disease and can eventually lead to a breakdown of immune functions, resulting in an inability to fight other ailments. The most common ultimate cause of death among AD patients is pneumonia.

The second most common neurological disorder is Parkinson's disease, with 60,000 new cases a year. This disease interrupts the nervous system's ability to appropriately control muscles. Researchers believe the disease affects the basal ganglia that are responsible for the production of the neurotransmitter dopamine, which signals the part of the brain in charge of movement. Early symptoms include tremors, rigid muscle reactions, and an inability to perform precise fine motor activities. The disease is progressive but slow and often takes many years to completely incapacitate an individual's mobility. Like AD, patients suffering from Parkinson's typically die from the breakdown of related biological functions. The most common ultimate cause of death is pneumonia.

There are no cures for either Alzheimer's disease or Parkinson's disease, though there are several prescription medications available to treat secondary symptoms or to slow their development. Both diseases are strongly linked to age, with very rare incidents of Parkinson's disease before the age of 50 and an average diagnosis at age 62. Despite considerable medical research devoted to discovering the cause and development of these diseases, there is no cure, and scientists remain unable to reliably identify risk factors. As far as science is able to determine, these diseases develop because we grow older—there are no other obvious causes. For this reason, these and other neurological diseases pose perhaps the greatest frustration for antiaging researchers. The general public has few assurances that they will not be listed among the victims of these and other similar diseases. The threat of the myth of Tithonus always looms ahead as we find cures for some of the most pressing diseases, and yet we still have no answers for those that might have the most immediate impact on our personal identity.

CONCLUSION

Another category of problems associated with old age is the general breakdown in immunity, which renders older adults more susceptible to death by pneumonia or influenza. The immune system is slower to respond and often mistakenly attacks tissues that are healthy or fails to attack tissues (like cancer) that are sick. The body does not heal as quickly from cuts, scratches, bumps, and bruises. More importantly, the body does not always know when it is sick, and so it is incapable of sending the appropriate corrective measures to heal itself.

The breakdown of general immunity is perhaps one of the most significant obstacles to extended life span. Even if medical scientists were able to discover the cures for heart disease, cancer, and respiratory illnesses, the basic infrastructure of the body may still be frail and fragile. It may remain predisposed to each successive wave of maladies that rise to attack it. In this way, the constant battle to defeat every source of mortal disease may be unending.

Part of the hesitancy in predicting whether general immunity disorders can be cured in the same way as other age-related diseases involves the difficulty of distinguishing between "condition" and "disease." The antiaging advocates argue firmly that all of these age-related problems stem, at one point or another, from a biological disease. It may originate at the molecular level and reside within a genetic corruption, or it may be more systemic as a problem with the larger feedback response mechanisms. Wherever it may reside, antiaging advocates argue that it is biological in nature and therefore can be cured just as any biochemical interaction can be adjusted and fixed.

The more traditional gerontologists disagree. The basic premise of the entropy theory of aging is that biochemical reactions are bound to move from order to disorder. As an organism develops, it becomes less ordered and less efficient, and in time, it simply ceases to be able to repair itself. This debate is not ended. At present, neither side is obviously more right than the other.

Both sides are willing to pursue any effort to find cures and solve the problems associated with the conditions of older age. And no matter which side of the issue they find themselves, there is also a great deal of excitement about the potential for new discoveries that may lead to remarkable results. Around the turn of the 20th century, the discovery of germ theory led to dozens of new treatments for childhood diseases. Infant mortality declined significantly, and as a result, the average life expectancy nearly doubled from 38 years to 70 years in about a century. Biomedical scientists of the 21st century are hoping to cross a similar frontier, perhaps finding cures for diseases that have afflicted older adults for millennia. From this perspective, it is not unrealistic to hope for another jump in the average life expectancy from 75 years to 150 years. Most of the optimistic news stories that cover the antiaging research use figures such as 150 years as a benchmark for the new normal.

There remain some significant critics to this optimism. The biodemographer S. Jay Olshansky calculated that even if science successfully eradicates all forms of cancer, the resulting impact on the average life expectancy would not exceed three years. Olshansky has repeated this claim for more than a decade, but he also admits that certain types of breakthroughs may challenge his statistical presumptions. Most antiaging advocates hope that the elimination of age-related diseases will contribute to an improvement of general health—perhaps solving the general immunity problem that seems to affect older adults after the age of 75. If scientists can cure the "diseases" of old age and also address the "conditions" of old age, then genuine changes in life expectancy might be possible. For the more traditional gerontologists, that solution is not only preferable, but absolutely essential. Failure to treat the conditions of old age would render the fears of the myth of Tithonus all too real. As the political economist Yoshihiro Francis Fukuyama warned, if medical science does not cure aging, we may face a "national nursing home scenario, in which people routinely live to be 150 but spend the last 50 years in a state of childlike dependency on caretakers."

The debate remains strongly divided and fundamentally boils down to whether you believe the human life span is fixed or changeable. As long as Jeanne Calment maintains the record of longest recorded life span (122 years), it also remains largely an academic debate. There are no examples of anyone breaking the long-held limit of 120 years (more or less), and so there is no way to prove with certainty whether that limitation is fixed by biology or by current circumstances. The debate is also closely tied to faith and philosophy. Why 120 years? Is this a limit imposed by God, or is it an arbitrary limit imposed by the necessities of evolution? Again, as long as no evidence exists to refute or prove the existing limitation, these questions will be argued based on hypothetical evidence only.

Chapter 11

What Can We Do Now to Extend Our Lives without a Prescription?

Searching for the fountain of youth is, at heart, a reflection of mankind's desire to overcome sickness and disease and somehow evade the power of death. Since ancient times, such promises of eternal youth have always been just beyond our reach. Not since the first millennium of Taoist China have we seen people in popular culture so willing to believe that the elusive fountain of youth was potentially and practically possible. Yet, today, the modern antiaging movement of the 21st century is convinced that a revolution in biomedicine is at hand, and popular culture seems to embrace that optimism.

In 2003, the Methuselah Foundation was cofounded by Aubrey de Grey, who explained, "Scientists are on the threshold of the development of genuine anti-aging drugs—pharmaceutical and genetic therapies that, jointly, can rationally be expected to postpone and even reverse age-related degeneration in humans, thereby markedly extending healthy lifespan." Since then, he has repeatedly speculated that the first human to live to 1,000 years is alive today. This view was echoed two years later by Ronald Klatz (cofounder of American Academy of Anti-aging Medicine (A4M)), who wrote, "We have now reached the cusp of immortality." Michael Rose, Ray Kurzweil, and a host of other scientists, medical researchers, and philosophers have now made similar predictions of practical immortality by the year 2045—not by discovering a magical fountain of youth but through discoveries from the modern wonders of science alone.

Despite this optimism, these same individuals all admit that, as of this writing, there are no successful or proven antiaging treatments. There are myriad new technologies, exciting therapies, and potential lifestyle changes that promise to improve the rate of aging and potentially reverse some age-related conditions. Yet, to date, none of these have scientifically been shown to be successful. At best, the most popular theoretical and biological options are supported only by in vitro research or correlational studies of large populations. No direct causal scientific connections have been made between particular treatments and the rate of aging in living human subjects. Nevertheless, the field of antiaging medicine researchers and the business of antiaging remedies are both increasing every year.

Antiaging researchers hope that one day soon science will make a breakthrough and one or more of these antiaging remedies will prove successful. The potential market for that treatment would be astonishing—truly revolutionizing the world. It is that hope that propels both the research and the industry. This chapter and the next will discuss some of the more popular antiaging recommendations that are available now as well as some that will potentially be available in the future (at least in theory).

The sheer number of potential antiaging remedies makes it difficult to categorize them all. For purposes of convenience, this book arranges them into three groups according to the level of involvement required by the medical community: (1) those treatments that do not require a doctor's oversight; (2) those treatments that do; and (3) those treatments that require some future technological innovation, which may not yet be possible (or legal).

The first category includes all those options that do not require a prescription. They are generally labeled as *defensive biochemistry* because they require a minimal amount of risk and yet still reflect the deliberate intention to extend a healthy life span. Some of these options are as simple as making lifestyle changes and following particular dietary models. This section discusses what science knows about promising "superfoods" as well as a broad collection of over-the-counter vitamins and nutritional supplements. This chapter also includes some discussion of the debate between traditional and nontraditional sources of medicine as they relate to the antiaging movement.

The second category includes all those recommendations that do require a doctor's oversight. There are labeled collectively as *proactive biochemistry* because the patient must follow treatments that require a prescription and a physician's oversight. These options involve greater risk of side effects. Some of these include hormone therapies and other forms of genetic manipulation, which are not yet proven to be either practical or effective. The theoretical research often sounds promising, but many of these treatment options are speculative at best—and some may currently be illegal. Nevertheless, they dominate the cutting-edge discussions in the antiaging movement.

In the final category, we consider some hopeful remedies of the future that only optimistic technological innovations could ever make possible. Transhumanism, virtual immortality, and the promise of a seamless technological and biological nexus are a dream for some antiaging advocates and a nightmare for their cultural critics. As they are not currently possible, we can only speculate on their positive and negative potential. These latter discussions will consume the next chapter.

DEFENSIVE BIOCHEMISTRY

No prescription is necessary to begin an antiaging treatment plan. Some of the simplest steps involve making healthy lifestyles choices and following recommended dietary plans. Antiaging consumers may choose to go further and purchase over-the-counter herbal remedies and nutritional supplements, or they may pursue other nonprescription treatments. Almost all reputable authorities recommend seeking the advice of a certified physician before undertaking any of these antiaging regimens, but the truth is that most of these do not require any doctor oversight at all.

Sources of Antiaging Remedies

There are thousands of antiaging Web sites that recommend tips to make you look younger and possibly live longer. The sheer number of information outlets can be both a blessing and a curse. Consumers can be overwhelmed by what seems to be an endless supply of products and treatment options. Unfortunately, the Web sites that are most accessible to the lay public are often the ones with the least verifiable information. Similarly, the sites that are most credible in scientific circles, such as peer-reviewed journals, are often very difficult for the lay reader to understand. For example, João Pedro Magalhães coauthored a 2016 article titled "Reductions in Hypothalamic *Gfap* Expression, Glial Cells and α-tanycytes in Lean and Hypermetabolic *Gnasxl*-deficient Mice," which was published in *Molecular Brain*. It is an interesting article that identifies certain genetic traits in long-lived mice, which may be relevant to understanding long life in humans, but it is not an easy read for the general public. By contrast, the *Huffington Post* featured an article titled "7 Anti-aging Treatments That Won't Break the Bank," by Cindy Augustine. It was much easier to read, but it included considerably less verifiable research.

In some cases, the Web site may sound too perfect. A search for "miracle supplements" may lead to the Master Miracle Supplement (MMS) Web site, which promises to cure any number of viruses, bacteria and other germs by utilizing "Ancient Wisdom combined with 21st Century Technology." The Web site claims that MMS cures cancer, AIDS, malaria, hepatitis, Lyme disease, asthma, and the common cold. Unfortunately, the Web sites that advertise "antiaging miracles" and sound like they have been endorsed by official doctors often have the least credibility. In this example, the Department of Justice convicted the manufacturers of MMS in 2015 for selling a toxic chemical to the public. The supplement included industrial bleach (sodium chloride) and water. Unfortunately, unless the supplements are actually toxic and pose an immediate danger to the public, there is very little oversight to ensure that Web-based claims are verifiable. There are no Internet police to monitor truth in advertising on the Web, so the consumer should be warned to be skeptical. If the treatments are being sold by a commercial site as an herbal (nonprescription) remedy, there is also no FDA oversight. As the adage reminds us, if a product or promise seems too good to be true, then it probably is.

LIFESTYLE CHANGES

The most accessible recommendations for antiaging are perhaps also some of the more difficult ones to follow. It is easy to take a pill or visit a doctor and take an injection. But lifestyle changes require self-discipline, and that is sometimes the most difficult task of all. In terms of general health, the these are the three most common recommendations: (1) if you smoke, quit; (2) if you have a drug or alcohol dependency, end it; and (3) if you are overweight, lose it. These are so easy to recommend, but they are often very difficult to carry out.

The most effective antiaging treatment to date is simply to live healthy. And the most proven effective method for healthy living is an active lifestyle that includes proper diet and exercise. Within the antiaging community, the most common and popular recommendations involve lifestyles changes that are very similar to what any doctor would recommend for maintaining health. Get your exercise, relax, get enough sleep, and eat a balanced, nutritious diet.

Exercise

As discussed in chapter 10, the most common prescription for almost every age-related condition and disease is exercise. Not only does it help to maintain a healthy weight, but exercise also triggers metabolic changes that build muscle and help the body repair itself—both of which are uniquely tied to youthful biology. More than a dozen studies from 2006 to 2012, studying thousands of older adults aged 60 and above, found that regular exercise reduced the effects of age-related inflammation. Ironically, acute exercise—which means exercising only once in a long while—can increase inflammation and cause some muscle tissue damage. That just means that exercise needs to be routine, and not just once in a while. It is common and expected to feel sore and out of shape at the start of a new exercise program, especially if we rarely exercise. Once started, however, regular exercise (five hours of moderate exercise a week) can reduce inflammation and increase antioxidant biomarkers. Chronic inflammation is a symptom of decreased immunity and has been linked to cardiovascular disease, kidney disease, osteoarthritis, diabetes, obesity, and Alzheimer's disease. Frequent, regular exercise can be one of the easiest antiaging treatments available.

The exercise does not have to be overly intense. In fact, a 2016 study found that high levels of intense exercise can actually hurt cardiovascular health. Athletes who engage in long-term endurance training can sustain structural changes to the heart muscle, making them more prone to abnormal heart rhythms. Marathon runners, in particular, are more prone to muscle and tendon damage and other immunity issues due to the continually harsh stress on the muscles and joints. For antiaging purposes, intense exercise routines are unnecessary. The goal is to engage in regular exercise of moderate intensity that increases the heart rate and blood flow and leads to a more active lifestyle overall. Simply getting up, moving, and being active on a daily basis is enough to trigger a positive metabolic response.

Happiness and Stress Relief

In addition, there are other antiaging recommendations that require a new way of approaching life. Avoiding stress and a habitually stressful lifestyle and maintaining a positive outlook on life all promise to reduce or limit many of the more common age-related conditions. Numerous correlation studies in the

21st century have shown that the deliberate pursuit of a "happy disposition" can add up 8 to 10 years to your life.

To this end, doctors again recommend regular exercise as a significant contributor to psychological health and well-being. A Finnish study in 2000 examined more than 3,400 adults between the ages of 26 and 64 and asked them to perform 20–30 minutes of exercise on a daily, weekly, or monthly schedule. Researchers found that those who engaged in routine exercise had lower incidents of depression, especially among the older adults. In addition, participants who exercised also showed benefits in other areas, scoring lower on anger scales, stress scales, and other scales that measured their sense of personal control in their lives. In all these measures, the older adults experienced greater results than the younger ones.

A similar study conducted in 2000 examined only older and sedentary adults with an average age of 65 years. Half the adults were assigned to an aerobics program, and half were assigned to a stretching program. Researchers found that in both groups, those who broke free from their sedentary habits experienced greater increases in "satisfaction with life" and general decreases in the feeling of loneliness. Quite a large number of later studies affirmed the findings that even mild exercise of 20–30 minutes at a time, three days a week, will have a significant impact on quality of life.

Most studies on "happiness" require participants to self-report their findings, but there are some clinical studies that take a more quantitative approach. One study conducted by Elizabeth Blackburn (who won a Nobel Prize for her work with telomeres) and Dean Ornish at the Preventative Medical Research Institute at the University of California, San Francisco, in 2013, examined the telomere length in the blood cells of men who had engaged in lifestyle changes that emphasized stress relief through regular exercise, low-fat high-carbohydrate vegetarian diets, and regular meditation routines with related support groups. What made this study unique was the addition of meditation and stress reduction as a factor in cellular health. It seemed that lifestyle changes alone may increase telomere length, which is responsible for the rate of cellular death. Many other antiaging remedies rely on potential genetic treatments to artificially modify telomere length, but this study suggested lifestyle changes may produce similarly positive results without any medical intervention. Critics note, however, that the study was conducted on a small cohort of only 10 men, and its results have not yet been duplicated. Others also noted that the telomere lengths of peripheral blood vessels have little impact on generalizations about the telomere length of cells in more critical regions, such as the heart or nervous system.

Stress relief can be found in many ways, including prayer, singing, massage therapy, or any activity that provides a temporary escape from daily demands. It also involves time management, social engagement, healthy communication and expression, and avoidance of the sources that cause anxiety. Stress relief is not the same as being stress-free. As discussed in chapter 9, humans need to have some daily demands to provide a focus for their lives. The lack of daily physical activities or other tasks that require frequent problem-solving skills may be a source of psychological stress in itself. In this context, *stress relief* refers to a temporary retreat from daily demands. It means simply relaxing at least three or four times a week by taking time out to find peace and tranquility in an otherwise busy schedule. The Ornish study suggests these sorts of stress relief can change our cellular biology, which may lead to longer lives.

Sleep

When asked about their secrets to longevity, one of the most frequent comments made by centenarians is that they "get enough sleep." The antiaging movement strongly stresses the importance of sleep, and medical science seems to affirm this recommendation. Research indicates that older adults need less sleep on average (7 to 8 hours) than younger adults, but only by an hour. It is not the quantity of sleep, though, but the quality of sleep that matters most.

There are five stages in the sleep cycle: drowsiness, light sleep, two stages of deep sleep, and REM (rapid eye movement) sleep. The first stage may last for only 15 minutes, and the remaining stages will repeat themselves in cycles of 80–100 minutes all night long. Light sleep involves relaxed muscles, while heavy sleep sets the body in a state of near-paralysis with deep breathing. At its deepest point, the REM cycle involves accelerated breathing, twitching muscles, and dreams. It is the REM stage that researchers believe is essential for proper psychological health because it provides an opportunity for the brain to unravel the problems of day.

There are numerous theories as to why we need sleep. One of the more popular theories is that healthy sleep gives the body necessary time to repair itself and function properly. Science has yet to fully understand exactly what sleep does, but it is clear that sleep is essential to health. Numerous studies dating back to World War II have shown what happens when the body is deprived of sleep. Frequent and extended sleep interruptions increase daily stress, memory loss, and otherwise impair concentration and other cognitive functions, including mood and judgment. Sleep deprivation is also linked to obesity, diabetes, sexual dysfunction, cardiovascular disease, and early death. In clinical studies, animals that have been deprived of all sleep will lose immune function and die within weeks. Human studies have shown that extended wakefulness for three days or more leads to hallucinations and a gradual breakdown of the immune and nervous systems. One theory that researchers use to explain the need for sleep is that sleep "cleans out" our neural system. The neurons in the nervous system produce the hormone adenosine, which builds up over time. As we sleep, the body clears away adenosine to restore and rejuvenate proper neuron functioning.

In terms of antiaging, sleep is viewed as a necessary process to ensure daily rejuvenation of the entire body. Routine and uninterrupted sleep, with frequent REM cycles, not only ensures proper physiological health but also promotes psychological health and well-being. If these two conditions are met, the body has a better than equal chance of repairing itself to fight other age-related conditions. One of the most apparent benefits of sleep is cosmetic: the skin heals more quickly and is less prone to fine lines and wrinkles. Other less visible benefits include improved immune functions that contribute to overall healing. Finally, an alert mind also protects people from making poor choices that could have debilitating effects later—not only in terms of physical accidents but also in terms of other lifestyle choices.

One of the problems facing older adults is that many of their age-related conditions and drug treatments for age-related diseases can disrupt normal sleep cycles. Medications that help people fall asleep or are used to treat insomnia often induce an incomplete sleep cycle. Patients taking sleeping pills may reach stage 2 or 3 in the sleep cycle, but they often avoid REM sleep. This can increase the risk of mood disorders and depression. As is the case for stress relief and happiness, the most common nonprescription recommendations for sleep are to avoid caffeine and to exercise frequently.

SUPERFOODS

Proper "diet and exercise" are two of the most commonly repeated words in any health plan. The problem is that a "proper" diet is not always easy to identify. Which foods are healthy, and which foods should be avoided? The popularity of particular foods often rise and fall according to cultural fashion and are tied to anecdotal observations and wishful thinking. Yet, some of these ingredients do have clinical evidence to support their fame. The antiaging movement has identified *superfoods* as those that are highly nutritious and are linked to long life. This section focuses on those foods and their popularly described benefits as well as any scientific evidence to support those claims.

Red Wine (Resveratrol)

The health effects of red wine first came to the attention of the public when observers noticed that people living in France tended to have low incidents of heart disease, despite engaging in high-risk cardiovascular health activities, such as heavy cigarette smoking and eating high-fat diets. The oldest recorded human life span is a French woman, Jeanne Louise Calment, who smoked until she was 117 years old and ate a typical French diet that included heavy sauces, olive oil, red wine, and chocolate. She lived to be 122 years old. This seeming contradiction of high fat and strong heart health has been called the "French paradox," and researchers have been studying what other correlations might explain the seeming contradiction. Besides heavy sauces, the French are also known for their red wine, and that triggered a wave of research studies into its active ingredient.

Red wine contains resveratrol, which is a phytoalexin, an organic substance produced by a plant as a natural defense mechanism against invading parasites. It is found in a number of berries and other plants, but it is most common among grapes and is found in greater concentrations in red wines than in white wines. Resveratrol is an antioxidant, meaning it reduces the number of free radicals caused by oxidative stress, which reduces inflammation within the cells.

A Life in History

Jeanne Calment was born in Arles, France, on February 21, 1875—the same year that Leo Tolstoy published *Anna Karenina* and a year before Alexander Graham Bell filed for a patent on his new telephone. She married at the age of 21 to a man 7 years her senior. They lived happily together for 46 years, until he died at the age of 74. Jeanne was in her forties when World War I broke out and in her sixties when World War II erupted. She lived through the depression of the 1930s, and the post–World War reconstruction and boom of the 1950s and 1960s. In 1965, when Jeanne was 90 years old, she made a deal with her lawyer that he would pay her 2,500 francs a month (approximately $500) for the rest of her life in exchange for the right to own her apartment after she died. He died 30 years later, in 1995, at the age of 77, while Jeanne Calment (at the age of 120) continued to live on. He paid twice the value of the flat and never took possession. Jeanne's famous quote was, "In life, one sometimes makes bad deals." She finally died in 1997 at the age of 122 and 164 days. Her parents both lived long lives: her dad died at the age of 94 and her mom at the age of 86. Yet, her genes were not necessarily destined for long living; her daughter died at the age of 36.

Why did Jeanne Calment have such a long life? That is the question that gerontologists have been asking ever since. She did not follow healthy lifestyle choices: she smoked, ate sugars, and was no more (nor less) active than anyone else of her generation. Jeanne's explanation was that she never stressed herself: "If you can't do anything about it, don't worry about it."

Numerous studies have linked the compound to significantly longer life spans among certain insects and small varieties of fish. No clinical studies have identified a causal connection between resveratrol and long life in humans, but the general theory is that any antioxidant will help avoid age-related cellular stress. That also remains a theory.

In addition to the French paradox, other large population studies have linked red wine to a general decrease in the risk of heart disease. A 2015 study at the University of Missouri found that resveratrol changed the immune system in dogs—though not entirely in positive ways. The inflammation capacity increased, but the ability to fight off bacteria decreased, which suggests that both resveratrol and the immune system in advanced mammals are more complex than originally thought and "immunity boosts" likely require more than a single ingredient. Another 2015 study at the University of Leicester found that small doses of resveratrol (the amount typically found in one glass of red wine) were more effective than large doses. This was an important revelation because other studies have shown correlations between high alcohol intake and increased incidents of cardiovascular disease and cancer risk. It is not the alcohol in red wine that is healthful, but the resveratrol. Unfortunately, it is difficult to extract the active ingredient in red wine without including the alcohol. The Leicester study seems to suggest, however, that a daily glass of wine is healthy if consumed in moderation.

Other related superfoods include blueberries, acai berries, cranberries, pomegranates, and their juices. It is fairly safe to say that most berries include similar antioxidant properties and are generally recognized as being healthful, though it is difficult to establish a causal relationship to longer life spans. Fresh berries have the advantage of being consumed without alcohol, but researchers at Tel Aviv University in 2013 suggested that alcohol may enhance the effect of resveratrol. Researchers found that a minimal amount of daily alcohol intake may be healthful because it can protect and promote telomere length. In this way, red wine is seen as an extra-superfood for combining the two agents in a single drink.

Dark Chocolate (Epicatechin)

The other favorite food of Jeanne Calment was chocolate. She reportedly consumed about two pounds a week, until her doctor recommended giving it up at the age of 119. Researchers believe that the active antioxidant ingredient in chocolate is epicatechin, which is a polyphenol that includes flavonoid compounds. In terms of biochemistry, catechins belong to a group of compounds called *flavonoids*, which are part of a large biochemical group called *polyphenols*, all of which have antioxidant properties. In antiaging literature, the terms *polyphenol*, *catechin*, *flavonoids*, and *antioxidant* are often used interchangeably, depending on the precision of the research argument. In chocolate, epicatechin is chemically similar to insulin and seems to protect the cellular membranes that are most prone to oxidative stress. It is found in cocoa beans, tea, and grapes.

In addition to Jeanne Calment and the French, the first historical record of using cocoa for medicinal purposes dates back to the 1500s, when Hernan Cortez found the Aztecs drinking the concoction for religious and physical well-being. More than 500 years later, certain indigenous populations in Central America continue to drink cocoa in high quantities, particularly the Kuna people living on a group of islands near Panama. A Harvard Medical School study found that the Kuna have lower risks of cardiovascular disease, diabetes, and strokes as compared to other natives of the same ethnic profile that live on the mainland and do not regularly consume cocoa.

Other studies suggest dark chocolate may increase the blood's antioxidant power by as much as 20 percent. In a 2009 study in the Netherlands, researchers found that older adults (men 60 years and older) who ate the equivalent of one-third of a chocolate bar per day lowered their blood pressure and their risk of death. Numerous other population studies seem to affirm the positive connections between chocolate and heart health. Epicatechin is found in all chocolate, but it is more concentrated in dark chocolate than in milk chocolate and is not found at all in white chocolate (which is not technically chocolate because it does not contain any cocoa powder).

Green Tea and Coffee

Other polyphenol-related foods include "super drinks" such as green tea and coffee. Similar to dark chocolate, green tea is linked to lower risks of cardiovascular disease because it helps to lower LDL (bad) cholesterol levels and raises HDL (good) cholesterol. It also lowers the blood's tendency to clot, which lowers stroke risk. The catechin in tea has insulin-like properties that help to protect the body against insulin resistance (diabetes) and control blood-sugar levels. When combined with caffeine, the polyphenols may help to burn fat, which may also protect against obesity (though clinical studies on this benefit are mixed).

A host of correlational population studies have linked daily consumption of both tea and coffee to lower incidents of neurodegenerative disorders such as Alzheimer's disease, Parkinson's disease, and dementia. It is not clear whether the decreased risks are due to the antioxidants or to the caffeine. Nevertheless, the research indicates that coffee consumption can improve muscle coordination, concentration, and memory, and it lowers the risks for skin cancer, cirrhosis of the liver, and depression. It also improves exercise performance, which explains why caffeine is so common among certain sports and energy drinks.

There are mixed opinions, however, on the benefits of caffeine alone. Some researchers have found a link between caffeine and the production of cortisol, which is a hormone that can decrease the biochemical pathways of sex-related hormones, from dehydroepiandrosterone (DHEA) to estrogen and testosterone. These links have not been affirmed, but a 2013 study conducted by researchers at the Human Nutrition Research Center on Aging at Tufts University found that it does not appear to be the caffeine in coffee but the coffee itself that improves nervous system functions. The research showed that the motor and cognitive behavior (including memory) of rats improved when given a diet that included the equivalent of 10 cups of coffee per day, as compared to those that were given no coffee at all. In the same study, though, rats that were just given the equivalent doses of daily caffeine, but without the coffee, did not experience any improvements in motor or cognitive behaviors. This suggests it is not the caffeine alone in coffee but somehow the mixture of caffeine with the other bioactive compounds in the coffee that provide the healthful results.

The Tufts' research suggests that other caffeine-enhanced drinks, including specialized sports and energy drinks, may not have any particular antiaging benefits. Energy drinks often include caffeine (70–200 mg per can), sugar, taurine (a mild inhibitory neurotransmitter), guarana (a densely caffeinated bean from South America), a variety of B vitamins, ginseng, L-carnitine, and a host of other ingredients that have become popular for their ability to enhance energy and metabolic processing, including glucuronolactone (DGL), yerba mate, creatine, acai berry, inositol, L-theanine, milk thistle, ginkgo biloba, quercetin, and other antioxidant supplements. In some cases, the energy drink is marketed as a multivitamin as well as a stimulant. Unfortunately, the artificial supplements do not necessarily interact in quite the same way as when found in their natural mediums (such as coffee, tea, fruits, etc.). The growing popularity of energy drinks prompted researchers to study their effects on other aspects of human health, and their conclusions were not positive.

The most common side effects of overuse of caffeine-based energy drinks are increased anxiety, insomnia, and a greater likelihood of headaches and migraines that follow caffeine withdrawal. Several studies conducted between 2009 and 2016 have also shown significant increases in cardiovascular health risk associated with energy drinks, especially among younger adults (ages 18 to 40), who are the most common consumers. Specifically, the combination of compounds added to energy drinks raises blood pressure and increases the risk of irregular heart rhythms, which may lead to heart attacks or strokes. The energy drinks were shown to improve athletic performance, but long-term use suggested negative effect on heart health.

By themselves, tea and coffee consumption appear to have positive health effects, especially for their antioxidant properties and their mixture of caffeine with other natural bioactive ingredients. Green tea tends to have more polyphenols than white and black teas, but no tea types seem to be absorbed well by the body. The positive effects of green tea required long-term consumption of multiple cups (10 to 12) throughout the day for weeks before blood levels of catechins increased. Catechin absorption increases when tea is combined with citrus juice (vitamin C) and when consumed away from food. For coffee, research suggests that dark roasts have lower levels of polyphenols than light or medium roasts. Adding milk does not appear to have any impact on the body's absorption of catechin in either tea or coffee.

In addition to internal consumption, the retinol compounds found in tea leaves have been shown to reduce the appearance of wrinkles and to help moisturize skin. Some fashionable cosmetic salons apply tea leaves (and in some cases ground coffee) as an antiaging skin treatment. These treatments, however, can only promise to provide temporary relief because, as discussed in chapter 8, there is no effective cure for wrinkles.

Asian Cuisine: Turmeric, Ginger, and Ginseng

Moving from Europe to the Far East, researchers have been studying common health trends among Asian populations since the 1980s. The Asian diet consists of rice, green tea, vegetables and fruits, fish, whole grains, nuts and beans, soybeans, and spices. There is much less consumption of red meat, and portion sizes are traditionally smaller than in the West. Vegetarians have been drawn to Asian ingredients because they provide a variety of proteins without the need for meat. In addition, Asian population studies find lower incidents of many chronic diseases that afflict Westerners, including cardiovascular disease, diabetes, obesity, and certain cancer types, especially breast cancer.

One of the popular superfoods in Asian cuisine is turmeric, which is a spice used in curry dishes and other rice-based recipes. It has a bright yellow-orange color that also made it popular as a fabric dye before the industrial age. Turmeric is a potato-like root that is related to ginger, and in its natural form, it looks like a cross between ginger and a sweet potato. Since ancient times, it was used both as a spice (with a peppery flavor) and as a medicinal herb to treat joint pains and digestive issues in India and China. In the modern era, scientists have isolated curcumin as the primary active agent in turmeric.

In addition to its general antioxidant effects, modern research has studied curcumin's ability to treat or prevent Alzheimer's disease and other neurological diseases. Current dementia treatments seek to inhibit the misfolding and aggregation of monomeric Aβ peptides (called beta-amyloid fibrillation). Several clinical trials suggest turmeric may act as a beta-amyloid inhibitor. A 2014 study also linked turmeric to an increase in telomerase, which may increase telomere length. All of these studies examined turmeric in vitro and not in humans. At least two studies have found no benefits at all from using turmeric as a treatment for Alzheimer's disease.

Related to turmeric, ginger has been strongly associated with overall health. Ginger and ginseng have similar names, but they come from completely different families of plants, though both ingredients are often lumped together as related superfoods. Like ginger, ginseng also enjoys a long association as a medicinal plant in traditional folk remedies. Much of their popularity in the West may be due to their exotic nature. Though ginseng is found in the Americas, both ginger and ginseng are mostly associated with Asian folk remedies and Asian cuisine. In traditionally Asian medicine, ginger was used to treat digestive disorders, nausea, and joint pain, while ginseng was used to improve almost everything, including immunity, impotence, strength, wisdom, and long life.

Modern research has affirmed that ginger has some antioxidant properties and that it can provide some mild relief for nausea. Studies have not, however, shown conclusive results on its ability to treat joint pain. Similarly, modern research has not found conclusive evidence to indicate that ginseng can cure most of what its folk remedies suggest. Some studies have found potential in improving immunity, and it may help to lower blood sugars (as most antioxidants do). But these results have not been consistently demonstrated in clinical trials.

Like coffee and tea, however, turmeric has also been studied for its potential cosmetic benefits. A 2010 study found that turmeric-enhanced facial creams may help to reduce age spots. Ginger and ginseng have also been added to some skin creams to enhance the appearance of "radiance." It is difficult to determine whether these ingredients were added for their chemical benefits or for their marketing potential.

Asian Cuisine: Soybeans

Apart from Asian spices, a significant source of nutrients in Asian cuisine comes from both the food fibers and the oils that originate in soybeans. Soybeans are the primary source of tofu, which may be used in a variety ways to produce different flavors and textures in food, and they constitute a significant part of the Asian diet. During the 1980s, tofu became popular in the United States as substitute for meat, and in the 21st century, soy extractions have become very popular as a substitute for milk and other dairy products. Soybeans are unique in that they contain all the essential nutrients necessary for human metabolism. (An essential nutrient is one that the body needs but cannot produce on its own and must be obtained through diet.) The biochemical versatility of soybeans also made it desirable for modern scientists, who use it for a wide variety of purposes. Since the early 2000s, more than 12,000 soy products have been developed, with the majority of soybeans grown, harvested, and exported from the United States being used for their oils and as a protein meal in animal feed. Since the 1980s, the popularity of soybeans as a potential superfood for human use has fallen in and out of favor several times.

From a biochemical perspective, soybeans are high in chemicals that act like estrogen (phytoestrogens). As estrogen is a precursor to other sex-related anabolic steroids (such as testosterone), soybeans are usually viewed as a healthy supplement for maintaining positive hormonal balances in both men and women. Soybeans also have no cholesterol and low saturated fat. They are a major source of protein, and soy extracts have become very popular among bodybuilders who hope to combine the testosterone precursors with elevated protein levels to promote muscle development. On the downside, soybeans also contain compounds that block the body from absorbing certain nutrients. In particular, soy can inhibit the body's ability to dissolve and process calcium, zinc, and iron. It may also inhibit digestion, and for some individuals, soy can trigger allergic reactions.

Soybeans may contribute to a nutritious diet. Most of the negative criticisms of soy come from its use as an exclusive dietary supplement; soy is often marketed as a substitute for meat and dairy. In practice, soybeans are best as a dietary accessory. Even in Asian cultures, soybeans do not constitute a dominant source of protein, so most nutritionists avoid recommending diets that are overly weighted toward soy products.

As an antiaging superfood, soybeans have lost much of their appeal. In the late 1990s, their relationship with estrogen initially made soybeans very popular among those antiaging proponents of testosterone and other anabolic steroidal hormones. By the start of the 2010s, though, the link between artificially enhanced anabolic steroids and certain cancers caused soybeans to fall out of favor. Beyond their hormonal properties, soybeans are potentially linked to decreases in LDL cholesterol. Several studies conducted since 2010 have failed to find any positive impact of soybeans on lowering cancer risks.

The Asian diet is not easily reduced to soybeans and spices. Some population studies have suggested that the decreased incidents of cardiovascular disease and breast cancer found in Asian countries may be due as much to genetic factors as dietary factors. Yet, a 2009 study of more than 1,200 Asian American women found that those who ate traditional Western diets in the United States, with high intakes of meats and starches, had higher risks of breast cancer compared to those who ate traditional Asian diets, with higher intakes of legumes, vegetables, and soy products. The Asian diet may hold some benefits, but it is not entirely clear in what way. The diet may not be reducible to one or more specific superfood ingredient.

Olives and Garlic

The last of the favored habits of Jeanne Calment was that she routinely and liberally doused her food with olive oil. Olive oil is not necessarily a major ingredient in French cuisine, but it is extremely popular in Mediterranean cuisine. Since the 1970s, ethnic demographers have questioned why the economically poor communities of Italy generally have lower risks of cardiovascular disease than the wealthier communities in the United States. Some nutritionists pointed to the Italian use of olive oil.

The active biochemical in olives is oleocanthal, which is another type of polyphenol compound called *phenylethanoid glycoside*. In plain language, it is another antioxidant, and it is linked to decreasing risks of LDL cholesterol. In addition, like turmeric's curcumin, oleocanthal is believed to be a beta-amyloid inhibitor. That means it is associated with decreased risks of Alzheimer's disease and other forms of dementia. As we discuss below, olive oil is also a major component of the Mediterranean diet, and in the antiaging community, it is often promoted as a cure for almost all age-related disorders. Clinical evidence is less optimistic. Some researchers have suggested a link between oleocanthal and the expression of genes that inhibit tumor growth, particularly in breast cancers. The research is not conclusive, yet neither is it refuted. Other researchers suggest a link between oleocanthal and osteocalcin, which is tied to collagen synthesis and bone formation. Again, the research was correlational in nature, and no proven causal connection has been established.

Another popular ingredient in both Italian and French cuisines is garlic. Though Jeanne Calment never indicated any particular preference for it, garlic is a staple in French cooking. More than 1,200 studies have been conducted on the cardiovascular benefits of garlic, and the consensus is strong that there is some positive benefit. There are numerous bioagents in the plant, but the most commonly studied is allicin, which is an organosulfur compound (which means it contains sulfur, the primary source of garlic's distinct odor). Popular testimonies claim that garlic reduces LDL cholesterol, increases HDL cholesterol, lowers blood pressure, and reduces blood clots, all of which lowers the risk of stroke and cardiovascular disease. Clinical studies indicate a fairly small reduction in total cholesterol over the short-term. Some correlative studies suggest a link between garlic and a reduction in cancer risk, but they are also not conclusive.

The Future

Some of the active bioagents in these superfoods have been successfully extracted in supplemental form, but research suggests that their benefits are often much less effective when removed from their original mediums. Garlic extract does not provide any added health benefits as compared to eating garlic through food. Similarly, resveratrol, epicatechin, and caffeine have not been shown to have the same effects as extracts outside of the food in which they naturally occur (red wine, coffee, and tea). However, researchers may have found a potential solution to this problem. In 2015, scientists at the John Innes Centre developed a way of producing industrial quantities of polyphenols by genetically enhancing tomatoes. Using a common variety of tomatoes found in gardens throughout England, researchers were able to cultivate a tomato with a skin that contains the nutritional equivalent of 50 bottles of red wine and 2.5 kilograms of tofu. As tomatoes are easily grown in very high yields per acre, this innovation potentially opens the door for drug companies to find ways for more efficiently extracting the active bioagents. There is also potential for consumers to enhance their antioxidant intake by eating raw vegetables that are grown to be super superfoods. The developers, however, offered no comment on how these genetic changes affected the taste. Moreover, as with any extract, there is a strong risk that the active ingredients might lose their effectiveness when removed from the other less-pronounced bioactive compounds of the original plant.

ANTIAGING DIETS

There is no formal antiaging diet plan universally promoted by the antiaging movement. Most recommendations focus on one or more superfoods that people should incorporate into their daily routines. But there are a wide variety of unique diet plans that have been promoted by individual antiaging researchers or that have become popular among antiaging clinics. The four most commonly cited plans are dietary restriction, regional diets, the paleo diet, and detox diets. Most of these diet plans include some promise of weight loss, but for the most part, they are popular for their antiaging properties and the promise of extended life spans.

Dietary (Calorie) Restriction

The dietary restriction model was first published by Richard Weindruch and Roy Walford in 1988, and it was received with considerable fanfare by the antiaging community (see chapter 5). Using a variety of insects and rodents, the researchers found that restricting the total caloric intake by 25 percent could extend the life span by as much as 50 percent. For obvious reasons of time and ethics, no research was conducted with humans, and so the dietary restriction model remains theoretical. Nevertheless, Weindruch and Walford advocated strongly that the theory most certainly applied to humans, and they began calling for policy changes to accommodate the dramatic increase in average life expectancy, which they anticipated would follow implementation of the model. Roy Walford died of Lou Gehrig's disease at the age of 79, but he had continued to advocate for the dietary restriction model up until his death. He argued that he would have died sooner from the disease if he had not practiced a restricted caloric diet. Richard Weindruch was Walford's student, and he continues to promote the model at LifeGen Technologies, which he cofounded in 2000.

Since 1988, the dietary restriction model has undergone considerable adaptation as a result of subsequent clinical studies. It is now known by at least three different names and is not so much a "diet" as it is a guideline that all diets can follow. There are no suggested superfoods to include and no recommended approaches to eating or cooking. The three branches of the model are (1) caloric restriction (CR), (2) caloric restriction combined with exercise (CE), and (3) dietary restriction (DR). The essential argument of the original model is found most in the CR variation. Caloric restriction involves a 20–40 percent decrease in caloric intake taken from any or all food types. Most antiaging diets strongly recommend smaller portion sizes and a goal of total reduced caloric intake, regardless of what the particular prescribed food groups might be. The CR model is the most common element found in all antiaging diet plans.

The term *dietary restriction* was first used in 1988 by Walford and Weindruch when they published their research. Since then, the term has been redefined to refer to a diet that reduces caloric intake mostly from one or more macronutrients. A macronutrient is one that is specifically required in large quantities for metabolic growth; these include carbohydrates, proteins, and fats and oils. A common DR diet might allow for carbohydrates but be low in protein (such as a vegan diet that emphasizes fruits and vegetables and avoids meats, eggs, and fish). Low-protein diets are not commonly recommended, except for people with kidney disorders and those who might have philosophical objections to eating animal by-products.

Conversely, a DR diet may also eliminate carbohydrates but retain other nutrients. For example, the popular Atkins diet allows participants to eat meat, cheese, oils, butter, and eggs but few to no carbohydrates (bread, potatoes, or pasta). It was very popular in the 1990s as a weight-loss model. The Atkins diet would not qualify as an antiaging model unless the participants also planned to significantly reduce the total caloric intake. Critics of the Atkins diet argued that the high levels of proteins and fats were harmful for cardiac health. In 2002, the founder of the diet, Robert Atkins, suffered a heart attack at the age of 71 and died a year later. He and his attending physicians argued the attack was a result of a viral infection that had nothing to do with his diet. But the controversy remained, and the popularity of the diet declined (though it was quickly repackaged the following year as the South Beach Diet by Arthur Agatston, with a focus on particular heart-healthy proteins to counter the criticisms). In both diets, though, the focus was on weight loss and not antiaging.

Oddly enough, the DR model does not necessarily require an overall reduction of calories; it only requires a reduction of one of the macronutrient groups. In this way, the modern DR model does not really satisfy the original DR theory proposed by Walford and Weindruch in 1988. In fact, subsequent research has found little evidence to indicate that the low-carbohydrate, or low-fat diets have any effect on extending life span. There is some indication, though, that a reduced protein diet might increase life span by as much as 20 percent due to the reduction of oxidative stress. Low-protein diets emphasize the high consumption of fruits and vegetables, most of which tend to have greater antioxidant properties. It is not clear whether the reduced calories or the antioxidants are responsible for the life extension in insect and rodents. In either case, none of these variations have demonstrated causal evidence of life extension in human subjects.

The CE model is most commonly recommended by physicians as a generic approach to any healthy lifestyle. Diet and exercise are routinely suggested as necessary remedies for most age-related conditions. The difference with the CE model and other traditional recommendations is that CE is also promoted as a preventative measure for maintaining youth and health. In theory, young adults who adhere to the strict discipline of an overall reduction of calories combined with routine, moderate-exertion exercises should be able to avoid many of the age-related conditions before they develop. Not only is daily caloric intake reduced, but daily caloric expenditure is also increased—you take in less, and you burn more. The added benefit is that the caloric reduction of the CE model does not have to be as extreme as the 20–40 percent required by CR. This helps to offset the potential side effects of listlessness, lack of concentration, and constant cravings that can accompany the CR model.

None of the three forms of dietary restriction have been studied with any consistency in human populations. Beginning in 2006, the Comprehensive Assessment of Long-term Effects of Reducing Caloric Intake (CALERIE) program was launched by the National Institute on Aging. From this program, human studies have been conducted for periods of 6 to 12 months over 2 years and up to 6 years. None of them have been able to follow human subjects for the entirety of a single life span (nor is it likely to ever be able to collect such data as ethical considerations would prevent infants and youth from being tested in that way from birth).

Most studies rely on certain biomarkers that attempt to measure the rate of aging. These are also problematic as science is still not certain how or why people age, much less how to measure the aging process. Nevertheless, data gathered from these studies indicate that the CR and CE models show some potential for improving cardiovascular health by lowing cholesterol, blood pressure, and heart muscle thickness. They also seem to improve the body's ability to regulate insulin and blood-sugar levels as well as verbal memory performance.

On many levels, the caloric restriction with or without exercise shared many of the same benefits. There were, however, some differences. A simple reduction of caloric intake did not appear to have any impact on reducing the rate of age-related muscle loss (sarcopenia) or bone density (osteoporosis). By contrast, the addition of routine exercise did seem to improve both bone density and muscle strength. This held true when the overall caloric intake remained the same: for example, the CR model of a 25 percent decrease of intake had the same results as the CE model that combined a 12.5 percent reduction of intake plus a 12.5 percent increase of caloric expenditure. Research suggests that the combination of diet and exercise adds more to the general health benefits than simple diet alone.

Religious Fasting as a Form of Caloric Restriction

Three religious traditions emphasize regular fasting as part of their annual observances. Orthodox and Catholic Christians often require limited fasting of certain types of foods during Advent, Lent, and the Feast of the Assumption. Islamic Ramadan requires 40 days of fasting during the day. Jewish traditions include a day of fasting as well as a "Daniel Fast," described in the book of Daniel in the Bible as a 21-day vegetarian diet with only water to drink.

The impact of each of these traditions has been tested under clinical conditions. Research suggests that the Christian fasts may result in weight loss as well as an overall reduction in cholesterol. The Ramadan fasts do not appear to have consistent results, but research suggests that this might be due to other factors related to the wide variety of cultural conditions during which these fasts are undertaken. Finally, the Daniel fast appears to provide noticeable impact on lowering blood pressure (suggesting a lower risk of cardiovascular disease), increasing insulin sensitivity (suggesting lower risks of diabetes), and reducing oxidative stress. However, none of these studies extended these religious fasts beyond the relatively short periods of time mandated by the traditions.

Regional Diets

The idea that certain geographic regions enjoy greater (or lesser) degrees of health due to the environment is as old as superstition and modern science. At the turn of the modern era, many Western scientists from the 13th to the 17th centuries routinely cited cases of lands where people lived hundreds of years. Roger Bacon (1214–1292) believed that people who lived in colder northern climates lived longer than those in hotter southern climates, and those who lived in moist climates lived longer than those in dry ones. This was repeated by Francis Bacon in the mid-1600s. Both men cited cases of far-off lands (mostly India or China) where people might live to be 300, 400, or even 600 years old. By the end of the 1900s, these stories had all been dismissed as legends.

Nevertheless, modern statistics resurrected the idea that some regions of the planet provide better conditions for long lives than others. Beginning in the 1950s, sociologists began comparing the relative health statistics of various regions in relation to their most common lifestyle patterns. They found that some regions, such as the Far East and the Mediterranean, had lower instances of certain diseases. By the late 1970s, health-conscious consumers began to adopt these regional diets to avoid those diseases. As the antiaging movement grew to maturity during the late 1990s, and the confidence that science might be able to extend the human life span increased, these diets shifted from being generically "healthful" to being "age-defying."

Mediterranean Diet

The first popular regional diet was launched in the 1970s by the sociologist Ancel Keys, who had spent 20 years tracing the relationship between various health trends and regional diets. His research included Finland, Holland, Italy, the United States, Greece, Japan, and Yugoslavia. According to sociological theory, the poorest country, Greece, ought to have had the worst health trends because it did not have the sociopolitical infrastructure to guarantee proper health care, nutrition, or preventative medicine. In practice, however, Greek populations had generally lower blood pressure rates and decreased risks of cardiovascular disease. Keys concluded it was the diet that was responsible, and he published another book promoting the "Mediterranean diet" as the cause.

Since the 1970s, the Mediterranean diet has been reduced to the region's primary emphasis on bread, olive oil, and red wine with a high intake of fruits, vegetables, and seafood and a low intake of red meats. In addition, the lifestyle includes a tradition of regular exercise, lots of sun, and the generally slower pace of living—all of which transform the modern Mediterranean diet into an antioxidant-rich nutrition plan. Originally, the correlational evidence of the diet focused primarily on decreasing risks of heart disease. In 2012, however, the University of Palermo studied Italian centenarians and found there were four times as many people (as a percentage) aged 100 and older in the mountainous regions of Sicily, where people most often eat a Mediterranean diet, than among those who lived in other regions of Italy, where the diet has been changed by other modern cultures. Other recent studies of genetic markers also suggest that the diet may delay cellular senescence. A long-term population study begun in 1976 on nurses in the United States provided data for a report published in 2014, which indicated that those middle-aged women who ate a Mediterranean diet tended to have longer telomere lengths than those that did not.

It is important to note, however, that these and other similar population studies rely on correlational evidence and do not imply a causal connection. Critics suggest that there may be a variety of other genetic or historical cultural causes for the seeming health benefits of Sicilian living.

Okinawan Diet

Following the academic trend set by Ancel Keys, researchers also studied sociological and medical factors that may contribute to the lack of heart disease in the Asian diet. In the process, they discovered that the inhabitants on Okinawa have the highest life expectancy in the world, with the lowest rates of cardiovascular disease and cancer, and one of the lowest stroke rates. Okinawa is not part of the main Japanese island. It is located about 500 miles south, in a chain of islands called the Ryukyu archipelago, which is located roughly between Japan and Taiwan. The Ryukyu Islands maintained their own kingdom for 400 years before they were taken over by the Japanese in the late 1870s. They were a major trading port during the time of Japanese isolation, and as a result, they share a culture that is distinct and yet influenced by China, Japan, and the Americas. Their diet is unique in the region, consisting primarily of vegetables, fish, and some minimal amounts of pork. The traditional staple of Asian cuisine is rice, but the sweet potato was introduced to the islands from Central America in the 1600s and now constitutes about 93 percent of the traditional Okinawan diet.

In 1975, Dr. Makoto Suzuki, a local cardiologist and geriatrician, launched the Okinawan Centenarian Study (OCS) as a long-term population study examining the possible causes of their health and longevity. He used verifiable data gathered from the family registers (*koseki*) of each village, city, and town to identify the centenarians and other older adults on the island and then studied their nutrition and other lifestyle routines. Since 1975, the OCS has examined more than 900 Okinawan centenarians and thousands of older adults aged 70 and above. By the 1990s, the study had found that Okinawans not only live longer but appear to be stronger, thinner, and less prone to traditional age-related conditions and diseases. During the 1980s and early 1990s, Okinawa was mostly viewed as a model for healthy lifestyles. After the turn of the 21st century, though, Okinawa became a model for prolongevity, and the Okinawan diet was promoted as a major contributor to the long span of healthy years. The OCS team eventually included Makoto Suzuki and two brothers, Bradley and Craig Wilcox. In 2001, they published *The Okinawa Program: How the World's Longest-lived People Achieve Everlasting Health—And How You Can Too*. This was followed up in 2004 with *The Okinawan Diet Plan: Get Leaner, Live Longer, and Never Feel Hungry*. Both books were best sellers, and the Okinawan diet became very popular both as a weight-loss program and as an antiaging model.

The basic features of the diet combine nutrition with exercise and a philosophy of meditation and relaxation. The nutritional components emphasize the purple sweet potato, which is very high in fiber, vitamins C and B, calcium, and potassium. Most recipes include leafy greens, fermented tofu, and seaweed (particularly *konbu*, which is high in essential fatty acids and other precursors to anabolic steroidal hormones DHA). Both seafood and meat is used sparingly and usually as a side to the meal and not as the main dish. Pork and goat meat is most common, with little red meat. Almost all portions of the animal are eaten, including the internal organs and the joints, which are high in collagen and elastin, though most fat portions are removed prior to cooking. The result is a diet that is very high in antioxidants, low in fat, and low in calories.

In addition to the bare nutritional components, the Okinawan diet also includes particular lifestyle habits. Food portions are small, and the culture promotes less eating rather than more, with a goal of eating until you are 80 percent full, not completely full. The result is a daily caloric intake of about 500 fewer calories than typical American cuisine. As the recipes tend to include a lot of water, Okinawans often eat more in volume than Americans, but most of the volume is calorie free. Finally, the Okinawan lifestyle includes daily work outside, with less reliance on mechanical conveniences. This reflects a much older animistic tradition that links food with spiritual balance so that the habits of daily life, including the methodical process of cooking, are revered as acts of metaphysical warfare against the agents of material corruption and disease. Researchers in the OCS and other studies attribute the generally lower levels of stress to these and other lifestyle practices.

Since the 2000s, new genetic discoveries following the completion of Human Genome Project provide additional explanations for Okinawan longevity. The OCS identified several "human longevity genes" that are linked to lower risks of inflammation and autoimmune diseases. Other data from the long-term population study suggests that long life runs in families, and siblings often share similar life spans. This suggests that genetics may provide a necessary predisposition to good health, which the cultural lifestyle choices take strong advantage of. It also raises a question of whether it is the diet, the genetic predisposition, or the culture that is most responsible for Okinawan longevity. Separating the diet from the culture may not produce the same results. All of the research associated with Okinawa is based on correlational population studies. There is no causal evidence to tie the diet to extended life spans in humans.

Paleo Diet

The antiaging movement added new dimensions to dieting plans that moved beyond simple weight loss. In the early 1990s, an ophthalmologist and antiaging specialist, Michael Rose, from West Hollywood published a book titled *Evolutionary Biology on Aging*, which proposed a new explanation of aging based on evolutionary theory. The book was unusual because it did not refer to molecular or cellular senescence to explain why people aged. Instead, Rose argued that aging and death are entirely a product of evolutionary forces of natural selection. His surprising conclusion was that the process of aging actually stops after a certain age. Using demographic data, Rose later argued that humans who live to the age of 90 have a higher survival rate than those who are only 70 or 80. He called that point the "immortal age" because it was then that humans could potentially live without aging at all. During the remainder of the 1990s, Rose presented these theories with the hope of finding some way that medical science might lower the age of immortality from 90 to around 40, when the individual is still healthy and strong. At age 90, each additional year of life is a 50/50 gamble because the body is already so frail and weak. At age 40, though, the likelihood of successfully surviving an additional year is much higher; therefore, the likelihood of living very long lives would increase significantly.

Michael Rose stimulated considerable debate within the community of antiaging researchers, but it was little noticed by the general public. Nevertheless, the popularity of the antiaging movement after the turn of the new millennium brought some of these ideas into the domain of the lay consumer. In 2002, health and exercise science professor Loren Cordain published *The Paleo Diet*, which used evolutionary theory to justify a new approach to diet and nutrition. Though loosely based on research conducted by Boyd Eaton and other authors who wrote about "stone age" diets in 1970s and 1980s, Cordain's contribution was unique because he tied the diet to a broad evolutionary model. In brief, he argued that human digestion mostly evolved during the span of several hundred thousand years when the species lived as hunter-gatherers before the Neolithic revolution when agriculture and domestication of animals emerged. As such, human metabolism responds best to those types of foods that were present before the invention of agriculture (around 8000 BCE), and he explained that many of our common ailments are a result of our digestive system reacting to foods that it had never fully adapted to. The paleo diet consists mostly of meat, fish, raw vegetables, fruits, and nuts and absolutely no vegetable oils or other processed foods. According to the theory, cereal grains (wheat, oats, rice, etc.—anything derived from grain or grass) and dairy products (anything from the udder of a cow) inhibit the natural immunities and muscle development that hunter-gatherers relied on to survive.

Cordain's book was not immediately a best seller, and the paleo diet did not become fashionable until 2010. For the first decade after its release, the paleo diet was marketed as another diet to maintain health and lose weight. Its popularity changed significantly, however, after Michael Rose embraced it as a potential anti-aging lifestyle choice. Rose argued that the age of immortality might be lowered to age 40 if we adopted the hunter-gatherer lifestyle and diet that our metabolism is most suited for. Rose distinguished himself from Cordain by arguing that the metabolism of adults in the prime of reproductive age (35 years and younger) had successfully adapted to the agricultural revolution, and he recommended they adhere to a Mediterranean or Okinawan diet. After age 35 or 40, however, Rose argued that the physiology of European people falls back to their ancestral tendencies of hunter-gather lifestyles. For these ages, he recommended the paleo diet.

In addition to a paleo diet, Michael Rose also argued that successful antiaging requires frequent use of modern medicine. Hunter-gatherers died young because they lived in hostile environments. Rose argued that modern humans can live to their full potential by taking advantage of the available technologies to protect human life, while at the same time maintaining a nutritional plan that reflects their hunter-gatherer origins. Michael Rose is a strong supporter of genetic cloning to replicate existing cells to repair those damaged by age-related conditions and diseases. He also supports ample use of vitamins, supplements, and any antiaging drugs that may be developed in the future.

The success of the paleo diet is primarily based on the theoretical explanations that justify its effectiveness. On paper, the diet is very logical. In actual practice, there has been very little clinical evidence to support the theory. Swedish researcher Staffan Lindeberg conducted several population studies of an island community near Papua New Guinea (Kitava) that continued to subsist off a hunter-gatherer lifestyle. He found lower rates of obesity, heart disease, and stroke. Other studies examined the health changes of Australian Aborigines who left their native communities to live in Western cities and found increased rates of obesity and diabetes. Other small-scale population studies (10 to 12 people) from 2008 to 2012 found some correlations between paleo diets and lower blood pressure, cholesterol levels, and insulin resistance. It was not clear, however, whether the changes were a result of the paleo diet or a reflection of the relative decrease in daily intake of sugar and relative increase in antioxidant-rich vegetables. There is strong correlational evidence to suggest the paleo diet can lead to weight loss as compared to no particular diet at all. There is, however, no causal evidence to indicate that the paleo diet will end or slow down aging or in any way extend the human life span.

Detox Diets

There is a category of antiaging diets that claim to remove toxins from the body so as to rejuvenate and revitalize the body as a system. These are particularly popular among amateur homeopathic Web sites that promote practical remedies that often rest on popular presumptions of human physiology that may not be supported by clinical research.

Many of these plans can be traced back to the Popular Health Movement of the 1830s and 1840s, which combined new scientific discoveries (of the era) with personal philosophies of the perfectibility of man. Sylvester Graham was a Presbyterian minister who invented the graham cracker as a simple food to promote simple living and moral self-restraint. By removing the excess foods in your life, Graham believed you could also remove any added temptations. In addition to his graham breads, he also advocated a strict vegetarian diet. His contemporary Dr. John Harvey Kellogg was heavily influenced by Graham's writings and developed a health resort in the 1860s based on his own lifestyle philosophy of personal restraint, exercise, and a diet based on whole grains, fruits, nuts, and beans. Kellogg and his brother eventually invented Corn Flakes as a special health food. Dr. Kellogg touted numerous procedures for cleansing the body of its toxins. He believed most illnesses were due to toxins built up in the stomach and bowels, and he advocated frequent yogurt enemas to clean out the intestines.

Kellogg's theories were not unique, and they were adapted later by the famous zoologist, Nobel Prize winner, and father of the science of natural immunity, Élie Metchnikoff, who wrote several books on the lower intestines as the source of "putrification" and the ultimate cause of all aging and disease. Rather than enemas, Metchnikoff promoted a diet of probiotic yogurts to help foster the phagocytes in the blood that are responsible for identifying and ingesting harmful foreign particles and other bacteria (most white blood cells are phagocytes). Metchnikoff earned his Nobel Prize for discovering the existence of phagocytes.

In the 21st century, Kellogg's and Metchnikoff's theories of latent toxins built up in the large intestines have mostly been disproved with the more developed understanding of the complex interrelationships of the endocrine system. Nevertheless, the popular conception that constipation and blocked bowels lead to increased vulnerability to aging and disease remains strong in the popular theories of *detox diets*. Most of these diets include foods that promote frequent bowel movements and include heavy amounts of water intake intended to cleanse the bloodstream and liver of harmful toxins. Usually, they also involve a special supplement designed to facilitate the process.

There is very little clinical evidence to support the claim that the body is being poisoned by excess fecal matter in the intestines. There is, however, considerable evidence to suggest that conditions related to irritable bowels are tied to an overactive immune system response to the normal bacteria found in the digestive tract. These conditions can lead to great discomfort among patients, including abdominal pain, constipation, or diarrhea. There is no evidence to suggest that the existence of fecal matter is the primary cause of this disorder. In fact, in 2014, doctors at the Farncombe Family Digestive Health Research Institute at McMaster University studied the effects of transplanting the fecal matter from healthy adults into the digestive tracks of patients suffering from irritated bowels. The fecal microbiota transplantation (FMT) is facilitated through a simple enema. In this case, the addition of a donor's fecal matter was found to provide some relief. There is no indication that FMT provides any antiaging benefits.

Several clinical studies support the idea of detoxification at the cellular level. The majority of superfoods are promoted due to their antioxidant properties. Foods that include active biochemicals that promote the elimination of free radicals within the mitochondria of each cell are viewed as a sort of cleansing agent. But these work within the endocrine system and require manipulation of particular hormones and other enzymes to produce the biochemical changes at a molecular level. They do not rely on the physical movement of matter through organs and pathways that are designed to hold such materials.

In general, any diet may be considered "antiaging" as long as it includes a majority of superfoods (fresh fruits and vegetables), promotes a plan for low calorie consumption, and includes recommendations for routine exercise. The theoretical basis for such diets fits into the general expectations of a healthy nutritional lifestyle. There is no evidence, however, that any particular diet will actually evade the onset of age-related conditions or delay the onset of age-related diseases.

SUPPLEMENTS

Depending on the interview, the director of engineering at Google, Ray Kurzwiel, is said to take anywhere from 100 to 250 supplements a day. In addition, he is also reported to take an intravenous injection of other supplements five times a week (the injection directly into the bloodstream avoids the problem of inadequate absorption through the gastrointestinal tract). Kurzwiel believes the age of practical immortality will occur within his lifetime, and he takes advantage of every available technological advancement to ensure he is part of the biomedical revolution.

Though the average consumer is not as aggressive as Kurzweil, dietary supplements are very popular. Americans spend more than $37 billion on them each year. In 2015, *Consumer Reports* found that 68 percent of adults take one or more supplements a day, and there is an 84 percent confidence rating among those who take them. The market is very competitive, with no company achieving more than a 5 percent share each year. Thousands of options are available, but the questions remain: Are any supplements effective? Will they prolong human life? Can they ensure a healthy life? Currently, scientific research can offer no guarantees, and the clinical evidence is mixed. As with dietary recommendations and the list of superfoods, the medical community does not have enough evidence to state with certainty that over-the-counter supplements help to avoid age-related conditions or diseases. Typically, most doctors will say, "They cannot hurt."

Natural Sources of Vitamins

Most nutritionists recommend trying to obtain the proper amount of vitamins and minerals through a healthy and balanced diet. The word *vitamin* was first coined by Casimir Funk in 1912 to describe those molecules that are essential to healthy living but which are not synthesized in the body and must be obtained through diet. The word comes from *vital amines*, or essential nutrients needed to cure particular diseases. His discoveries led to a cure of beriberi through the ingestion of thiamine (from polished rice). By the 1920s, Funk had helped to launch a vitamin movement, which included the discovery of more than a dozen vitamins before World War II.

Vitamin A (retinol) was one of the earliest vitamins to be discovered and synthesized as a supplement. It is necessary for healthy vision, immunity, and bone growth and is critical for reproduction because of the role it plays in cell division and cell differentiation. Beta-carotene is a compound that the body uses to synthesize vitamin A. As too much retinol may lead to bone loss, the National Institutes of Health recommends eating foods high in beta-carotene and letting the body synthesize only as much vitamin A as it needs. Natural sources of beta-carotene include most dark green leafy vegetables (spinach) and fruits and vegetables that are deep yellow or orange (carrots, sweet potatoes, peaches). Vitamin A can be found in poultry products, red meat, and dairy.

Vitamin B was the first vitamin discovered by Casimir Funk, but since then scientists have discovered eight variations that are sometimes distinguished by a number but most often identified by their chemical names: B_1 (thiamine), B_2 (riboflavin), B_3 (niacin), B_5 (pantothenic acid), B_6 (pyridoxine), B_7 (biotin), B_9 (folate, or folic acid), and B_{12} (cobalamin). The collection is often referred to simply as the *vitamin B complex*. These are essential for the production of red blood cells and are often credited with providing added energy and enhancing mood. Since the 1990s, many professional baseball players have taken injections of vitamin B_{12} to enhance their performance without violating antidoping rules that prohibit anabolic steroids. In terms of antiaging, they are mostly a source of rejuvenating healthy cells.

- Thiamine (B_1) helps break down simple carbohydrates to create new cells. It is found in beans, peanuts, whole grains, wheat germ, spinach, and molasses.
- Riboflavin (B_2) is an antioxidant necessary for the production of red blood cells. It is found in almonds, milk, eggs, spinach, soybeans, and brussels sprouts.
- Niacin (B_3) helps to reduce LDL cholesterol and is found in red meat, milk, eggs, beans, and green vegetables.
- Pantothenic acid (B_5) is a precursor to anabolic steroids and helps to break down fats and carbohydrates for the production of new cells. It is found in yogurt, eggs, meat, beans, and avocados.
- Pyridoxine (B_6) lowers the risk of heart disease and also promotes the natural synthesis of serotonin, melatonin, and norepinephrine, all of which

contribute to regular sleep rhythms and stabilizing mood. It can be found in poultry meats, fish, cheese, lentils, sunflower seeds, carrots, and brown rice.

- Biotin (B_7) helps strengthen hair, skin, and nails. It is also essential for proper fetal development during pregnancy and can be used to lower blood glucose levels. It is found in pork, chicken, and fish as well as eggs, cauliflower, potatoes, barley, and nuts.
- Folic acid (B_9, or folate) is highly recommended for pregnant women and is associated with reducing birth defects. It also helps cognitive functions such a memory and mood. It can be found in dark leafy greens, asparagus, beets, milk, salmon, wheat, and beans.
- Cobalimin (B_{12}) supplements iron in its ability to produce red blood cells. It is only found in animal products such as red meats, pork, fish, mollusks, and dairy products.

Vitamin C (ascorbic acid) is one of the more popular vitamins. At one point, the double Nobel Prize–winner Linus Pauling believed that huge doses of vitamin C could cure cancer and the common cold—neither or which proved to be true. Nevertheless, vitamin C has been shown to help immunity by aiding in the production of collagen, which is used to repair skin, tissues, ligaments, and bones. It is also necessary for the enzymes that transport lipids to the mitochondria, which produce cellular energy. Natural sources of vitamin C include oranges (and most other fruits), peppers, kale, broccoli and cauliflower, and brussels sprouts.

Vitamin D is a nonhormonal secosteroid that is necessary for the metabolism of calcium. Deficiencies can lead to soft bones, which was a common affliction of malnutrition in the 1800s known as *rickets*. In adults, it can lead to osteoporosis. Vitamin D is very easily synthesized by passing cholesterol under ultraviolet (UV) light. Harry Steenbock developed a process by which milk could pass under the UV light, resulting in vitamin D–fortified milk. This process helped to eliminate rickets as a national problem among children during the 1920s. Vitamin D is also believed to stimulate the immune system. In addition to bone density, deficiencies in vitamin D are also linked to increased cancer risks (breast, colon, and prostate); heart disease; depression; and obesity. In addition to fortified milk, vitamin D is easily obtained from 15–30 minutes a day of direct exposure to the sun. Most glass windows, sunscreens, and other forms of UV protection will block the synthesis of vitamin D. The best natural source is to walk outside with exposed arms and skin for short durations.

Vitamin E (tocopherol) is primarily an antioxidant. It is brought to the liver after being absorbed in the intestines and then resynthesized into a variety of different forms. It is most important in limiting the creation of free radicals when lipids are transformed into energy in the mitochondria. It may also reduce risks of stroke and increase immunity. Among some cosmetically focused antiaging advocates, vitamins C and E are touted as especially critical antioxidants for avoiding wrinkles because they protect against the cellular damage caused by free radicals. In 2015, however, a study conducted by Michael Velarde at the Buck Institute for Research on Aging found that excessive amounts of free radicals in younger mice promoted healthier skin than for those with normal or reduced levels of free radicals. His research suggested that vitamin E may be less useful as a preventative measure against wrinkles for adults under the age of 50. After age 50, the oxidative stress caused by free radicals may be more harmful. Vitamin E may be found naturally in nuts, seeds, vegetable oils (especially wheat-germ oil), and spinach.

Natural Sources of Minerals

Like vitamins, nutritional minerals are compounds that are necessary for healthy metabolism. They differ from vitamins in that they all originate in the soil and are not created by plants or animals. Nevertheless, they remain essential to human nutrition. Plants get their minerals from the soil in which they grow, animals get them from the plants they eat, and humans can get them from both plants and animals. The most essential minerals are calcium, cobalt, iodine, iron (and copper), manganese, magnesium, phosphorus, potassium, selenium, sodium (and chloride), sulfur, and zinc. Most minerals are found in abundance in fruits, vegetables, and animal sources. It is rare for humans to be mineral deficient, especially for manganese, phosphorus, and selenium. In most cases, because it is used so much in preserving and processing foods, people often have far more sodium than they need. Also, as iodine is added to table salt in developed countries, iodine deficiency is also very rare (though it can be quite harmful when it occurs, especially among pregnant women). The remaining minerals (calcium, chromium, iron, copper, zinc, magnesium, and potassium) may be less abundant in unbalanced diets.

Potassium is a natural element found in leafy greens (spinach), grapes (raisins), blackberries, bananas, oranges, grapefruit, carrots, and potatoes. It is an essential mineral because it stimulates the electrochemical charge across cell membranes and is critical in helping muscles contract, which is especially important for cardiovascular health. There is also a link between potassium and lower blood pressure. It also serves to maintain normal water balances between cells and other body fluids and is important for moving nutrients into cells and waste out of cells. Antiaging researchers who believe in the waste accumulation theory of aging place a lot of attention on potassium because it is believed to clean up the unwanted compounds that can collect in older cells. Having too little potassium may lead to muscle cramps and irregular heartbeats. Too much potassium may also lead to irregular heart rhythms (including cardiac arrest), though it is very difficult to take in too much through natural food sources because the kidneys easily flush it out through the urine. Excess potassium levels are usually a sign of kidney disease.

Magnesium keeps bones strong and is critical to metabolic functions, particularly in regulating muscle and nerve functions, blood sugar, and blood pressure. The mineral is most often found in chlorophyll from green leafy vegetables (spinach), nuts, seeds, and whole grains. It is also found in most milk products. Magnesium can be age dependent, with men over the age of 70 and teenage girls most prone to deficiency. Too little magnesium can lead to mood disorders, muscle cramps, migraine headaches, and abnormal heart rhythms. There do not appear to be any harmful side effects of too much magnesium when ingested from natural foods. However, excessive amounts from extracted supplements may lead to heart disease, including irregular heartbeat and cardiac arrest.

Calcium is the most abundant mineral in the body and is critical to bones, teeth, muscle, blood, and the nervous system. It is so important that the body will ensure a constant supply for ordinary metabolic function regardless of dietary intake. If the diet does not provide enough calcium, the body simply takes what it needs from the bones, which means that calcium deficiency usually leads to osteoporosis. Up to 99 percent of calcium is stored in the bones and teeth, and the process of adding and extracting calcium in bone tissues is continual. In older ages, the extraction of calcium tends to outweigh the addition of calcium, which is why older adults (especially postmenopausal women) tend to be more vulnerable to osteoporosis. Calcium is found naturally in milk, yogurt, cheese, tofu, salmon, cabbage, and rhubarb. Deficiencies usually occur in conjunction with vitamin D deficiency because the vitamin is essential for the absorption of the mineral. Getting too much calcium from natural food sources is rare, but the high-volume extracts found in supplements may lead to increased risks of kidney stones, prostate cancer, and cardiovascular disease.

Iron, copper, and zinc are all trace minerals, which means the body needs very little of them to function. They are, nevertheless, very critical to proper health. Iron is especially important for the transmission of oxygen to the tissues and organs through the bloodstream. An iron deficiency results in anemia, which leads to shortness of breath, dizziness, and a general feeling of fatigue because the oxygen is not nourishing the cells at the level the body requires. Long-term side effects can include cardiovascular disease because the heart is forced to beat more rapidly to transmit sufficient amounts of oxygen throughout the body. Iron is found naturally in most meats and seafood as well as spinach, nuts, seeds, chocolate, and soybeans. Vegetarians and vegans need twice as much iron as meat eaters.

Copper works closely with iron to help form the red blood cells that carry oxygen through the body. Very little copper is needed, and most people easily obtain the mineral through natural dietary sources. Too much copper can be toxic to the brain, kidneys, and blood.

Zinc is important for protein synthesis that supports immunity, and it can be found in mollusks, clams, oysters, lamb, pork, and red meats. Zinc deficiency may lead to impotence in men as well as hair loss, weight loss, and difficulty in healing (skin and wounds). The side effects of too little zinc helped to create a popular theory that the mineral is a general immunity booster. The symptoms of zinc deficiency are similar to those of many age-related conditions. Research indicates, however, that too much zinc over an extended period of time can lead to similar symptoms as too little, particularly lower immunity, nausea, and loss of appetite. Mega doses of extracted zinc supplements may be as harmful as having too little zinc.

Ray Kurzwiel: Inventor and Transhumanist

Raymond (or Ray) Kurzweil was born to immigrant parents who had fled their Austrian homeland during Hitler's rise. His parents were both artists. Frederic Kurzweil was a musician, and his mother was a visual artist. Ray was born in New York City among the baby boomers who defined the 1950s and 1960s. While still in high school, he worked with his uncle at Bell Labs, where he designed a software program that could identify patterns in classical music and then recreate new compositions based on those patterns. He won first prize in an international science fair. Ray Kurzweil moved on to the Massachusetts Institute of Technology (MIT), where he developed another software program that could help place students in the most suitable college. He sold the company for more than $100,000 in 1968, before reaching his junior year. Over the course of the next decade, Kurzweil used his skills in pattern recognition software design to invent optical character recognition (OCR) and text-to-speech devices for the blind. He started and sold several technology companies and eventually moved into music synthesizer technology. Ray Kurzweil earned dozens of honorary doctorates and other science awards, including the National Medal of Technology, which he received from President Clinton in 1999.

When Ray Kurzweil was 35 years old, he was diagnosed with glucose intolerance, which typically leads to type 2 diabetes if left untreated. In response, he made significant changes to his diet and exercise habits and became increasingly interested in the power of technology to improve and enhance health and potentially extend life span. He began writing books on the subject in 1990 and published *The Age of Intelligent Machines*. The 20 books he has authored or coauthored include *The 10% Solution for a Healthy Life* (1993), *The Age of Spiritual Machines* (1998), *The Singularity Is Near* (2005), and *How to Create a Mind* (2013). In 2012, Kurzweil was selected as Google's director of technology. He is a member of the Alcor Life Extension Foundation and plans to have his body preserved cryogenically after his death.

Chromium has been found to be critical to insulin resistance and is linked to lower risks of diabetes. The body usually takes in more than enough chromium through normal diets, but these levels may be reduced by high-sugar diets, infections, pregnancy, or lactation. When chromium levels decrease, the risk of diabetes increases. There is some evidence to suggest that chromium levels decrease naturally with age. Some antiaging advocates believe chromium may help control diabetes, lower weight, and improve muscle strength. Unfortunately, it is difficult to determine chromium levels with any certainly because there are no reliable biomarkers to point to. Yet, chromium deficiency is strongly linked to the onset of diabetes. No clinical studies have examined the effectiveness of chromium supplements on counteracting age-related diseases, particularly diabetes. Other studies have found no improvement in body mass or composition. At the same time, there is also little evidence to suggest that too much chromium is harmful.

Vitamins, Minerals, and Herbs as Supplements

Most supplements come in a pill form, but there are a variety of options that include capsules, softgels, liquids, chewable tablets, bulk powders, and hard lozenges. Consumers often form strong opinions about one format over another, but research indicates that as long as the digestive system is working properly, all forms are likely to break down with sufficient efficiency. The difference is mostly in the speed of digestion. Typically, there is no more than an hour's difference between the absorption of a liquid versus the absorption of a solid tablet, and that delay will not result in any significant nutritional difference. However, This does not mean that all supplements will be equally absorbed into the metabolism. This problem is more a function of the active ingredient in the supplement than it is a problem with the particular form that enters the body. The supplements may enter the bloodstream, but the body may not use them in equal proportions. If the body already has sufficient amounts, the excess will simply be flushed away through the urine stream.

But do they work? There is a strong consensus within the medical community that the best way to achieve healthy levels of vitamins and minerals is through a balanced diet. Supplements may potentially address certain deficiencies, but in most cases, they do not noticeably add to health if they are taken when no deficiencies are present. Most of the research on the subject is negative. In 2013, in response to an increasingly growing supplement industry, the United States Preventative Services Task Force met to evaluate the health benefits of supplemental vitamins, minerals, and herbs. In their report, they did not recommend regular use of vitamins, though they found little evidence that they caused any harm. There were, however, some exceptions. They explicitly recommended not taking herbal supplements because it is a completely unregulated industry; the consumer does not always know what is in the product. Moreover, they recommended consumers not take beta-carotene or vitamin E. Beta-carotene is a precursor to vitamin A, and excessive levels can diminish the absorption of calcium and lead to bone loss (osteoporosis). Similarly, too much vitamin E is harmful because it has been linked to increased risks of prostate cancer and may lead to digestive problems, fatigue, and slow healing. Sufficient amounts of both of these vitamins can be obtained through healthy diets, and they seem to be processed more efficiently that way than the extracted versions.

There were other exceptions. Vitamin B_{12} does not seem to be absorbed as easily through natural foods for adults over the age of 50. In addition, vegetarians and vegans will not likely take in enough of this vitamin because they avoid meats. Also, pregnant women require more folic acid (B_9) than is typically found in normal diets. The Task Force recommended supplements for pregnant women and women who are planning to become pregnant. Finally, vitamin D supplements are recommended for adults over the age of 65, especially for those at risk of falling (and who may need to heal).

A 2011 Iowa Women's Health Study examined 38,000 women over a period of 20 years. They reported that women who took daily vitamins tended to die sooner than those who did not. This study requires some caution. It was a correlational population study, and there was no evidence to establish a causal link between vitamins and increased death rates. One possible explanation is that those with compromised systems were also more likely to take daily vitamins, in which case it was the preexisting disease and not the vitamins that influenced death rates. Nevertheless, the general consensus among health practitioners is that a proper diet is the best way to ensure balanced nutrition. Supplements will not offset a poor diet.

Part of the problem with supplemental extracts of vitamins and minerals is that the critical ingredient is removed from its biological context. The multitude of bioagents found in a raw vegetable (spinach, for example) are far more complex than a collection of individual vitamins. Spinach includes vitamins K, C, E, and B_1, B_2, B_6, and B_9. Its minerals include manganese, iron, copper, calcium, potassium, phosphorus, and choline. Yet they are all meshed together in a dietary fiber that contains significant proteins, calories, and other bioagents that are unique to spinach. A single multivitamin may include some or all of these vitamins and minerals, but they would be removed from the fibrous package of the spinach leaf. More importantly, the combination of each vitamin affects the absorption of the others. For example, the high oxalate content in spinach binds the heavy calcium levels, resulting in an absorption rate of about 5 percent of the total calcium in the plant. That may seem like a drawback, except that the body does not require equal amounts of each vitamin and mineral. The particular combination in spinach ensures a proper balance for human consumption. A multivitamin may include a wide variety of these with no natural balance, resulting in potential excesses.

Traditional versus Alternative Medicine

Needless to say, there is considerable debate over this subject. The sheer number of supplements taken by Ray Kurzweil indicates that at least some antiaging advocates believe that the natural diet cannot provide the ratios of particular nutrients needed to overcome the traditional limitations of cellular decline and disease. Among the general public, there is often a debate between traditional medicine, which is sometimes viewed as motivated primarily by financial and corporate interests, and alternative medicine, which is sometimes described as more natural or legitimate. In this debate, the pharmaceutical companies are grouped in with traditional medicine because their products are heavily regulated by the Food and Drug Administration (FDA). By contrast, the supplement companies do not require any regulatory oversight. Rather than being viewed as a negative, the lack of FDA regulation of nontraditional medicine is often described as a freedom from corporate pressures. The fact that both the pharmaceutical companies and the supplement companies are large corporations does not necessarily change the argument for the general consumer.

In practice, the pharmaceutical companies frequently describe supplements as potentially dangerous due to the absence of regulatory oversight, while the supplement companies describe prescription medicines as potentially dangerous due to the clinical sterility of corporate research. The debate has done little to limit the popularity of either side. As of 2015, there were 65,000 supplements on the market. During the same year, there were more than 4 billion prescriptions sold at pharmacies across the United States. More than 60 percent of adults took prescription drugs in 2015, which was up from 50 percent in 1999. The most common types of drugs sold in 2015 (80 percent) were those used to manage heart disease, high blood pressure, diabetes, and high cholesterol, all of which may be associated with age-related conditions.

Herbal Supplements

Alternative medicine may be defined as any remedy that is not based on biochemical science but instead relies on traditional explanations that often defy clinical research. Typically, alternative medical traditions owe their roots to Indian (called *ayurvedic*), Chinese (often called *TCM*, or *traditional Chinese medicine*), Native American, or medieval European practices that date back before the advent of the scientific revolution. In Eastern traditions, these remedies are based on an animistic belief that plants and physical movements in the material world can influence the more potent powers of the immaterial world. Similarly, in Western traditions, many of the nontraditional remedies were used as magical reagents that forced an immaterial solution to a material problem.

As these alternative remedies have been passed down into the modern age, most of the mythical explanations have been stripped from their descriptions. Instead, modern retailers tend to rely on ambiguous claims of historical authority. As one Internet retailer explained, "Where ancient wisdom meets modern medicine." Unfortunately, the historical record does not often justify the claims of authority. Most chronicles of Western doctors practicing in India and China during the 19th century describe rather gruesome conditions for local populations. Most internal maladies, such as fevers, cholera, and appendicitis, were treated with a combination of physical pressures and mystical incantations. Patients frequently died from septic reactions that only an understanding of germs and internal medicine would have prevented. In some cases, the use of mercury, lead, or arsenic poisoned the patient to the point of death. When these Western doctors (usually missionaries) entered into a region, they often faced local resistance. Very quickly, however, the resistance faded, and these Western clinics and hospitals were usually overrun with patients who found successful treatments for ailments that had long been untouched by their indigenous practices.

The reality of ancient remedies was far less romantic than modern marketing suggests. As herbal supplements do not require FDA certification, most of them do not have clinical research to support their claims of effectiveness. For this reason, herbal supplements and alternative medicine have become natural partners. Since 2010, the FDA does require that all supplements comply with "good manufacturing practices," but that only means that they should not be shown to be explicitly harmful. For the modern consumer, most herbal supplements have been divorced from their ancient roots in Eastern (or Western) mythology. Ginseng and ginger were both popularized as alternative remedies, but today they are viewed as somewhat exotic ingredients to be included in modern fusion recipes. The associated explanations from ayurvedic and TCM mythology are mostly forgotten, though their medicinal properties continue to be presumed, rather than demonstrated, by modern science. In part, this separation of herbal medicine from the mythological roots is reinforced by the fact that most grocery stores sell their herbal supplements right next to their vitamins and minerals. The packaging is usually very similar, and the average consumer does not necessarily distinguish the types of supplements.

For the purposes of antiaging, most supplements (vitamins, minerals, and herbs) are taken for their antioxidant properties. This reflects the growing dominance of the oxidative stress theory of aging, which argues that cells lose their ability to faithfully replicate and repair themselves as a result of the damage caused by excess free radicals within and outside the cellular membrane. The most common antioxidants among the vitamins are A, C, and E. Other critical antioxidant enzymes are superoxide dismutase (SOD), catalase, and glutathione peroxidase. The problem with taking these protein enzymes directly is that they tend to break down very quickly in the gastrointestinal tract.

One of the reasons why herbal supplements have become popular within the antiaging movement is that they are valued for their ability to carry antioxidant proteins past the stomach to facilitate the production of SODs. Some of these supplements include milk thistle, ashwaganda, and bacopa—each of which owe their initial popularity to ayurvedic medical traditions. As a large portion of antiaging researchers are clinically based in traditional scientific methodology, there have been a number of research studies on each of these ingredients. As with ginger and ginseng, the results have been mostly mixed. Some benefits were apparent in small measures during in vitro tests, but they could not easily be distinguished from the benefits that might be expected from any other antioxidant.

A significant segment of the antiaging community are not scientists but lay consumers who are convinced that the combination of modern technology and medicine (in whichever form it takes) will find a successful solution to age-related conditions and perhaps even death itself. These might be called amateur antiaging enthusiasts. For these consumers, the dichotomy between traditional medicine and alternative medicine seems to mirror the other dichotomy between traditional gerontologists who believe in a fixed life span and the progressive antiaging researchers who believe that the human life span is indeterminate. From this comparison, the potential for alternative medicine to find an elusive cure that may have been ignored by traditional Western medicine is appealing. The added claims of "ancient wisdom meeting modern science" can be very compelling.

The perceived value of these non-FDA-regulated supplements is further enhanced when they are derived from chemical compounds that are found in human metabolism. In these instances, it is not the mythological traditions of ancient wisdom but the modern tradition of common sense that makes an herbal supplement popular; science identifies the compound, and amateur antiaging literature explains why they *should* work. Many of the most popular antiaging supplements combine traditional ingredients with modern chemical compounds, which reflects the very essence of "antiquity meeting modernity." The conviction that it is possible to extend life is often enough to build consumer confidence that one or more supplements will help to make that goal possible. In these cases, the fact that supplements are not verified by clinical research or medical practice makes little difference. Some of the more popular antiaging supplements include the following:

- Probiotic supplements are used for digestion and boosting immunity. Probiotics were initially identified and promoted by Élie Metchnikoff in the 1890s, based on his belief that all diseases originate in the stomach and intestines. As such, probiotics are believed to build immunity to other diseases because they boost the phagocytes in the intestines. It is, however, mostly based on Metchnikoff's 19th-century theories and not on modern research. In the 21st century, probiotics have been repurposed as an antiwrinkle agent for skin protection. A 2016 study provided some evidence that probiotics may lessen photoaging, improve hair quality, and limit oxidative stress on skin by restoring acidic pH balance. These effects relate to cosmetic antiaging, and there is no evidence that probiotics will extend human life span.

- Ginkgo (also known as ginkgo biloba) is used to improve memory and defer dementia. This is a legacy of traditional Chinese medicine and is associated as a treatment for asthma, cancer, digestive disorders, and irritable bowels. In the modern era, the aglucone flavone compound within ginkgo has been identified as an antioxidant and has mostly been studied for its effects on memory, autoimmunity, and general well-being. The clinical research was mixed. There was some evidence to support claims of mild improvements in memory and alertness, and it may improve circulation. A 2014 in vitro study from China found some evidence to suggest that ginkgo may improve immunity function. There were also studies from 2004 and 2005 that indicated people taking the supplement "felt better." Human results, however, were mostly self-reported, and the conclusions remained correlational and not causal. Large clinical studies conducted by the National Institutes of Health affirm that there is no evidence that ginkgo has any positive effect for treating or preventing Alzheimer's disease or other forms of dementia. There is also no conclusive evidence that ginkgo will extend human life span.

- Melatonin is a real hormone synthesized in the pineal gland that is involved with regulating sleep patterns. It is light sensitive and is mostly responsible for triggering sleepiness after it becomes dark. Melatonin does not initiate sleep; it only tells the body when to sleep. Most people who have difficulty sleeping are not melatonin deficient: their sleep disturbances are often due to other environmental or social stresses (caffeine, overwork, stress, etc.). Melatonin is available in relatively high doses (3–10 times the natural levels found in the body) as an over-the-counter supplement. Doctors may recommend it for people who work night shifts and need to adjust their natural sleep patterns. Research, however, suggests that higher doses may be less effective than lower doses and may have other unintended side effects as a contraceptive. Many countries outside of the United States have banned the drug without a prescription. For antiaging purposes, melatonin is used both for its antioxidant properties and as a sleep inducer, as sleep is recognized as an important part of healthy living and long life. Research does not support either indication, as melatonin does not initiate sleep and its antioxidant properties are minimal.

- Pycnogenol is derived from the bark of a pine tree. It is traditionally used for circulation problems, allergies, asthmas, tinnitus, high blood pressure, muscle aches, diabetes, ADHD, reproductive issues, erectile dysfunction, and as a virtual cure-all. In the modern era, there have been some studies to suggest pycnogenol may improve blood circulation and alleviate minor allergy issues related to trees. It is an antioxidant and has become popular within antiaging circles. From a biochemical perspective, the extract has generally not been shown to be effective for the wide number of cures that it is traditionally used for. Research suggests, however, that it is mostly safe, though long-term use may cause dizziness, digestion problems, headaches, and mouth ulcers.

- Echinacea comes from the purple coneflower and is part of the medicinal traditions of the North American native populations. The indications have changed. Originally used to treat general aches and pains, in the modern era, it has become more associated as an immunity booster. It is very popular both as a cure and a deterrent for the common cold and cancer. Numerous studies have failed to find evidence that it has any effect in either indication. Echinacea became popular within the antiaging community after a 2005 population study conducted at McGill University using mice suggested some extension of average life expectancy. Additional in vitro research suggested mild benefits for immunity, but there was little evidence of increasing animal life span. No studies have been directed using humans. The most common commercial use of echinacea is as a topical cosmetic for skin problems.

- L-theanine is an amino acid extracted from the leaves of gyokuro tea, which is popular in Japan. It was originally intended to promote sleep and relaxation and to boost concentration, which were the traditional medicinal uses of gyokuro tea in Japan. As the antioxidant properties of green tea became popularized in the early 2000s, L-theanine became associated with all the same benefits. Within the antiaging community, the supplement has been used to avoid and combat cancer, obesity, and Alzheimer's disease and to lower blood pressure. There is some evidence that large amounts of green tea may have antioxidant effects, but the research also suggests that the active ingredient does not have the same effectiveness when removed from the context of the green tea. In 2012, a population study of roundworms found potential for extending natural life expectancy. No research has been conducted on human life span or its effects on general health.

- Omega-3 is found in fish oil and has been a popular medicinal reagent in England since before the 1600s, especially in the form of cod liver oil. The active ingredients in fish oil are omega fatty acids, which contain eicosapentaenoic acid (EPA) and docosahexaenic acid (DHA) that thin the blood and reduce inflammation. It is often used as an anti-inflammatory, for anticancer, and as a general immunity and cognition booster. Omega-3 supplements became especially popular after the rise of the Mediterranean and Okinawan diets, which emphasize large portions of fish, as many large wild fish are susceptible to mercury poisoning and other toxins in the oceans. Subsequent research affirms that eating fish may reduce the risk of heart disease, but more than two dozen studies conducted between 2005 and 2013 indicated omega-3 alone does not affect cholesterol levels, reduce risks of heart attack or stroke, nor have any impact on cognitive disorders such as dementia or Alzheimer's disease. Despite the frequent reports of the relative ineffectiveness of omega-3, the sales of fish oil have continued to increase. Recent studies have suggested that excessive use of omega-3 may be hazardous if combined with blood thinners such as aspirin, leading to bruises and nosebleeds. By contrast, eating fish is still recommended because fish contains many other nutrients and not just omega-3.

- Coenzyme Q10 (also known as CoQ10) is a natural antioxidant found in every cell that helps in the conversion of lipids into energy. As a synthetic supplement, it is thought to help fight Parkinson's disease and heart failure, improve male reproduction, and boost immunity. Some research indicates that people who took CoQ10 within three days of a heart attack were less likely to have subsequent attacks. Also, it may help to lower blood pressure, but it usually requires extensive use (4 to 12 weeks) and is most often used in conjunction with other prescription medicines. There is no scientific evidence that it lowers cholesterol, improves immunity, or has any impact on diabetes or male reproduction. It is most valued by the anti-aging movement as an antioxidant and because it appears that the natural levels of CoQ10 decline with age. It is popular to assume that the effects of age-related conditions may be avoided by artificially augmenting the enzymes and hormones that naturally decline with age. Clinical research has not often affirmed this theory. Recently, researchers at McGill University have cast doubt on the antioxidant properties of CoQ10. Studies of the active compound in CoQ10 (ubiquinone) did not exhibit significant antioxidant properties. Nor is there any causal evidence to suggest CoQ10 extends human life span.

- Glucosamine and chondroitin sulfate were originally developed for veterinary medicine, but they have been marketed for joint pain relief since the 1990s. These enzymes are related to fatty acids found in fish oils and have been promoted as an anti-inflammatory. Most of the research has been conducted by the same company that originally marketed the supplement (Rottapharm). Clinical tests suggest these enzymes may provide relief for moderate to severe pain, but not for most mild stiffness or aches. They were embraced by the antiaging community as antioxidants, especially after a 2014 study affirmed antioxidant properties in an in vitro experiment. The population study also found some increase in the life expectancy among mice. No in vivo studies in humans have been conducted. Potential side effects include upset stomach, nausea, heartburn, and diarrhea. Otherwise, there is little harm in the supplement.

- St. John's wort is the nickname for goat weed, scientifically called *Hypericum perforatum*. It earned its popular name from an association with St. John the Baptist, who was believed to appear in the dreams of those who slept under the herb on the eve of his feast day and would give a blessing guaranteeing another year of life. It is part of the medieval reagent tradition in the West and was used to heal wounds and kidney problems and to protect against insanity and demonic possession. Like garlic, it was also used to repel vampires. In modern times, it is often used to combat depression. One clinical study conducted by the University of Maryland Medical Center suggests it is useful for mild to moderate depression. It may enhance moods, but it is ineffective for severe depression. It is often used by antiaging advocates as a general stress reliever based on the theory that a stress-free lifestyle enhances longevity. It is often used as an anti-inflammatory. When taken topically, St. John's wort is supposed to reduce wrinkles, but when taken orally, it actually makes the skin more sensitive to UV rays, which can increase wrinkles. No clinical evidence exists to support life extension or that it promotes general healthiness in humans.

- Saw palmetto was used by the ancient Mayans and later by the Seminole tribes of Florida as a general protection against diseases, particularly aches, pains, and infertility. It was also used to enhance female breast size, promote lactation, and prevent male impotence. In the modern era, saw palmetto has been used to treat and prevent urinary problems, prostate health, and male impotence (poor libido). It contains DHT, which is a precursor to anabolic steroids. Some population studies indicated improvement in urine flow for those patients with urinary problems. It was been used by antiaging advocates as a nonprescription alternative to anabolic steroids, which some antiaging advocates believe to be the key to longevity because they are age dependent. DHT is only a precursor hormone, though, and the body does not automatically synthesize testosterone just because there are elevated levels of DHT. As discussed in the next chapter, even if DHT did lead to an increase in anabolic steroid synthesis, there is little evidence to suggest an ultimate increase in life expectancy. As an herbal supplement, there is no clinical evidence to support claims of antiaging benefits.

CONCLUSION

Since 2006, several studies have suggested multivitamins and other supplements have no impact on health or other chronic age-related conditions unless the diet is already deficient (vegans). A National Institutes of Health study in 2006, called the Women's Health Initiative, compared 161,808 women aged 50–79 years and found no appreciable difference between those who took multivitamins and those who did not. Another study in 2011 examined 182,099 men and women aged 45–75 with similar results. A study of 14,641 physicians aged 50 and older also indicated no appreciable difference between those who took daily vitamins and those that did not. The essential vitamins and minerals are critical to health, but it is not clear that multivitamins provide more benefit than not taking any supplements at all. There is strong consensus among the medical community that the best way to maintain healthy nutrition is through a balanced and diverse diet.

Supplements cannot make up for an unhealthy diet, but they may be useful for older adults who are taking other prescribed medications and need to offset certain nutritional side effects. One problem facing consumers is that the lack of FDA oversight of herbal supplements raises concerns about purity and standardization. Some vendors may be unscrupulous, but even if they are completely honest, all supplements face an inherent problem of consistency. Part of the difficulty with single-ingredient supplements is that they do not often reflect the complexity of the original compound. In vitamins, for example, nutritionists usually refer to a family of compounds by a common name. Vitamin B helps energy. Yet, there are at least eight chemical variants in the vitamin B family, and each variant contributes in a slightly different way to the human metabolism. There are also at least eight variations of vitamin E. Often, biochemists have identified potential variants, but they cannot easily isolate them. The body synthesizes at least five variants of vitamin D, but scientists have great difficulty isolating them outside the body. The point is that supplements that mimic compounds in the body do not always include the chemical variations that the body relies on. In this way, supplements may not always provide the same efficacy in isolation and may lose some of their effectiveness as an extraction.

Another problem is that the vitamins and minerals found in plants and animal tissues are ordered by a natural balance that was determined by the organism's native metabolism. Humans absorb nutrients most effectively when they are combined with many other bioagents found in the original foods. For example, the ratio of minerals and vitamins in the muscle tissue of beef were determined by the cow's endocrine system, and it is unlikely that the compounds will interact negatively with each other. Commercially produced multivitamins, by contrast, are combined by artificial means and may not always interact consistently. For example, zinc lowers the absorption of copper, vitamin B_1 reduces the effectiveness of vitamins B_{12} and B_6, and both magnesium and zinc limit the absorption of calcium. Yet, all six compounds may be found in the same pill.

In addition, some vitamins are fat soluble (A, D, E, and K), while others are water soluble (B and C). Likewise, the effectiveness of some supplements changes depending on whether they are taken with food or on an empty stomach, or whether they are taken in the morning at the start of the day or at the day's end. Fat-soluble vitamins tend to last longer because they are stored in the tissues of the body and may become toxic, whereas excessive amounts of water-soluble vitamins are more easily flushed out through the urine, though even water-soluble supplements can build up in certain nervous tissues or may overwork the body's natural filters in the liver and kidneys. As many multivitamins include large doses of each compound, the upper limits of daily intake are more likely to be reached when they are combined with other fortified foods, such as milk, cereal, and many health snacks. The combinations and portions of each commercially produced vitamin and mineral is not limited to the ratios naturally found in dietary foods.

Not only do various vitamins and minerals interact with each other, but they can also interact with other supplements and with other medications. For example, combining fish oil with other anti-blood-clotting supplements (like ginkgo) may cause internal bleeding. Taking fish oil with artificial oral contraceptives may counteract the blood pressure effects. Calcium supplements limit the absorption of osteoporosis drugs and reduce the effectiveness of certain antibiotics. Vitamin D may negate the effects of cholesterol-lowering prescription drugs and may also enhance calcium levels, resulting in kidney stones. Physicians want to know what other supplements their patients are taking so they can be prepared for unexpected interactions. Often, these supplements are taken by consumers without physician oversight. Many herbal supplements do not include potential lists of interactions, and they may undermine the effectiveness of other drugs.

The Perfect Antiaging Elixir

There is always some concern that the marketing of any superfood, diet plan, or supplement may overemphasize the reported benefits. The nature of advertising and marketing is to set the product apart from others, and so it is understandable that vendors promote their products as the *most* healthful available. The term *superfood* presupposes that they are better than other foods, and it is easy to believe that one ingredient or one compound will cure all ills if taken regularly. The mixture of appeals to both tradition and technology is compelling, so manufacturers of certain supplements (such as ginseng, ginkgo, or echinacea) naturally describe each as "the oldest and most popular supplement on the market." Market promotions naturally compare themselves to other products, but clinical research rarely does. As a result, consumer expectations often exceed actual results. For example, gingko supplements have been shown to improve alertness, but there is no evidence that it does so more than a cup of coffee. Is St. John's wort more effective at enhancing mood than a bar of dark chocolate? Is glucosamine and chondroitin sulfate more effective than routine exercise?

As supplements are not required to list all possible side effects of interactions, it is often difficult for the consumer to weigh the health benefits and potential costs of taking them. Supplements are not medications, and no supplement has been proven to prevent or cure any disease or ailment. Ultimately, they cannot promise anything more than the ability to contribute to a generally healthy lifestyle. Further claims would trigger FDA regulations and require substantial clinical evidence to support the assertion, along with a comprehensive list of known side effects. Instead, they must rely on the consumer's willingness to believe in their potency.

Consumers should also be aware of the general theories upon which these diet plans, supplements, and other recommendations are based. Many of the recommendations of alternative medicine owe their origins to prescientific cultures that presumed a magical interaction between the material and physical worlds. These presumptions do not often hold today, and yet the popularity of their remedies remain. Even among the purely scientific recommendations, many treatments are based on theories of aging (or science) that have not been decisively proven. The paleo diet presupposes that humans evolved with no guiding purpose, and therefore modern agricultural diets are contrary to the nature of human digestive system. A critic who believes that God intentionally created humans with a purpose would argue that their digestive systems were intended for agricultural diets and not the other way around. Similarly, the value of antioxidants is mostly based on a single theory of aging, which argues that cells break down and decay as a result of too many free radicals.

There are several other theories of aging, and the free radical theory is only the most popular at the moment. At least two studies in 2015 have questioned that theory. In addition to the Michael Velarde study at the Buck Institute for Research on Aging, which suggested excess amounts of free radicals in younger mice may actually promote healthier skin, there was another study the same year conducted at the Memorial Sloan-Kettering Cancer Center in New York that found evidence that antioxidants might increase the metastasis of cancer in mice. It is possible that antiaging researchers have made incorrect conclusions about the purpose and presence of free radicals. In the 1990s, shortened telomere lengths were viewed as a negative process leading to cellular senescence and aging, whereas more recent research suggests they are necessary feedback mechanisms to prevent cells from becoming cancerous. Similarly, current theories argue that free radicals are the cause of oxidative stress, yet other equally recent research suggests that oxidative stress may be a function of other processes. Free radicals may have an unknown, but necessary, function in maintaining healthy cells.

Future research may refute the free radical theory, or it may affirm it. Medical science is always imperfect and is more or less constantly in flux. It takes a great deal of faith in current scholarship to blindly follow only one recommendation of today's leading authorities. Chances are likely that the recommendations in 50 years, or even 20 years, may be significantly changed as further research uncovers new and as of yet unknown processes.

At heart, the problem of relying on particular diet plans and supplements to maintain health and prolong life is that science still has no certain answers as to why we get old, why we develop age-related conditions, and why we contract age-related diseases. If we do not know the cause of Alzheimer's disease, we cannot take effective measures to prevent it. If we do not truly understand the biochemical chain of causation behind sarcopenia or autoimmune degeneration or even gray hair, we cannot hope to reverse these effects. Proper diet and exercise will help to maintain a healthy lifestyle, but there is nothing to guarantee that a healthy person will not succumb to any of these conditions or diseases. Scientific evidence does not support one kind of food over another, nor one collection of supplements over another, but the modern futurist is not driven by current scientific evidence as much as he or she is driven by the hope that science will one day find an answer. It is the increasing faith in material solutions as the only compelling force in determining health and life span that most drives the antiaging movement.

Chapter 12

What Can We Do Now to Extend Our Lives with a Prescription and Future Technology?

In 2007, Dr. Sanjay Gupta, the chief medical correspondent for CNN, published a book titled *Chasing Life* with the subtitle *New Discoveries in the Search for Immortality to Help You Age Less Today*. Gupta begins his book with an account of his visit to a Russian antiaging clinic run by Alexander Tepliashin, who promised the modern equivalent of the fountain of youth through periodic injections of a special elixir made from the client's own stem cells. The theory behind Tepliashin's treatments is not secret: he took stem cells from fatty tissues found in the abdomen or thigh and then multiplied the cells in vitro to create a serum unique to the individual to be reinserted in various areas around the body to rejuvenate aging skin, muscles, and general metabolism. He claimed to be able to treat age-related conditions and diseases, including Alzheimer's disease, heart disease, and wrinkles. Treatments cost anywhere from $12,000 to $30,000, and Tepliashin's clinic was full of customers.

Sanjay Gupta never wrote about whether Tepliashin's treatments actually worked, but he was clear that such treatments would certainly be illegal in the United States and in most countries of Europe. According to popular reports and published anecdotes, the stem-cell treatments seemed to work, and hundreds of wealthy customers testified to their effectiveness. At the same time, however, people who pay thousands of dollars per treatment most likely already believe in the theory, even before they take the product. Few people are willing to admit that they wasted such large sums of money on a placebo, or worse. Stem-cell clinics have opened up elsewhere in Central and South America, India, and China and any other region where enforcement of medical regulation is lax.

Not all the anecdotes are positive. There have been many cases of stem-cell therapies resulting in harmful tumor growths or triggering genetic mutations that lead to other diseases. Yet, the influence of the positive testimonials is often stronger than the less-publicized negatives, and the potential of hope is difficult to resist. The greatest power of these and other antiaging regimens lies in the faith of the consumer. Just as modern consumers are often easily convinced by the potential of supplements and programmed diets, so too a fair segment of the population has high confidence in the ability of science to significantly alter the human body in a way that defies its natural tendencies toward disease, decay, and death.

There is a difference, though, between the level of personal commitment required for special diets and supplements and the level required to take prescriptions that carry potentially harsh side effects and may be illegal. It is easier to believe that proper diet and exercise are both healthy and may add years to our lives. If the life-extension promise proves false, at least consumers can trust that their efforts contributed to a generally healthy lifestyle. But there is a thin line between pursuing a heathy lifestyle and chasing the potential fountain of youth that may carry significant financial, physical, and emotional risks if it fails. The level of commitment, confidence, and faith in these treatments is much higher.

This chapter examines options that require at least a prescription and, in some cases, the willingness of the consumer to violate existing laws. We begin with a look at some of the ethical concerns that might face patients, doctors, and pharmaceutical companies with regard to taking antiaging drugs. Then we look at the most popular prescriptions that have been used since the 1990s, with special attention to the changes in popularity of some drugs over others. The chapter closes with a discussion of future technologies that promise to combat aging and death. These not only include promising prosthetics but also the potential of shifting human consciousness from the body to a machine. The transhumanist movement is a natural outgrowth of the innate faith in scientific potential that underlies the antiaging movement. It is this shift of focus from an old faith in immaterial ends to a new faith in material potentials that drives the modern search for the fountain of youth.

PROACTIVE BIOCHEMISTRY

To be proactive means to make a deliberate effort to change conditions in a way that leads to favorable results. Rather than reacting to problems as they arise, a proactive position seeks out potential solutions and sets them in place before problems have a chance to develop. In terms of health care, a proactive approach focuses most on preventative medicine. Proactive biochemistry does not seek to cure an age-related disease as much as it seeks to prevent the disease or condition from ever forming. As the antiaging research community is still on the beginning side of this movement, their work also focuses on treating existing diseases (heart disease, dementia, and cancer) as a necessary first step in the approach. Ultimately, though, the successful antiaging treatment plan will no longer include the need to "cure"—only to "prevent."

The bulk of consumers who pursue antiaging treatments are not looking for cures for their existing ailments. Most are driven by a desire to prevent and evade the effects of aging. For this reason, the "success" of a particular treatment is often difficult to define. A patient may take a treatment for 10 years with no appreciable changes and believe that the treatment has been successful precisely because there have been no changes. In other cases, a patient may begin to feel the effects of age through a loss of physical conditioning or decline in energy, and he or she may take treatments to reverse these effects—and he or she may experience immediate positive results. Yet, it is difficult to determine whether the positive changes came as a result of the treatments or as a result of the patient's renewed commitment to change his or her lifestyle (a proactive approach to life). These ambiguities raise important ethical concerns for both the patient and the physician.

Black Market Therapy

There are currently no legally approved antiaging drugs. In fact, there are no drugs of any kind that can be officially prescribed to treat aging. This is because no medical regulatory body in the world recognizes "aging" as a disease, and therefore there is no basis by which to measure the effectiveness of any drug intended to treat it. In practical terms, that means that every drug that is used for antiaging purposes is being used "off-label"—which means it is used in a way that was not approved by the Food and Drug Administration (FDA). It is not illegal for a doctor to prescribe drugs off-label. It is illegal for retailers to sell pharmaceuticals for that purpose, and it may be illegal for consumers to use certain regulated drugs without a prescription (though the latter group is rarely prosecuted). Nevertheless, nearly one in five prescription drugs is legally prescribed off-label. The FDA only regulates drug approval and does not regulate drug prescription. Nevertheless, the entire market for prescription-based antiaging drugs is off-label, and therefore unregulated by the FDA or DEA, except indirectly.

That does not mean that research scientists may not continue to explore and discover potential antiaging remedies using any and every chemical compound available. The FDA does regulate drug approval. Research is restricted by extensive regulations that ensure proper safeguards for experiments that involve living subjects, whether they are animals, children, or consenting adults. Research that is conducted outside the oversight of institutional review boards is illegal in most developed countries. Their findings are generally excluded from publication, and they lose their source of legitimacy and credibility within the scientific community. Any drug that purports to have been developed completely in secret from any government oversight is either deceptive or is otherwise working in opposition to the recognized scientific community.

Within the antiaging marketplace, some retailers may claim to have access to "secret" or "miraculous" antiaging treatments that the established authorities seek to shut down. The element of conspiratorial science may be compelling for a certain segment of consumers, but such drugs do not hold a legitimate place in the antiaging movement. This chapter will only consider the prescription drugs that have followed legitimate scientific methodologies, even if they are often prescribed for off-label or illegal purposes.

The Ethics of Treating Aging as a Disease

What would happen if the medical community suddenly chose to classify the process of aging as a disease? There would be certain social consequences almost immediately. In chapter 9, we discussed the problem of age discrimination, which occurs when society treats age as if it were a disability. Older adults are treated as less able and less capable than their younger counterparts and are thus not recognized as fully contributing members of society. Yet, the antiaging movement is entirely based on the conviction that age is a disease that needs to be cured with all available resources. This raises ethical dilemmas, not only in terms of respecting the priorities of the antiageism movement but also in terms of medical practice. If the process of aging were a disease to be prevented, at what point is a physician required to intervene? At which point would a doctor's unwillingness to treat the disease be considered malpractice? When is it too early to start treatments? When is it negligent to postpone them? At what point is a treatment "therapeutic," and at what point is it "cosmetic" or "voluntary enhancement"?

A 65-year-old man may visit a doctor to request a prescription for testosterone because he is losing muscle strength and the television commercials warn him that he may be suffering from "low testosterone." It is a fact that adults lose muscle strength as they get older; it is called age-related sarcopenia, and it is a natural condition. Adult males also begin to have declining rates of testosterone after age 40, and it is an expected part of healthy aging. Is the 65-year-old man suffering from a disease, or is he experiencing the normal conditions of a healthy man his age? How should the doctor respond? In practice, the 65-year-old man may have exactly the proper levels of testosterone that are expected for a man his age, yet he is looking to maintain levels of testosterone expected for a man half his age. Does he suffer from a disease or a desire?

These questions have significant policy implications, and in a future world where age-related conditions become treatable, they may have serious ethical consequences as well. Currently, health insurance companies will usually not cover cosmetic or elective procedures. If the age-induced reduction of testosterone levels is not viewed as a disease, insurance companies will not pay for the treatments. If it is treated as a disease, what would prevent younger men from requesting the same treatment because they are not as strong as they would like to be or their testosterone levels are not as high as they would prefer? What would prevent competitive athletes from claiming that they need higher-than-average levels to maintain their elite levels of performance? And if insurance companies chose not to cover these age-related conditions, would the promise of a fountain of youth be limited only to those with sufficient economic means? The antiaging movement frequently speaks of pushing the boundaries of science for the benefit of all mankind, but what if only a small portion of mankind is allowed to enjoy its fruits?

The antiaging movement has been confronting these philosophical issues almost as long as it has drawn serious attention from the biomedical research community. Antiaging treatments are often indistinguishable from the treatments used for preventative care. Insurance companies generally do not cover vitamins and supplements unless there is a specific deficiency caused by a particular condition (such as a cancer patient taking iron supplements to offset the effects of radiation treatments). The differences in distinguishing therapeutic and elective needs lay mostly in the motivations of the patient and the physician. For the time being, almost all antiaging treatments that require the oversight of a physician are considered elective, or cosmetic, and must be paid for out of pocket—and must not be justified as a treatment for "aging." Mostly, this is because the process of aging and its age-related conditions are as yet incurable. There is no available treatment for being "old," and so there is no compulsion for society to provide financial support for it. If a reliable treatment is found, however, the ethical implications will be significant and will require considerable public debate over what, when, and how age ought to be treated.

Dangers of the Black Market

Most antiaging research is directed toward uncovering and understanding the obscure processes of molecular biology related to DNA transcription, cellular repair, and senescence. The reports in scientific journals speak mostly of chemical ratios found through in vitro experiments or of comparative interactions between a compound and the mortality rates of a population of organisms. A great deal of antiaging research has no immediate practical results except in contributing to a larger body of knowledge that science uses to direct and guide future avenues of experimentation. Practical application often starts with researchers examining the effects of certain chemical compounds on the mortality rates (or health statistics) of insects, worms, rodents, and other mammals. Human research tends to be limited to large population studies that examine correlational trends over time. So far, there is little question about the ethics of researching the process of aging and in identifying the conditions that might retard or accelerate its rate because no drug has been marketed and tested to "prevent" aging. Each new drug is tested to treat or prevent one of any number of age-related diseases.

The ethical gray area arises when physicians undertake clinical treatments of preexisting drugs off-label. Antiaging clinics exist not only in Russia, Mexico, and China, but they are also common in the United States. Legally, they are prohibited from promoting and marketing the use of drugs for purposes unapproved by the FDA, but it occurs nonetheless. Some very famous antiaging labs exist in the United States, including the Hammer Institute in Arizona; the Optimal Hormone Therapy Centers in Los Angeles; the HD Spa and Clinic in Chicago; Global Life Rejuvenation in New Jersey; the MD Longevity Clinics in San Francisco and New York; and Biogenesis of Miami. There are hundreds of clinics in all major cities and more than 500 in South Florida alone. Each clinic features growth hormone therapies as well as bioidentical hormone therapies for men and women (which include the use of testosterone, estrogen, and progesterone). These clinics are not hidden in dark alleys but are often housed in upper-class neighborhoods and post advertisements throughout the Internet. In every instance, when the doctors in these clinics prescribe and provide testosterone, human growth hormone, rapamycin, or other "antiaging" drugs, they do so off-label and outside of FDA regulations. The physicians may justify the prescription with a diagnosis of "hormone deficiency," but the FDA does not recognize age-related hormone deficiencies as a disease. So the practices clearly violate both the letter and spirit of the regulations.

The marketing campaigns of antiaging clinics always show beautiful men and women looking in the prime of health and enjoying each other's company. Everyone wants to be young, and some drugs provide the hope for finding that lost youth. With such images of health and vitality, what could the potential dangers of off-label usage be? There are two primary concerns: the first is methodological, and the second is practical. In terms of scientific methodology, patients who take drugs for purposes that the medicines were not originally intended to treat run a higher risk of experiencing unexpected side effects. Drug companies only measure side effects for patients that exhibit the targeted diseases; their effects on otherwise healthy patients is studied with less precision. Moreover, as treatments used for antiaging are given contrary to indication (which means they are unregulated), physicians and clinics usually do not collect or publish statistics on either the short-term or long-term results. Patients who take drugs off-label are essentially acting a test subjects without the benefit of an organized experimental moderator.

Perhaps most importantly, drugs used for antiaging purposes cannot (as of yet) be verifiably tested, even if there were large-scale clinical trials. Scientists have been unable to identify a reliable biomarker for aging, which means there is no way to quantifiably determine the "rate" of aging. There is no way to determine whether a drug is slowing down the effects of time on human biology or merely masking one of myriad symptoms of age-related conditions. Any claim that a product will "slow the rate of aging" is based on bold assertion alone. Science can identify many age-related conditions and symptoms, but it cannot mark with any precision the actual rate by which the biochemical compounds in a body age. Patients who trust in the marketing pitches of antiaging clinics do so based on their own faith in the salesmen. There is no clinical research to support the claims.

Second, there are also practical concerns with black market medicine. Ideally, we would like to presume that all physicians are humanitarian minded and would never prescribe a treatment unless they believed it was the best therapeutic option for the patient. In fact, however, there are numerous examples of consumer fraud in the medical community, just as there are in any other industry. Black market medicine has no regulatory protection. Patients typically only have legal recourse for malpractice in cases of extreme negligence resulting in noticeable physical harm. Prices for treatments range from $500 to $5,000 a month for routine procedures and medicines, and there are no other guarantees that the treatments will have any impact on the rate of aging or even on general healthiness. Perhaps more frightening, there is little guarantee that the treatment the patient buys is, in fact, what it claimed to be. Patients do not have the scientific equipment to test the quality and purity of the drugs they are receiving. Patient confidence is based purely on faith alone.

One horror story published in the *New York Times* reported on a man who paid more than $300,000 for treatments to multiple stem-cell clinics in Mexico, China, and Argentina in an attempt to reverse the effects of a stroke he had suffered in 2009. Six years later, his doctors found an aggressive tumorous growth on his spinal column. The tumor was a result of the stem-cell treatments, which clearly did not do what they were expected to do. More disturbing, however, was that later biopsies revealed that the tumor contained cells from other patients. He was told that the clinics were using his own stem cells, but they had lied.

Just as consumers should be cautious about purchasing prescription drugs over the Internet from unlicensed providers because the pills may be counterfeits, so too patients at antiaging clinics must maintain an equal degree of heathy skepticism. Patients have little assurance that the hormone therapy they are buying actually contains the hormone they expected. Antiaging clinics manage to build up patient trust (usually through high-end facilities and equally high-quality marketing campaigns), but they do so outside the benefits of officially sanctioned verification by federally recognized medical boards.

Hormone Replacement Therapy

In most traditional medical circles, "hormone replacement therapy" refers to the use of estrogen (an anabolic steroid) as a treatment for women over age 50 who are suffering from hot flashes, night sweats, heart palpitations, and other symptoms of menopause. In the antiaging community, hormone replacement therapy (HRT) means something altogether different. It refers to the use of anabolic steroids for both men and women as a general treatment for all age-related conditions. It was one of the first prescription-based treatments that was genuinely intended to stop the process of aging.

The antiaging version of HRT dates back to the rise of small, popular networks of enthusiasts during the 1960s and 1970s, who were drawn together by a common interest in health and longevity. They looked for any health food plan, dietary practice, or exercise regime that promoted healthy living and promised to extend life. Mostly made up of younger baby boomers, the health food movement was more willing to look for nontraditional sources of authority, and its participants were often self-educated and usually not physicians, though they often had some academic background. In 1982, Durk Pearson and Sandy Shaw wrote *Life Extension: A Practical Scientific Approach*, which was more than 800 pages of anecdotal commentaries on their experiences with various vitamins, supplements, and medical-testing programs. Sprinkled throughout were reports of obscure research undertaken in laboratories around the world. Reference was made to the theory of free-radical oxidative stress throughout the text, and the final list of recommended daily supplements included heavy doses of antioxidants as well as, with physician approval, "sex hormone replacement" (which was how they described anabolic steroids). Anabolic steroids were first developed about 15 years earlier and had become common among weight lifters and bodybuilders during the 1970s. By 1982, Pearson and Shaw were among the first who saw their potential as a tool for life extension.

The basic idea behind HRT as a potential antiaging remedy is based on the observation that certain anabolic steroidal hormones are age dependent. That means that they occur at very low levels in the body at younger ages and then increase naturally throughout maturation and early adulthood, only to decline during later ages. These are the hormones that are responsible for reproduction and secondary sex characteristics. As they decline with age, one theory is that the symptoms of age-related conditions are all caused by declining steroids. Instead of assuming that age causes the decline, HRT assumes that declining hormones cause the very process of aging itself. From this perspective, the secret to rejuvenation is to maintain constant levels of all age-related hormones and enzymes and thereby avoid all age-related conditions.

Perhaps the most famous advocates for the use of anabolic steroids and human growth hormone (hGH) are the founders of the American Academy of Anti-aging Medicine (A4M), Robert Goldman and Ronald Klatz. As discussed in chapter 5, Goldman and Klatz published their first book, *Death in the Locker Room*, in 1984, which recounted the dangers of ergogenic (performance-enhancing) drug use among athletes. At the time, they warned strongly against the use of anabolic steroids among athletes who put short-term benefits ahead of long-term pains. A dozen years later, though, the two men published *Stopping the Clock*, which completely reversed their position. The new book recommended exercise, diet (including many popular supplements), and the use of anabolic steroids, including estrogen, progesterone, testosterone, hGH, and the steroid precursor dehydroepi-androsterone (DHEA). They had joined the growing amateur antiaging movement and popularized it for their generation. Since then, HRT has become one of the dominant forms of antiaging treatments found in any clinic.

During the 1980s and 1990s, anabolic steroids were mostly associated with performance enhancement and used by competitive athletes (generically called *doping*). They were also used to build the massive muscular frames of Hollywood action heroes, such as Arnold Schwarzenegger and Sylvester Stallone, and of World Wrestling Federation (WWF) stars Hulk Hogan, Roddy Piper, and dozens of others. Looking back at the 1990s, when Goldman and Klatz began promoting their use in antiaging, it is difficult to determine for certain whether the public attraction to anabolic steroids was based more on the promise of eternal youth or on the promise of an unusually strong physique.

In many ways, the two options do not seem contradictory, so the promise of youth was often equated, in popular culture, with the promise of sexual virility and physical strength. Testosterone is a male hormone that is most responsible for facial hair, deeper voices, greater muscle mass, and more aggressive moods. It is synthesized by the male gonads and converted to dihydrotestosterone (DHT), which is used for building muscle tissue. If the drug is introduced artificially outside the testes, the hormone will still trigger all those same reactions—even if used by women.

Traditional HRT uses the female sex hormone estrogen to offset the natural side effects that follow when women no longer menstruate. The same theory applies for men using HRT. As men grow older, the natural levels of testosterone decrease as does general muscle strength. The difference is that, unlike women, men continue to be capable of reproduction throughout their lives, and testosterone levels have very little to do with male reproduction. Anabolic steroids will not make men more sexually virile. In fact, it can often cause both impotency and a decline in libido. Critics of HRT argue that it relies mostly on hormones that help build muscle mass and not the other hormones and enzymes that build cartilage, improve joint health, increase bone density, or address other age-related conditions that may be compromised by unusual development of muscle tissue. A 65-year-old steroid user may develop the biceps of a 25-year-old, but his joints, tendons, and bones will still be 65 years old and unaffected by artificial supplements of testosterone or DHT. Increased muscle tissues have no impact on the nervous system, memory, or the respiratory or digestive systems, which also impact age-related conditions.

Perhaps more significantly, the side effects of long-term steroid use include increased risk of cardiovascular disease, kidney and liver disease, and tumor growth, not to mention loss of libido, hair loss and aggressive mood disorders. Many of these side effects resemble the most common age-related conditions that HRT is intended to address. For these reasons, and others related to ergogenic abuse among professional athletes, anabolic steroids were classified as a Schedule III controlled substance in 1990 and may not be taken without a prescription. Moreover, physicians may be at risk of prosecution for prescribing them without demonstrable medical need. Nevertheless, steroids are popular among consumers who yearn to look young and are commonly found in antiaging clinics, but they are not favored by most antiaging researchers.

Human Growth Hormone

Three years after their first antiaging book, Goldman and Klatz published *Grow Young with HGH: The Amazing Medically Proven Plan to Reverse Aging*. In terms of biochemistry, the first artificially synthesized human growth hormone (hGH) was developed by Genentech and approved by the FDA in 1985 as a treatment for children afflicted with growth disorders, such as dwarfism. The hormone is a naturally occurring polypeptide synthesized by the pituitary gland and is responsible for new cell production and bone growth. It converts insulin into a growth factor (often called insulin-like growth factor 1, or IGF-1) for bones and other tissues. It also creates DHEA, which is a precursor to estrogen and testosterone, and may (with sufficient exercise) lead to a natural increase in the body's anabolic steroid levels. Prior to 1985, hGH had to be harvested from the pituitary glands of cadavers, and it was rarely used because it was linked with a fatal neurological disorder known as Cruetzfeldt-Jakob disease. The synthetic version of hGH alleviated that risk, and it provided hope for children suffering from growth disorders.

Human growth hormone is different from testosterone-based anabolic steroids because it is not sex dependent. Secondary male sex characteristics are enhanced with steroids, including muscle strength, but hGH is produced in the pituitary gland and responsible for growth and development of the human body regardless of gender. At the same time, it may still increase testosterone levels, but only as mandated by the body's natural endocrine system. That means that it does not carry some of the side effects as artificially administered testosterone, such as early-onset male pattern baldness and emotional aggressiveness that can create a psychological dependency. Human growth hormone does not create the massive muscle mass that weight lifters and Hollywood action heroes may be looking for, but it does promote the synthesis of new protein tissues needed for muscle repair and generally leaner muscle tone. It also promotes bone density and may actually increase bone strength and size. Anecdotally, it also tightens skin and helps prevent sagging muscles and breasts.

Almost as soon as it became available in 1985, hGH was used off-label by athletes who wanted a substitute for testosterone-based hormones. The International Olympic Committee began testing for steroids in 1984. But there was no reliable test for hGH until 2004, so athletes had a greater chance of using it without fear of detection. Also, hGH comes in a powder or a pill form and does not require an injection like most anabolic steroids. By the late 1990s, several drug manufacturers had joined the market, with Eli Lilly selling Humatrope in 1987, Novo Nordisk selling Norditropin in 1988, and Teva and Pfizer selling Tev-Tropin and Genotropin in 1995. The original childhood disease for which hGH was developed is extremely rare, affecting only 5 out of 10,000 people, and yet the market for synthetic versions of hGH increased more than 70 percent annually. It is estimated that more than 90 percent of all units sold were eventually used for cosmetic and antiaging purposes.

Officially, hGH is prohibited by competitive sports associations. But the National Football League did not begin initiating tests until 2015, and their testing protocols are fairly loose. In other noncompetitive venues, such as acting and modeling, hGH is very popular. In 2004, Suzanne Somers, the blonde actress from the 1970s sitcom *Three's Company*, published *The Sexy Years: Discover the Hormone Connection— The Secret to Fabulous Sex, Great Health, and Vitality, for Men and Women*. The book promoted the use of both anabolic steroids and hGH as well as other hormones as an antiaging treatment. Somers popularized the term *bioidentical hormone therapies*, which have become most popular in antiaging clinics around the country as a euphemism for HRT and hGH.

Reports from Hollywood newspapers routinely speak of the prevalence of hGH use among actors, actresses, and behind-the-camera producers and talent agents. Hollywood culture thrives on the appearance of youth and sexual vitality, and hGH appears to carry all the positive benefits of steroids with fewer side effects— especially the emotional instability, which can be costly in the high-pressure environment of the entertainment industry. Somers has written more than 20 books on diet, exercise, and beauty and is extremely popular as a speaker on antiaging issues. Her primary emphasis, however, is on cosmetic appearance and not on the biochemistry of life extension.

Critics point out that the science behind hGH is not as convincing as its popularity. Like anabolic steroids, hGH is more popular because of its potential cosmetic benefits and not because of its proven ability to slow or stop the process of aging. Most antiaging clinics combine chemical supplements with other related programs for cosmetic enhancement, including Botox, tummy tucks, liposuction, facelifts, skin resurfacing, and other surgical options. In this context, "antiaging" is less concerned with life extension and more focused on maintaining the appearance of youth. As a marketplace, the cosmetic side of the antiaging movement is far more powerful and dominant than the scientific side of life extension.

Little research has been conducted on the antiaging effects of hGH at the cellular level. Genentech originally developed (and procured FDA approval) for the drug as a treatment of childhood growth disorders. As such, the company did not evaluate the effect of hGH on adults aged 65 or older. Anecdotal evidence suggests there are fewer short-term side effects of hGH as compared to anabolic steroids, but the long-term effects have not been fully studied. Short-term effects include headaches, carpal tunnel syndrome, swollen joints, and increased risk of diabetes. In 2015, a longitudinal population study of 184 adults aged 90 and older conducted by the Institute of Aging Research at the Albert Einstein College of Medicine found that centenarians tended to have lower levels of IGF-1 (the hormone triggered by hGH), not higher levels. Researchers found that every nanogram *decrease* per milliliter of IGF-1 correlated with one more additional week of life. Other clinical tests

Suzanne Somers: Actress and Activist

Suzanne Marie Mahoney was born in California in 1946, just after World War II. She played small roles on television during the 1960s under the stage name Suzanne Somers and achieved national fame with her role as Chrissy on the television sitcom *Three's Company*, starring alongside John Ritter and Joyce DeWitt. In 1981, she was written off the show over a salary dispute and largely disappeared from public view.

Then, in the late 1980s, she became a spokesperson for an exercise tool called ThighMaster, which she promoted as the source of her attractive physique. At the time, she was over 40 years old and still looked very much like the pretty blonde character from *Three's Company*. The marketing program was very successful for Somers, and she landed a series of leading parts in later television shows, including *She's the Sheriff*, *Step by Step*, and *Candid Camera*. Her most enduring national popularity, however, came as an author and spokesperson for diet and health. She published a diet book in 1997 and followed it with more than 20 additional books over the next 20 years, including two biographies and a host of lifestyle and wellness books. She became involved with hormone replacement therapies and alternative medicines after she was diagnosed with breast cancer in 2001. At the time, she underwent surgery to remove the cancer but chose not to pursue chemotherapy. She turned 70 in 2016 and is still regarded as a sexual icon.

with rodents indicated that those that maintained higher levels of IGF-1 tended to have shorter life spans than those with lower levels. There is also some evidence to suggest links to increased risks of cancer and tumor growth. Many scientific researchers in the antiaging movement remain highly skeptical of its potency and do not recommend hGH or HRT for life extension.

Historic Fashions in Amateur Antiaging Medicine

The subculture of antiaging enthusiasts of the 1970s largely grew out of the health food movement of the 1960s. Rachel Carson wrote a book called *Silent Spring* (1962) that discusses the impact of DDT and pesticides on the ecology of food production. Carson and other authors such as Helen and Scott Nearing and Wendell Berry led a "back to the land" movement, with young baby boomers moving out to farms to grow food the natural way, without modern pesticides or other chemical additions. Popular culture described these people as "hippies" living in communes and adhering to more organic and "sustainable" lifestyles. The very early organic movement of the late 1960s not only helped stimulate a parallel environmental movement, but it also helped to sustain thousands of small cooperatively owned natural health food stores. Many of these stores evolved from distribution points for organic ingredients and later became virtual apothecaries for health food supplements. By the end of the 1970s, these stores remained physically very small and included very little actual food, but they nevertheless housed aisles of pills and powders containing traditional herbal supplements and other nontraditional cures. It was from this background that Drew Pearson and Sandy Shaw emerged.

In 1980, two health food enthusiasts named Saul Kent and Bill Faloon founded a mail-order supply company called Life Extension Foundation in South Florida dedicated to supplements that would promote healthy living and extend human life. They also produced a monthly catalog, which developed into a magazine that included articles on new antiaging products (as well as ordering information on how to purchase them). In 1994 and 1995, when the graphical version of the Internet was first becoming popularized with linked Web pages, the Life Extension Foundation became one of the first businesses to advertise directly online. Since then, Lifeextension.com has become a major source of antiaging articles and an outlet for antiaging products. In 1994, right around the time Goldman and Klatz formed their A4M association, *Life Extension Magazine* published a list of the top 10 most-effective antiaging drugs that were currently available. The list was ranked in reverse order of efficacy and included the following:

10. hGH: At the time, this was only recently being publicized as an antiaging drug, and Life Extension Foundation was unable to sell it directly. But they did provide a phone number that would refer customers to doctors who might be able to prescribe the drug. In 1994, the drug cost between $1,000 and $18,000 a month.

9. Piracetam: This is an analog of gamma-aminobutyric acid (GABA), which is a neurotransmitter. The product was developed in Europe and is not approved for sale in the United States. It is not considered a drug nor a dietary supplement, and it is not approved by the FDA to treat any disorders. Life Extension Foundation sold the product as a memory booster. The FDA issued numerous warnings to retailers who sold the product as an herbal supplement (including the Life Extension Foundation).

8. DHEA: In 1994, this precursor to testosterone and estrogen was touted as a treatment for diabetes, atherosclerosis, Parkinson's and Alzheimer's disease, and multiple sclerosis. In 2014, the Mayo Clinic affirmed that population studies showed a correlation between high DHEA levels and higher bone densities, though there was still no causal evidence to demonstrate that DHEA was responsible for the higher densities. Some evidence suggested usefulness for depression and weight loss, with moderate utility for treatment for lupus and erectile dysfunction. DHEA is still highly touted among amateur antiaging enthusiasts. Unfortunately, quality tests of DHEA supplements show that many brands do not contain any or all of the amounts claimed on the package.

7. Vinpocetine and Hydergine: Vinpocetine is an herbal supplement extracted from periwinkle and has supposedly been tested in over 000 research studies in Europe and Asia with amazing results promoting "memory enhancements, cognitive performance, cerebral circulation, and mental acuity." In fact, only a few clinical studies were published to secure drug approval in Germany. It is a vasodilator, which means it will increase blood flow to the brain, and in this capacity, it is sold by prescription only in Germany under the name Cavinton. It is used to reduce the chance of disability and death in stroke victims. The FDA does not allow it to be sold as a drug in the United States, but it does permit it to be sold as an herbal supplement. Unfortunately, as an herbal supplement, it is even less monitored. A 2015 analysis by the National Center for Natural Products Research at the University of Mississippi found that out of 23 vinpocetine supplements, more than a quarter did not contain any vicpocetine at all, and the remainder contained anywhere from 0.3 mg to 32 mg per serving—doses that range from insignificant to prescription strength.

Hydergine is a prescription drug approved by the FDA in 1982 for the treatment of significant symptoms of dementia (inability to care for oneself, loss of all motivation). During FDA trials, some minimal improvement in alertness was seen in patients with significant loss of cognitive functions. Side effects include nausea and stomach issues. There is no evidence that hydergine improves cognition or memory in patients without dementia, and there is no evidence that it has any impact on life extension. Most online sources sell generic versions that are illegal and not FDA approved, and, like vinpocetine, they probably do not contain any active ingredients.

6. GH3 (K.H.3): Invented by Romanian physician Anna Aslan as an antiaging drug in the 1950s, it claims to cure arthritis, dementia, heart conditions, arteriosclerosis, deafness, Parkinson's disease, depression, impotence, baldness, wrinkles, and will even restore natural color to hair. The National Institute on Aging reviewed all available literature as early as 1977 and found no evidence for any of these claims. Side effects, however, include low blood pressure, respiratory problems, and convulsions. A 2008 study by the Cochrane Review indicated that the side effects heavily outweighed any potential benefits. The FDA banned the product in 1982 and continues to send out warnings for products that are advertised as equivalents of GH3. Several companies, including Gero-Vita and Life Force Laboratories, were sued (and eventually fined) by federal and state authorities for selling the product.

5. Centrophenoxine: This was later named meclofenoxate and sold under the brand name of Lucidril. Its potency claims to be based on numerous life-span studies as a compound that removes lipofuscin, which is an auto-fluorescent pigment found in the cytoplasm of some long-lived cells. No evidence of these studies can be found in any legitimate medical publications. Lipofuscin is sometimes referred to as "aging pigments" because it appears to accumulate over time, though the actual process of accumulation is unknown.

Lipofuscin is found primarily in postmitotic cells (those that do not replicate themselves), such as those found in the neurons, the heart, and the optical nerves. In theory, lipofuscin is the by-product of oxidative stress, and many antiaging researchers believe that removing lipofuscin would be like clearing out the debris of age and worn cells, thereby rejuvenating the cells to the condition of a younger age. Lipofuscin accumulation in the retinal nerve is theorized as a major cause of blindness due to macular degeneration. These disorders are untreatable, which is why macular degeneration remains untreatable. (A 2014 research group at Columbia University proposed using beta cyclodextrins to bind retinal lipofuscin, but it remains only theoretical.) Nevertheless, numerous theories among amateur enthusiasts exist for potential lipofuscin removal options, including the use of intensely precise lasers, microscopic nanobots, or miraculous chemical compounds. Centrophenoxine is supposedly one of those mysterious compounds, though there is no reliable information outside of vendor-sponsored Internet ads.

As with most of these antiaging drugs, it was supposedly developed and tested in Asia and Europe and sold there in plenty. U.S. consumers are instructed to buy through local distributors (with an added import fee) to obtain these precious drugs. In fact, though, there is no evidence of their use in Europe or Asia. There are hundreds of Web sites that refer to ample research, and they often include a general tone of conspiracy between the FDA, the Post Office, and the U.S. Customs Service, who are bent on preventing consumers from gaining access to antiaging drugs that promote greater intelligence. In this case, centrophenoxine clearly is not a drug and does not exist as a legitimate pharmaceutical product (legal or illegal). Vendors who sell it are selling placebos based on a theory.

4. Phosphatidylserine: This is a soy-based extract that is intended to imitate the compounds extracted from the brain cortex of cows. In 2002, manufacturers of the compound applied for FDA approval of claims that it could treat dementia and other cognitive dysfunction. The FDA rejected the application in part because it rejected the claim that the soy-based molecules were equivalent to the cow cortex extracts. In part, the FDA also failed to recognize that either the soy-based or the cow cortex–based molecules were effective in treating dementia. None of the 10 studies that were included in the application met the necessary standards of legitimate scientific research. However, the FDA did allow that as the molecule was derived from organic compounds, it could be classified as a dietary supplement, provided it did not claim to treat any particular medical conditions. The FDA did not find it hazardous. The FDA warned, however, that use of the term *cognitive dysfunction* was not medically appropriate as it has no precise meaning.

3. Deprenyl: This is also sold as Eldepryl, which is approved by the FDA as a treatment for Parkinson's disease. It is described as a monoamine oxidase (MAO-B) inhibitor, which is essentially an antioxidant. It was originally developed by Joseph Knoll and used to treat depression in the 1960s. It is chemically similar to methamphetamine. In the 1990s, it was occasionally prescribed as a treatment for Parkinson's disease, with minor results. In the amateur antiaging community, the line between drugs that combat dementia and drugs that slow the effects of aging is often very thin. Deprenyl was often described as the "first antiaging drug" by supporters who believed it actually slowed the effects of aging based on studies (in Europe) that it extended the life span of mice. The FDA does not recognize any life-extension properties of Deprenyl and has successfully charged several individuals and businesses for fraud based on their distribution and marketing of Deprenyl without a prescription. In 2010s, it remains a popular underground antiaging treatment, though it is now also touted as an aphrodisiac (increasing sex drive).

2. Acetyl-L-carnitine: This is a naturally occurring amino acid produced by the liver and kidneys that help cells produce energy. The compound may also be derived from red meat. It is often advertised in amateur antiaging circles as a general cognition and memory booster. In the 2000s, it also became popular among bodybuilders, who call it ALCAR and use it as a potential appetite suppressant and energy booster. In terms of biochemistry, it is an antioxidant and may help reduce blood clots after a heart attack when used in conjunction with other approved drugs. The FDA has approved the use of acetyle-L-carnitine in patients with kidney disease who become deficient in L-carnitine as a result of hemodialysis treatments. There is no evidence that acetyle-L-carnitine holds any benefits for Alzheimer's patients or as an energy booster for general athletic performance. Some research indicated the potential for

preventing the age-related decline of energy in rats, but there is no research on humans. Side effects include nausea and stomach issues. Most acetyle-L-carnitine is imported into the United States from China and South Korea. The FDA does not classify it as a pharmaceutical, so it passes under the rules of a dietary supplement, which only requires evidence that it is not harmful. It does not seem to be toxic to humans, but it is toxic to dogs and cats.

1. Melatonin: This is a hormone produced by the pineal gland that regulates sleep patterns. As discussed in chapter 11, it is a very popular supplement that is taken for its antioxidant properties and for the mistaken belief that it will promote deeper sleep. In 1994, however, melatonin was described as "the most documented antiaging therapy in the world." It was reportedly used by physicians around the world in high doses to treat a wide variety of age-related diseases, with no toxic side effects. In the 2010s, melatonin has fallen out of favor as an antiaging cure-all, but it remains popular among amateur enthusiasts as a general health supplement.

One of the interesting patterns found within this top 10 list from 1994 is that the amateur antiaging community did not always distinguish between drugs that treat dementia and drugs that enhance cognitive performance. The general theory is that if a chemical compound can improve the mental functions of someone in cognitive decline, it must also improve memory and cognition even more for those that are healthy. These patterns may also reflect a touch of desperation among those who have loved ones who suffer from dementia and who have found no success from traditional medical sources.

Another pattern is that the vocabulary of the amateur antiaging community is self-constructed. The term *nootropic* is used frequently in modern Web sites to describe an entire class of antiaging drugs that are supposed to improve brain functions and brain health. The term is not recognized by biochemists, and it has no place among legitimate pharmaceutical research. Yet, it is referred to commonly by hundreds of Web sites that use the word to describe their special antiaging compounds. It is a reasonable assumption that if the Web site is using "nootropic" to describe a product, then the Web site is in some way related to an amateur anti-aging vendor (and is not an objective scientific source).

Along these same lines, the amateur antiaging community has become very adept at using the Internet to provide scientific legitimacy for its products (supplements and pharmaceutical). Dozens of Web sites use very official-sounding names to appear to be legitimate medical reference sites. Some of these include drugs-forum.com, www.worldhealth.net, dailyhealthanswers.com, and nutritionreview.org, among many others. These sites are not impartial, and they do not reflect scientific research from academic sources. Like the Life Extension Foundation and its related organ *Life Extension Magazine*, these Web sites are actually marketing arms of the various amateur antiaging vendors. In the 1970s, the products advertised in these forums would have been sold through independently owned health food stores or co-ops, but in the 2010s, they are mass marketed through the Internet.

Saul Kent and Bill Faloon: Amateur Antiaging Pioneers

Saul Kent was born in 1939, and Bill Faloon was born in 1954. Kent was one of the three people to form the Cryonics Society of New York in 1965, and though that venture eventually failed, he maintained a lifelong commitment to the technology. His friend Karl Werner coined the term *cryonics*, which is a mainstream version of the term *cryogenics*. In 2000, Kent explained in an interview, "My objective was not to be frozen and come back. What I really wanted to do was not to die at all."

Bill Faloon is 15 years younger than Kent and was in high school when he first heard about cryonics. He had little formal training, except a year at the Pittsburgh Institute of Mortuary Science, where he earned a mortician's license. Faloon and Kent met in the 1970s, when they formed the Florida Cryonics Association (later changed to Life Extension Foundation, Inc.). Around the same time, the two partners began importing supplements from overseas to make them informally available to other antiaging enthusiasts. They also published a newsletter that contained the latest news and developments in antiaging therapies and also promoted their supplements. In 1982, after an appearance on *Merv Griffin*, they formed a more formal retail outlet for antiaging products. They launched a mail-order business in 1983.

Their success drew attention from federal agents, who raided their offices and searched for illegally imported pharmaceuticals that were not approved for sale in the United States. After four years of investigation, a federal grand jury indicted the pair on more than two dozen charges related to conspiracy to import dangerous drugs. The case fell apart in 1996, and the charges were eventually dropped. Both men have contributed millions of dollars from the Life Extension Foundation to cryogenics research and other antiaging projects.

Current Hopefuls

Not all antiaging drugs are promoted by amateur enthusiasts. Among the more scientifically based researchers, there is almost equal enthusiasm for potential antiaging drugs from existing medications taken off-label. In 2009, clinical trials of a new family of medicines called *rapalogs* were found to boost immunity and extend the life span of worms, fruit flies, and mice. The primary drug in the family, rapamycin, was originally developed by Wyeth Pharmaceuticals as an immunosuppressant used for organ grafts and kidney transplants and as a coating for stent implants during heart surgery. The compound was originally isolated from soils found on Easter Island and is a polyketide similar to resveratrol, in that it is created by bacteria to increase survival rates. It has been studied for its ability to suppress autoimmune reactions, which may be promising in fighting certain cancers. In 2015, it was used to extend the average life span of dogs.

Another drug from the same family is called *everolimus*, and sold under the brand name Afintor. Like rapamycin, it is an mTOR (mammalian target of rapamycin) inhibitor and was originally developed by Novartis to treat various cancers, including breast, kidney, pancreatic, and other gastrointestinal tumors. Part of the reason why rapalogs drew the attention of antiaging researchers is that the increase of mTOR suppressers is also associated with calorie-restricted diets. One of the original goals of the research in caloric restriction was to find the chemical compound that triggers the cascade of cellular rejuvenation that reduced-calorie diets induce. Everolimus and rapamycin were exciting because they could potentially trigger that cascade of reactions without the need for drastic restrictions of caloric intake. It would be like taking diet and exercise in a pill form.

In addition to the rapalogs, another potential antiaging drug, metformin, was also originally developed for other purposes. It is extracted from a French lilac (often called "goat's rue") and was used during the Middle Ages as a folk remedy for diabetes. The active ingredient was first isolated in 1929, and it was successful at lowering blood-glucose levels in animals but was found to be toxic in humans. A French researcher named Jean Sterne developed a biochemical analog that was better tolerated in human subjects. The synthetic version was used during the 1950s to treat type 2 diabetes, but it fell out of favor due to an association with lactic acidosis, which is a side effect of diabetes in some patients. However, a 20-year longitudinal population study launched by United Kingdom Prospective Diabetes Study (from 1977 to 1997) found that diabetics who used metformin had fewer heart attacks and generally lived longer than those taking other drugs. Since then, metformin has become very popular. Like rapamycin, it was also studied on animals and found to extend the life expectancy of yeast, fruit flies, and roundworms. In 2015, Nir Barzilai, the director of the Institute of Aging Research at the Albert Einstein College of Medicine, applied to the FDA to begin clinical trials to test metformin for its potential in reducing the rate of aging in humans. It was approved as the first clinical trial to test for potential antiaging effects on humans.

Both rapamycin and metformin have become very popular within the antiaging research community. During the early 2000s, S. Jay Olshansky and Steven Austad were both vocal critics of amateur antiaging enthusiasts who claimed to have found "cures" for aging (see chapter 5). Yet, both men were present in Washington, D.C., in late 2015, when Barzilai presented his proposal to the FDA for the first clinical trial of metformin. At the time, Olshansky said it was "a fundamental sea change in how we look at aging and disease," and Austad described it as "a groundbreaking, perhaps paradigm-shifting trial." At the same time, however, the application to the FDA did not actually use the word "antiaging," and Olshansky was clear to explain that the goal was to extend "the period of healthy life." He said emphatically, "We're not arguing—and we've never argued—that we're trying to achieve life extension." It was a distinction of semantics because Barzilai as project director was equally clear that his goal for the trials was to determine whether drugs could "delay aging." Whether the human life span is ultimately fixed or flexible is another issue.

In addition to rapamycin and metformin, the Barzilai group also planned to test the effects of low-dose aspirin, acarbose (another diabetes drug), 17-alpha-estradiol (a female anabolic steroid), and nordihydroguaiaretic acid (an extract from the creosote plant). They were not planning on testing supplements that have already been demonstrated to have no impact on life extension, including fish oil, green tea extract, curcumin, or resveratrol. The primary result of the FDA approval was that this study opened the door for future drugs that might be allowed to treat aging itself as an FDA-approved indication. If this ultimately proves successful, antiaging drugs may not always be off-label or black market.

While the Barzilai group plans to adopt traditional scientific-based clinical trials, their results will necessarily remain mostly correlational rather than causal. Large populations (about 3,000 adults) will be given various compounds in double-blind studies, and all the routine safeguards will be adhered to. Nevertheless, the final results will remain correlational in nature because they can only measure effects after the compounds have acted. There is no practical way of identifying exactly which biochemical agents are causing which reactions that result in healthier life spans. More importantly, there is still no objective way for quantitatively measuring the rate of human aging, so researchers will be unable to prove decisively if these drugs are effective.

Ultimately, like the amateur antiaging enthusiasts, scientists also appear generally willing to believe in the power and efficacy of antiaging drugs, not based on scientific evidence but on the hope of scientific potential. In essence, their belief is based on a strong faith in mankind's eventual ability to combat the forces of nature and determine its own order on the material world.

FUTURE TECHNOLOGIES

The technologies of the future do not have to involve robots and artificial intelligence. Many future technologies dreamed of by medical researchers are more subtle and yet are still theorized to result in significant improvements in general health and well-being. For most antiaging advocates, the true potential of extending the human life span requires some degree of technological innovation to achieve ultimate success.

Of course, at the other end of the spectrum, the transhumanist movement envisions a society filled with robots, digital consciousness, and entire worlds that exist only in virtual reality. The final result of what the technologies will look like in the transhumanist world is not clear, but many advocates argue that the future is much sooner than most people realize—closer to 20 years rather than 200 years. Similarly, the full social, political, and economic implications of these technological changes are difficult to fully imagine, but the ethical considerations can be hypothesized, even without the existence of any current applications.

For both the subtle and the extravagant, theories of future technological innovation all rely on a basic presumption (perhaps faith) in human achievement to make changes to life and the material world that have hitherto been impossible. While that is arguably true for any new invention, the changes required for the realm of antiaging involve changes of a different order of magnitude. In some cases, they might require changes in metaphysical nature.

Genetic Manipulation

The dream of genetic manipulation might potentially come from several options. The first option, therapeutic chemistry, is the one most commonly attempted in current biomedical research. Doctors prescribe a medicine that is intended to inhibit or encourage the expression of certain genes. The problem with this approach is that chemistry rarely alters the original DNA sequence and must rely on the existing genome (defects and all) to facilitate cellular healing. Technological innovation through this option requires more detailed understanding of which genetic sequences are involved in the metabolic activity of each organ. This has been an ongoing process of discovery since the first transcription of the Human Genome Project and has resulted in new innovations appearing frequently in scientific journals. It is, however, also a relatively slow process with no precise end date for completion.

The second source, direct genetic editing, is one that is currently in its infancy. Even before the Human Genome Project was complete, scientists around the world were considering ways of manipulating the sequences of genetic codes to potentially alter the genome. A Spanish scientist, Francisco Mojica, was the first to identify a potential pathway for genetic manipulation in 1993. It was not until 2010 that Canadian researcher Sylvain Moineau successfully cleaved the double-strand DNA strings at precise locations. Over the next two years, researchers in Lithuania and Berkeley, California, independently discovered ways of precisely joining DNA strands of diverse origins and also of fusing them together. By 2013, Feng Zhang, a Harvard scientist, had applied all these processes to demonstrate genome editing. In theory, the human genome can be edited to facilitate almost any genetic alteration.

When scientists speak of direct genetic manipulation, in which parts of the DNA strand are replaced with others, they often refer to CRISPR, which is an acronym for clustered, regularly interspaced, short palindromic repeat technology. The scientific articles often refer to "using CRISPR" to edit a particular gene. In this context, it sounds like CRISPR is a giant computer that takes in cells, manipulates the DNA strands, and then spits the edited cells back out. In truth, CRISPR is not a device, but a process that uses biochemical interactions of bacterial "repair templates" of guide RNA to manipulate replication of particular DNA sequences. It is more complex that it sounds, and the actual "editing" occurs using known properties of particular biochemical reactions. The molecules involved are so small that they often change only small clusters of particular atoms. There is very little physical manipulation involved in gene editing, and particularized editing of specific sequences at will remains a future goal.

There is considerable debate as to whether direct genetic manipulation (even if accomplished consistently and efficiently) would lead to significant antiaging breakthroughs. A significant number of geriatric researchers argue that aging is not entirely, or even mostly, a function of cellular action or genetic expression. For example, the wear-and-tear theory of aging argues that the molecular structure in human biology simply begins to break down over time. Manipulating genetic processes will not fix those parts that have already begun to degrade.

There are others, however, who argue that age is a result of genetic mutation, when the DNA strands lose their integrity and begin to be replicated imperfectly. For this latter group of scientists, the dream of precise genetic manipulation would allow doctors to reformulate the DNA strands back to their original sequences at birth, thereby refreshing the entire body. It is this part of the dream that requires future technological development. Scientists would need to figure a way by which the perfected DNA strands could somehow be replicated throughout the more than 37 trillion cells estimated in the human body, in all their variations. In theory, only those core cells for each organ that provide the source material for future replication would require editing.

Another form of genetic manipulation that is very popular among antiaging researchers focuses on the telomere length found at the end of each DNA strand. There is some research already on chemical processes that might extend telomere length, but, unfortunately, they mostly exist in peripheral systems (such as blood cells) and not in the more critical systems, such as the heart muscle or the neurons of the brain. The same problem exists for telomeres as it exists for direct genetic manipulation: how do scientists make changes to the older existing cells that are in most need of change? In theory, solving this problem would result in revolutionary medical breakthroughs in many areas, including cancer research. If doctors could kill only those individual cells that are destructive and protect those cells that are beneficial, there would be no more cancer. Unfortunately, the process of replicating healthy cells, with healthy telomere lengths, remains a technological hurdle that has yet to be solved.

Bioprinting

For many amateur antiaging enthusiasts, the future of genetic manipulation involves the purposeful and precise placement of living cells into the exact arrangements needed for medical use. Based on the same theory of 3-D printers, the "bioprinter" creates three-dimensional objects with living tissues so that exact copies of human organs (or other enhanced versions) would be made to order. These solutions are imaginative, but there are some substantial hurdles to be overcome before that technology could have practical application.

Bioprinting does not manipulate specific molecules, and it cannot create life where none already exists. There are certain limitations of quantum physics that prohibit scientists from physically manipulating specific atoms into particular arrangements. Nevertheless, there are experimental bioprinter prototypes that follow the model of plastic-based 3-D printers to create forms within which living cells may be inserted like drops of blood. The biggest hurdle to using bioprinters for medical applications is that the body is composed of at least 200 different cell types, and complex organs involve hundreds of different combinations. Bioprinters do not produce coherently living organisms but are more akin to carefully sculpted and arranged boxes that contain living tissues. Several companies in Japan and the United States have invested money in the technology, including Organovo and Invetech. Their goals are to create platforms from which to construct synthetic bones, skin grafts, or possibly entire organs.

The promise behind bioprinting technology is that biological life will simply adapt to whatever form it is inserted. If the right kinds of cells are placed in the right kinds of formations, they should grow on their own. There are some considerable obstacles that remain. A printer-like machine might be constructed that would assemble cells as precisely as might be needed to recreate tissues in particular arrangements, but there are other limitations faced by all living organisms. Living tissues act as a whole, not as individual cells. Yet, cells do what they are programmed to do both by biochemical interactions and by their genetic DNA blueprints. Physically forcing cells to lay next to each other will not guarantee that the cells will join together or that, once joined, they will work as a coherent organism. Simply printing individual cells in a precise order most often results in an organic mess. Cellular tissues grow; they are not built. Even with bioprinting technology, there is an assumption that the cells will need time and resources to grow into place or they will simply die.

Bioprinters are frequently referred to as a future technology that will revolutionize and solve the problems of aging, disease, and human longevity. If a human part wears out, scientists could simply print out another one. The practical likelihood of complex organ development is, currently, well beyond the possibilities of known physics, chemistry, and biology. Nevertheless, when used in conjunction with particularized gene editing, the potential of synthetic organs becomes at least theoretically possible. Rather than printing organic tissues, scientists can grow tissues from genetically modified sources.

The most common scenario conceived is using gene editing technology to develop "designer babies" that are free from any perceived defects. In practice, the DNA from the father's sperm and the mother's ovum would be manipulated prior to an in vitro fertilization. There are considerable ethical concerns with this technology. While the prospect of healthy children is welcomed, the fear is that those children who did not benefit from the genetic manipulation would face strong social discrimination for being handicapped. In the worst-case scenario, our imperfect knowledge of every genetic sequence might lead to the creation of new and even deadlier diseases with more lethal results. Such human experimentation could result in an increase of mortality rather than longevity.

Stem Cells and Cloning

Closely related to the conceptual promise of bioprinters is the promise of using stem cells to create generic tissues that could be transformed (or cultivated in a lab) into customized organs. Stem cells are cells that have not yet differentiated into particular types and which potentially can be replicated indefinitely into any other type of cell. Stem cells reached popular culture through news reports in the early 2000s, when President George W. Bush issued a national speech setting forth national parameters for using the tissues from fertilized human embryos for experimentation. These embryonic stem-cell tissues came from aborted babies, and the specter of encouraging abortion rates to facilitate experimentation on human organisms raised considerable ethical debate from both sides of the political and moral spectrum. Since 2000, scientists have discovered that stem cells may be found in numerous sources, including the fat tissues of mature adults. This resolved many of the ethical concerns related to abortion, and many antiaging scientists place great hope in using stem cells to repair and rejuvenate existing cells in adults.

Despite the promises made by various unregulated antiaging clinics around the world, the technology for reliable medical treatments using stem cells is still far away. In theory, the goal of successful stem-cell therapy is based on the fact that every cell contains a complete set of blueprints for every other cell (and biochemical process) as contained in the DNA. Scientists would like to extract an undifferentiated adult cell and then force it to transform into the type of cell that is afflicted by disease (such as a heart cell or a liver cell). Using cloning technology, these cells can be replicated in vitro and then specifically cultivated to develop particular organs or parts of organs that could be used to graft or replace diseased tissues.

In theory, treatments could be accomplished in one of two ways: the first is to physically transplant the engineered tissues back into the body, and the second is to somehow create the conditions by which the stem cells could force renewed rejuvenation of diseases cells within the living body. It is the promise of the second option that draws hopeful patients to supposed stem-cell clinics around the world. Unfortunately, in terms of biomedical science, the second option is the least likely to be successful in the current state of technology.

The first option of in vitro development of organs and tissues has much greater potential, and some researchers have been successful with small-scale applications of animal tissues. In 2016, scientists at the Tokyo and Kyoto University successfully grew a human ear on the back of live rat using stem-cell technology. Scientists in London have used a similar technology to grow a nose on a patient's arm, and another was grown on a patient's forehead. In 2016, researchers at Washington University were able to use stem cells to grow synthetic cartilage for hip replacements. These experiments involve only sculpted cartilage and are not in any way as complex as growing an organ. Cultivating organs would require particularized DNA editing combined with the development of suitable environments in which the tissues could develop. Finally, it would require more advanced transplant procedures to accommodate any nerve-intensive organ (such as the eyes).

In essence, cloning involves a chemical copying of DNA from one host to another. The concept in its most basic form was understood as early as 1885, when Hans Dreisch successfully created twins from a sea urchin by shaking the embryos when in very early development. It was not until the 1950s that Robert Briggs and Thomas King successfully transferred the nucleus of a tadpole embryo into a frog egg. From those beginnings, Ian Wilmut and Keith Campbell successfully cloned a sheep in 1996 by taking a nucleus from a sheep's udder and inserting it into an enucleated egg (one where the nucleus had been removed). This technology opened the way for similar transference of particular genetic material into the potential replicating cells of another host medium.

These breakthroughs opened a theoretical pathway for in vitro organ development, but significant hurdles remain. As of yet, cloning technology still requires the use of an egg to stimulate reproduction. Scientists have not been able to force tissue growth from mammals without the basic ingredients of sexual reproduction. Another dream of researchers is to figure a way for organs to regenerate outside the normal processes of reproduction. Like a salamander that regrows its tail, humans might be able to regrow a limb or an organ. That technology also remains far in the future. There is an added obstacle, though, that even if adult stem cells are successfully replicated outside the natural process of development from an egg, the new cells would begin with shortened telomere lengths. This problem has not been resolved, but telomere researchers such as Michael Fossel are hopeful that the solution is relatively close at hand (see chapter 5).

The future hope of antiaging researchers is that patients may be able to grow their own organs in vitro to be used for perfectly matched transplants. This future seems rather near for bone and cartilage transplants. For some antiaging advocates, the hope of in vitro organ cultivation may replace the need for chemical drugs. Instead of taking medicines that interfere with the body's endocrine system, future physicians might strive to maintain a steady biochemical balance and use transplantation to repair most diseases. There are numerous biotechnical obstacles to be overcome. If it is possible at all, this technology remains far in the future.

Ethics

In addition to technological hurdles, there are a great many ethical concerns that underlie these future technologies. Mostly, they begin with questions about when and how life begins. The primary objection to embryonic stem-cell research was that scientists were potentially experimenting on living human beings, even though very young. The prospect of cloning hundreds, or thousands, of human embryos for the sake of experimentation on various tissue samples and body parts stirs up memories of Nazi experimentation on Jewish concentration camp victims during World War II. The ultimate fate of those embryonic experiments would be destruction. From the point of view of some medical researchers, the human embryos were so young that they were hardly distinguished from the biological cells they routinely experiment on when using single-celled organisms or other nonhuman life-forms. From the point of religious critics, all human life is sacred regardless of age, and experimentation at one end of the life span is no different than experimentation at the other end or at any point in between.

Fundamentally, the ethical question deals with the exceptional value of human life as an intrinsic end in itself. If human life is not regarded as unique, then the door is opened for any number of other ethical dilemmas. What would prohibit the cultivation of an entire human body, without a brain to be used by the donor as a source for "spare parts"? And if, as the strict materialists suggest, the biological tissues of human life are really no different than the biological tissues of any other animal, then why not develop a fully functioning cloned human being with the purpose of using the brain to maintain the constant health of all the biological parts? The clone could be kept unconscious so as to be unaware of its condition, because the ultimate purpose of the body would be to harvest organs as needed by the donor host. Would the clone ever have any individual rights to life, liberty, or its own pursuit of happiness? This is not an easy question to answer, as many of the same ethical principles are also involved in the question of abortion and infanticide, and society has not arrived at a clear consensus on that issue either.

In a related issue, what happens when medical experimentation on living tissues fail? One of the controversies surrounding in vitro fertilization is that so many human embryos are required to guarantee at least one or two successful fertilizations. Depending on the age of the client, doctors may transfer up to 5 or more embryos, which means that if all are successfully implanted, the mother may carry up to 5 babies. In some cases, doctors have implanted 10 or more embryos, which means that many embryos fail to implant, or some are later destroyed to ensure at least 1, 2, or 3 live births. Many European nations have mandated that only 1 embryo may be transferred per procedure, but these mandates have been resisted in the United States and other nations.

The Catholic Church opposes in vitro fertilization because it usually involves some form of abortion, either in vitro or in vivo. Other supporters of in vitro fertilization do not believe that human life begins in the embryo until after the baby has been intentionally delivered. In terms of antiaging in vitro organ development, or cloning, there is always a prospect that human life may be transferred and destroyed at some point during the research process. Experimentation on human life, at any stage, involves serious ethical considerations. Some critics would argue that experimentation on any life, including animals, involves similar kinds of ethical dilemmas. Modern society generally accepts experimentation on animal tissues, provided that the animals do not needlessly suffer, but there is more hesitation to permit experimentation on human tissues that have potential to grow on their own accord. There is no clear consensus on these issues.

Finally, there are also ethical concerns about the preservation of original genetic genomes. This has become controversial in agricultural sciences, where certain strains of high-protein grains have been developed in vitro in such a way as to prevent farmers from using seeds of existing crops to plant future harvests. The ethical concern is that farmers in developing nations would become continually dependent on the agricultural suppliers from developed nations to be able to grow the food needed to sustain themselves. If the original protein grains become extinct, the natural ecology of the agricultural system would be permanently compromised.

In a similar way, there are ethical concerns of breeding genetic mutations in animals and humans that might permanently alter their respective genomes. What would become of the nonenhanced versions? Would social policies need to be developed to ensure the same legal protection for nonenhanced genetic profiles as is provided for the enhanced versions? If genetic enhancements lead to life extension, would social policy likewise mandate (or provide the option for) equal access for all people? Would some people be allowed to resist the enhancement, and if so, would they face negative consequences (social or political or economic) for doing so? As is evidenced by the continued debate with regard to organic food, it does not appear that a national consensus on these issues has been achieved.

Cryonics

Many of the really powerful antiaging technological innovations remain in the distant future. The headline of a 2005 article in *LiveScience* read, "Hang in There: The 25-year Wait for Immortality." Inside, Aubrey de Grey predicted that the first real changes in antiaging technology would begin sometime around the year 2030, after which each successive decade of life extension may well create a window for new innovations that would extend it even longer. The key would be to live until the start of that sequence of technological development.

For some people, however, 25 years may be too long to wait. It is for this reason that cryonics was developed, at least in theory. Robert Ettinger published a book in 1962 titled *The Prospect of Immortality*, in which he outlined a plan to immerse a body that had only moments before being declared legally dead into a liquid nitrogen solution that would keep the body indefinitely. The goal would be to preserve the body until such time that science would be able to repair the vital organs needed to revive the patient back to life. This was based on the theory that some aspects of the body, particularly the primary functions of the brain, may continue to be "alive" even after the heart has stopped beating. In theory, it is the same principle behind organ transplants, as the tissues remain alive even after the donor has died. The prime difference is the presumption that human consciousness is somehow stored in the physical biological tissues of the brain, and if the biological functions of the rest of the body could be restored through some future innovations, the person could be revived—even after death.

There has been considerable success in overcoming many of the technological hurdles of freezing a body, but more work remains. Originally, the goal was to freeze tissues to −320 degrees Fahrenheit (−196 Celsius), which would essentially slow down molecular activity to the point of being almost stopped. The theory of cryonics is that they are not "freezing dead people" but providing long-term care for critically ill patients who, for all intents and purposes in the modern world, may appear to be dead, but for whom later technology may be able to later revive. The key is to freeze the brain within the short window between when the heart has stopped and before the brain tissues become irreversibly dead. The problem is that the process of freezing usually creates crystals that can destroy the delicate cell membranes, which is a problem as the body is composed of 50–65 percent water. During the freezing process, blood is slowly replaced with high concentrations of glycerol to reduce ice formations to prevent damage during freezing.

These methods significantly reduce ice damage, but the damage risks are not zero. More recent research is focused on a new process called *vitrification*, which would allow for greater preservation, even among the delicate tissues of the brain's nervous system. These processes are under continuous development, and in 2015, researchers were able to reignite some electrical activity in a rabbit's head that had been frozen in a cryonic state. The brain remained quite dead, but the electrical activity demonstrated that the synaptic connections were undamaged. No similar experiments have been successful with human heads.

The practice of freezing organisms to preserve them for later study has become commonplace since the mid-1980s. In some cases, animal cells and human embryos have been preserved for more than 30 years. Certain roundworms are routinely frozen and then revived. Animal transplants of organs that have been frozen have been successful for sheep, rodents, and rabbits. The real difficulty, however, is not in the freezing of human bodies or human tissues, but in the revitalization after they have been frozen. At this point, scientists have been unable to revive dead tissues of any sort.

The theory of cryogenics asserts that the bodies and brain tissues are not really dead, but as far as all the evidence of modern science is concerned, they are dead. No one has been able to restart life after it has been extinguished in an

Alcor Life Extension Foundation

Robert Ettinger died in 2011 at the age of 92 and was frozen at his Cryonics Institute in Clinton, Michigan (with 130 others). James Bedford was the first person to be cryogenically frozen in 1967, but it was another six years before a full-scale facility was created to house bodies. The Alcor Life Extension Foundation was established in 1972, followed by the Cryonics Institute in 1976. Since then, each facility has accepted about 130 people. A Russian cryonics facility, KrioRus, was started in 2005 in Moscow, which holds around 50 people and many animals. A fourth facility, Oregon Cryonics, was opened in 2016; it specializes in preserving heads only—based on the theory that when the time comes for reviving these people, the technology will be available to clone a new human body from a cell found in the head.

The procedure of freezing only the head triggered a murder investigation after Dora Kent died in 1987. Her son Saul (the cofounder of Life Extension Foundation in South Florida) rushed her to the Alcor facility after she came down with pneumonia and it was clear she was unable to recover. She died at the facility without a doctor present. The coroner later arrived to discover a headless body, and though he initially accepted the conclusion that she had died of pneumonia, later pathological evidence suggested she may have been alive when her body was frozen. The coroner asked for permission to test the head, but Alcor refused. Though several Alcor members were initially arrested, all charges were eventually dropped. The case remains unresolved as long as the head remains absent. There is no official confirmation that it is under preservation at Alcor.

organism—no matter how small. Dr. Frankenstein's dream of reanimating dead tissues certainly has a long history, but there has been no success in that area of research. As such, if it is possible at all, the promise of reviving the tissues of cryogenically frozen bodies and heads remains far, far in the future.

Needless to say, the theory of cryonics requires a great deal of confidence in the potential of natural science to restore life to a body that has been legally declared dead. It also involves a great deal of confidence that all the people who are caring for the frozen body will continue to do so during the time span between when the first death occurred and the restored life begins. The first three cryonics institutions (Cryo-Care of Phoenix Arizona, Cryonics Society of New York, and Cryonics Society of California) all went bankrupt. All but one of the 18 bodies frozen between 1966 and 1974 were eventually thawed and buried due to the financial collapse of the institutions. Only the first body, James Bedford, remains frozen at the Alcor Life Extension Foundation in Arizona.

Transhumanism and Computerized Prosthetics

Perhaps the most popular form of antiaging technology shown in movies and in television is bionics and enhanced prosthetic devices. Beginning in 1973, the ABC television network launched *The Six Million Dollar Man*, which lasted for five seasons and inspired a spin-off, *The Bionic Woman*, from 1976 to 1978. The premise of both shows is that a secret government agency spent millions of dollars to attach advanced prosthetics on the main characters, who had suffered terrible accidents. The new mechanical implants (legs, an arm, eyesight, and hearing) were indistinguishable from ordinary human flesh. Not only were the main characters saved from disability, but their new (albeit expensive) prosthetics allowed them to take on nearly superhuman responsibilities.

Though clearly fiction, the television shows inspired real-life research into advanced prosthesis technology. Several companies around the world specialize in making mechanical limbs equipped with miniature motors that are controlled by sensors that attach to the nerve endings remaining at the ends of amputated limbs. While certainly not indistinguishable from real flesh, and with significantly less power than human muscle, these devices can provide limited functionality as mechanical limbs. As computer processing technology becomes more powerful and robotic technology becomes more graceful, it is not impossible to foresee a time in the very near future when prosthetic limbs and other artificial organs might be used to substitute for natural appendages. This is the germ from which transhumanism has become most popular.

Transhumanism is a philosophical outlook that foresees humanity transcending its natural biological limitations through the use of technology. It is much older than the 1970s, and the term was first coined by Julian Huxley in a 1951 essay titled "Transhumanism," which was later included in his book *New Bottles for New Wine* (1957). Huxley envisioned a time when the process of evolution could be permanently stopped by the rise of human ingenuity. He wrote, "It is as if man had been suddenly appointed managing director of the biggest business of all, the business of evolution." Huxley was advocating for a new religion based on scientific awareness, and he believed that a united consciousness of mankind's mastery over nature would result in taking "the human species [to] the threshold of a new kind of existence, as different from ours as ours is from that of Peking man. It will at last be consciously fulfilling its real destiny." Huxley was only original in his use of the term, but the concepts and arguments could be traced even further back to Friedrich Nietzsche (1844–1900) and his theory of the "Superman" who transcended his moral environment through deliberate act of conscious will.

Many Christian writers, including G. K. Chesterton and C. S. Lewis, were explicitly opposed to the idea and goals of humanity ever claiming total dominance over creation, and they often likened the idea to the biblical stories of the Tower of Babel and the serpent's promise to Adam and Eve. Despite the resistance among traditional religious voices, the spirit of transhumanism remained popular throughout the latter half of the 20th century.

Between the 1960s and 1990s, transhumanism transitioned from being a philosophical outlook to an actual political movement. In 1965, statistician I. J. Good predicted a time when "ultraintelligent machines" would become so powerful that they would take over the planning and organization of human society. It would be created by mankind, but it would eventually come to be the source for all future technological innovation. That moment was called the "singularity." In popular culture, this moment is usually described in very negative terms. It was the subject of the 1984 science fiction movie with Arnold Schwarzenegger, *Terminator*, about a time when computers have taken over the world and launched a war against humanity. The same theme dominated *The Matrix* and its sequels, beginning in 1999, which are about a future world where the majority of humanity is forcibly locked into a virtual reality by machines who secretly control the earth. Though Hollywood generally fears the prospect of technology eliminating human free will, there are many philosophers within the modern transhumanist movement who believe it is the pathway to immortality in the future.

At heart, transhumanism rests on a theory that machines can develop an artificial intelligence that can rival or even surpasses human intelligence. When that happens, humanity would actually benefit from artificial intelligence because they would be evolving to match a superior state that is above the limited biological conditions created by evolution alone. In 1989, a philosophy professor at the New School for Social Research in New York, originally named F. M. Esfandiary, led a group of "UpWingers" in a movement to promote a transhumanist revolution (the name was intended to distinguish their group from left or right political groups). Esfandiary later legally changed his name to FM-2030 and was one of the first people to receive the new vitrification preservation process for cryogenically maintaining his brain after his death (in 2000).

By 1992, philosophy professors Max More and Tom Morrow had cofounded the Extropy Institute, as a public policy think tank for transhumanism ideas. ("Extropy" is the opposite of "Entropy Theory," which argues that nature naturally decays over time.) The goal of the movement was to encourage social awareness of the need for substantial public and private support for any technology that can enhance human life and surpass natural human limitations. Since the 1990s, the transhumanism movement has become both a philosophical ideal as well as a political movement. In 2016, Zoltan Istvan became the first presidential candidate under the Transhumanist Party.

The Singularity

Among modern transhumanists, the singularity is the point at which mankind may potentially achieve immortality, if not through biological life extension, then through a fusion of biological and technological bionics. One of the critical developments required for the future singularity is molecular nanotechnology, which would be used by robotic machines to synthesize more complex robotic machinery in the future to facilitate a perfect fusion of human biology and technology. Nanotechnology involves very small machines that are invisible to the human eye. They could be inserted into the human bloodstream or in other biological mediums to repair biochemical structures. Molecular nanotechnology would be so small that these machines might be able to manipulate atomic structure (the key ingredient missing from any practical bioprinter). Using a common communication system of bioelectricity, the synthetic technologies could be virtually indistinguishable from biological technologies—not necessarily in terms of appearance but in terms of function. A robot may be made to look human, but, more remarkably, a human could be made to look like a robot. And a robot could be made to act, think, and behave like a human—regardless of what shape it adopted.

In the ultimate transhumanist world, humans will not only rely on enhanced prosthetics that replicate natural body parts (limbs, muscles, eyes, ears, etc.), but they will also create new senses that humans do not currently possess. An integration of technology and biology would allow humans to be implanted with electronic chips that could insert memories directly into the human brain. Not only would this resolve issues of cognitive decline, but it would revolutionize education, as information would be uploaded directly into the brain instead of requiring years of training through visual and aural sensory input. Similar sorts of chips could include communication networks that would allow people to speak directly from one mind to another without the need for verbal or written communication. In this new world, human life would transcend into a sort of biotechnological synthesis.

Ray Kurzweil has written more than a dozen books on a wide variety of transhumanist concepts, such as the importance of artificial intelligence, nanotechnology, and virtual immortality. In his 2006 book *The Singularity Is Near*, Kurzweil predicts a very near future (within 40 years, around 2045) in which the power of computing technology will become so pervasive in society that human civilization, and even biology itself, will undergo an irreversible revolution resulting in a new synthesis of technology and humanity. Specifically, he predicts the creation of artificial intelligence that can so closely mimic human intelligence that the two might become interchangeable. Once the computer platform is prepared, humans could upload their consciousness and achieve a sort of virtual immortality.

This storage would only be a first stage for recording a past life. The next stage would involve an ability to transfer the consciousness into a new avatar (or robotic body, or series of bodies) that could provide additional sensory perceptions to allow continued growth of that consciousness. At that point, humanity would have achieved immortality on earth because it would no longer depend on physical bodies. It would no longer matter whether the biological body remained intact because the virtual consciousness would be able to transcend any medium to live forever in a virtual world (a little like *The Matrix*, except on a voluntary basis).

Kurzweil is known for making hundreds of predictions, but his theories are as much a symptom as they are a cause of a larger transhumanist movement. Along with other intellectuals, such as physicists Michio Kaku and Dirk Helbing, writers such as William Gibson and Paul Roberts, and computer scientists such as Christopher Alberg and Aubrey de Grey, Kurzweil both echoes and leads a growing following of like-minded people. Some of these include many economic leaders in technology, such as Peter Thiel (cofounder of PayPal), Larry Ellison (founder of Oracle), Larry Page and Sergey Brin (cofounders of Google), Mark Zuckerberg (founder of Facebook), and Sean Parker (founder of Napster and first president of Facebook). These young billionaires became interested and invested in antiaging during their thirties and have dedicated millions of dollars of their own money, plus billions of dollars of investment money, into antiaging research, development, and technology. There is little question that part of the reason for the growing popularity of the antiaging movement in the 21st century (and its growing funding) is largely due to their vocal and financial support.

The transhumanist movement is a subset of the antiaging movement, but it also goes beyond it. The antiaging movement hopes for biological immortality, whereas the transhumanist movement would be content with virtual immortality. As with many transhumanists, Kurzweil and others tread along the border between both movements. In addition to promoting futurist technologies, he also advocates strongly for any medical innovation that helps to extend the human life span. Technology will lead to an upcoming singularity, but it will also lead to biological life extension. This latter goal will require all the previous technologies discussed: chemical supplements to maintain consistent metabolic balance within the body; genetic manipulation to ensure continual functioning of cells; cloning and bioprinting to create synthetic replacement parts as needed; and nanotechnology and artificial intelligence to create enhanced prosthetics that ensure ultimate human abilities at all stages of life. For Kurzweil and others in the movement, the general benchmark of reaching the singularity is when most individuals in society prefer to live with artificially enhanced prosthetics over their naturally formed human body parts.

Utopia or Dystopia?

Hollywood mostly portrays a future singularity as the beginning of the end of humanity. Most science fiction films portray the future of humanlike artificial intelligence as the start of a war between humans and machines. Perhaps projecting past human trends on future computer personalities, Hollywood presumes that the virtual agents of intelligence will be just as quick to resort to violence and physical force to ensure a properly ordered society (much like Stalin, Hitler, or Mao Tze Tung, and others who believed scientific reason justified their dictatorial governments).

Hollywood is not alone in this skepticism. Jaron Lanier is a computer scientist who first popularized the term *virtual reality* as he developed many of the software constructs, such as immersive digital environments and the use of avatars to represent participants. Several of his technology firms were later purchased by Oracle, Adobe, Google, and Pfizer (for medical applications used for surgical simulation). Despite his history as a pioneer in developing virtual-reality technology, Lanier does not support Kurzweil's view of a coming singularity as either a practical reality or a positive goal. Two of his books, *Who Owns the Future?* (2014) and *You Are Not a Gadget* (2010), argue that human exceptionalism will never be replaced by human inventions, including imitative technologies. He has described the dream of a future singularity as "cybernetic totalism" and "digital Maoism" because it takes a theoretical ideal and imposes it as a single solution for all mankind. In the process, it ignores the reality both of actual computing potential and human individuality. Computers only do what they are programmed to do, and individual humans remain the only source of genuine creativity.

In the Utopian model of the singularity, mankind eliminates the vices and problems of human society by curing disease, aging, death, and other fundamental problems of human miscommunication and material scarcity. Once aging and disease have been defeated by biotechnology, only social conflicts remain. People can overcome individual prejudices by intimately joining one another in a common consciousness that transcends the limitations of speech and language. The need for material necessity can be overcome by the instant construction of virtual reality where there is no scarcity of anything. Long-held fears of overpopulation are overcome because biological bodies become less important than virtual identities, and there is an infinite amount of space in a digital landscape. A postsingularity society would raise ethical issues regarding the rights of virtual identities as well as the rights of human clones and biotechnological avatars. There would be a need for more regulatory oversight of biological reproduction because the physical bodies would not be allowed to outstrip the natural resources. But in a truly postsingularity society, all new births would be conducted through in vitro fertilization and planned according to social need, thereby eliminating the fear of overpopulation.

In the dystopian model, all the aforementioned benefits might be viewed as an ultimate assault on those characteristics that make humans human. Aldous Huxley, less optimistic than his brother Julian, wrote a dystopian novel of a technologically planned society in *A Brave New World* (1932). At the time, he was reacting to the growing sociopolitical philosophies of scientific determinism that were becoming dominant in Europe and which resulted in Soviet Communism and German National Socialism. For modern critics of a future singularity, the prospect of sterile efficiency would be viewed as an oppressive dictatorship if it eliminated the unpredictable randomized accidents and genius of individual free will. Even if computers were able to imitate human intelligence, their decision making would be based on detailed analysis of probability and outcome and not on the conviction of creative imagination that looks outside the realm of past experience to develop genuinely new ideas.

Jaron Lanier is not alone in his criticism of the potential for a future singularity. Nor is he alone in his belief that it is simply not a practical reality. Colin McGinn, a British philosopher specializing in mental cognition, argued that artificial intelligence only resembles human intelligence in its ability to recognize patterns, but computers cannot develop new ideas that are outside of these patterns. In this regard, human intelligence is unique. These criticisms were also echoed by Pulitzer Prize–winning philosopher Douglas Hofstadter, who described it as "a very bizarre mixture of ideas that are solid and good with ideas that are crazy." Like Lanier, other computer scientists are also skeptical for many of the same reasons. Paul Allen, one of the cofounders of Microsoft and a multibillionaire in his own right, argued that artificial intelligence is not simply a matter of building faster computers but about building software systems that reflect the "billions of parallel neuron interactions [that] result in human consciousness and original thought." Unlike Hofstader and McGinn, Allen does not dismiss the possibility of such artificial intelligence, but he argues it is so far in the future that we do not have enough information to even make a guess as to when it may occur—but certainly not anywhere near 2045. It would be akin to scientists discovering a technology that defies gravity: it is not necessarily impossible, but it is so far advanced that there is no way of predicting when (or if) it might be developed.

Perhaps the greatest criticism of the practical reality of a future singularity comes from religious quarters. The basic premise of transhumanism is that the biology of mankind evolved arbitrarily in reaction to its natural environment. As the creation of human life was arbitrary, the direction of evolution was equally arbitrary, except as a reaction to basic laws of nature. There is nothing preventing evolution from changing as humans decide. Once humans became conscious of their environment and masters of their environment, mankind also became masters of the evolutionary process itself, and all subsequent technological innovation is defining that process. Transhumanism, then, reflects man's conscious ascendency as the master of evolution and, in effect, creation. Immortality, then, becomes both a natural and an inevitable choice. This argument, and its premises, contradict any sense of religious belief that assumes mankind was deliberately created with a purpose outside of arbitrary chance.

By contrast, such geneticists as Michael Denton and the Discovery Center Institute of Human Exceptionalism based in Seattle, Washington argue that humans are exceptional because they were deliberately created by God and endowed with intelligence that is unique in the animal world. Likewise, Francis Collins, the director of the National Human Genome Research Institute at the National Institutes of Health, and author of *The Language of God*, has also argued that humans are exceptional among all living organisms. They have a unique potential of answering "why" we are here because humans were created with a particular kind of intelligence that comes from outside the created world (God).

Computers can never develop that intelligence because they owe their origins from the material world alone; as such, they can do nothing more than what humans program them to do. Computerized models are incapable of considering anything original and can only act through reference to preexisting ideas. Only humans can come up with new ideas. Other emotional virtues, such as love, compassion, empathy, humility, and courage (as well as their opposite vices), are also uniquely human traits and are critical components for understanding human intelligence. In these and other criticisms, there is a belief that human life is more than a collection of biochemical impulses, and the human consciousness exists outside the physical realm and as such cannot be replicated or transferred into material or digital mediums.

From a religious perspective, human identity exists from the soul and not from the bioelectrical impulses stored in the brain. Even if technology were to be developed that could capture those impulses, the "person" would not transfer with the digital copying process. It would remain tied to the body, just as life remains tied

Public Opinion and Artificial Human Enhancement

According to a Pew Research survey of 4,700 American adults in 2016, most people remain opposed to the prospect of using technology to improve human abilities. The survey also included six small focus groups of 47 people and asked their opinions on gene editing (to create "designer babies"), brain chip implantation, and the use of synthetic blood (to improve athletic performance). A large majority of respondents agreed that medical technology should continue to pursue innovations to "help the sick," but an equally strong segment opposed innovations intended to enhance otherwise healthy people. More than two-thirds (68 percent) said they were "somewhat worried" or "very worried" about using gene editing on human embryos to reduce the chance of contracting certain diseases. Such technology does not currently exist, but the potential is not unrealistic. Similarly, 69 percent of respondents said they were "somewhat" or "very" worried about brain chips to improve cognitive abilities, such as memory, and processing. The greatest reason for opposition was the fear that the technology would create inequitable social divisions between those who could afford the technologies and those who could not. Only 63 percent of respondents were concerned about synthetic blood that may enhance physical abilities by increasing potential oxygen intake. Mostly, the concerns were that the blood would undermine legitimate athletic competition.

to a physical organism. Science cannot create or transfer life from one substance to another, and so it cannot imbue virtual identities with real personhood into a computer hard drive.

For their part, transhumanists strongly reject these religious views. In 2016, Zoltan Istvan wrote an article for the *Huffington Post* titled "To Ensure a Future of Transhumanism, Atheists Should Confront the Deathist Culture Religion Has Sown." The title essentially states his thesis. Istvan's argument is that religion promulgates a belief in life after death, which provides an incentive for ignoring the potential and priority of pursuing an antiaging transhumanist agenda. Religion promotes a culture of humble acceptance of a divine will outside of human agency. It is the faith that there is something beyond this material world that interferes with full-scale investment in solutions that might perfect the conditions within this earthly realm. For transhumanists, that sort of faith contradicts the presumption of human sovereignty.

CONCLUSION

The practical goals of radical life extension do not require immediate solutions. The goal is not to create a 1,600-year life span by 2045, but rather to extend the expected life span merely 20 years by that time. If adults routinely lived to between 120 and 150 years, there would be more time to push the barrier back even further. Once the fixed life span of 120 has been broken, the natural evolution of medical advancements ought to gradually extend the limits each decade—from 150 years to 250 years, and from 250 years to 350 years, and so on, until virtual immortality is reached. Those who catch the initial wave of innovation might potentially become the first humans to live to that 1,000-year benchmark that Aubrey de Grey predicted. This is, however, not a new strategy. It was precisely the same strategy advocated by the Taoist masters during the second century in China.

Despite the often overoptimistic promises of existing drugs and the fantastic possibilities of future technology, most people in the antiaging movement are quite realistic about the reality of aging, age-related conditions, and death. In a 2013 interview, Aubrey de Grey explained, "At the moment, we are treating the diseases of old age as if they were curable. But actually, because aging is a side effect of being alive in the first place, of course they can't be cured." As a result, he warned that society places "far too much emphasis on treatment and far too little on prevention." The problem is that reactive medicine is always too late because by that time, most of the damage is already done. Damage from aging occurs most by affecting the body's ability to repair itself. Once that function has been crippled, the conditions of aging become irreversible.

For Aubrey de Grey, the solution, then, is to develop technologies that repair the seven major sources of cellular damage that inhibit the body's natural repair mechanisms. These include cell loss (tissue atrophy); cancerous cells; mitochondrial mutations (corruption of DNA during replication); death-resistant cells; extracellular matrix stiffening (hardening of cells); extracellular aggregates (accumulated waste outside cells, such as arterial plaque); and intracellular aggregates (accumulated waste inside cells, such as free radicals). For many antiaging advocates, the solution to defying age is to cure the causes that lead to age. It is no more than a mechanical solution to a mechanical problem.

On the other side of the aisle are critics who maintain that the human body is more than a biomechanical machine. Repairing its parts may improve healthy living and enable a more active lifestyle, but eventually the core of individual life includes an intellectual, emotional, and spiritual existence that transcends the physical body. In this regard, the purpose of life and its associated will to live is more significant than the biomedical machinery that permits it. The meaning of life is not simply to live, but to live with a reason. If all sickness, disease, and other effects of aging were resolved, and yet there was no underlying purpose behind life, then the extended years may well be viewed as much as a curse as it is a blessing. The critics of the antiaging movement do not oppose the goal of increasing health and well-being for the living, but they do not see it as an important enough goal to offset other spiritual and emotional priorities that constitute human fulfillment.

Zoltan Istvan argues that religion is a distraction to the antiaging movement and to the transhumanism movement because it builds on a future life in heaven, which renders mortal existence less important. Similarly, religious advocates such as Leon Kass (of the American Enterprise Institute) and Wesley Smith (of the Center on Human Exceptionalism) argue that the antiaging movement and transhumanism are a distraction to the more relevant goals of spiritual identity, which include increasing moral virtue and character development. Each side rests on fundamental presumptions that are contrary to the other. On one side are those who believe nothing exists outside the material physical realm and that all notions of an invisible immaterial world are wishful creations of human imagination that do not exist. On the other side are those who believe that there is an immaterial realm where the fundamental truths and causal agents upon which the spirit of life depends exist. For them, the immaterial realm enlightens and ultimately provides meaning for life. The belief in an immaterial realm requires a great deal of faith because there is no quantifiable evidence to support it. At the same time, however, it is equally clear that the belief in a strictly material realm requires at least an equal amount of faith.

In terms of antiaging, all the proposed remedies require more faith than the available scientific evidence provides. Chapter 11 identified a number of lifestyle changes that provide a better-than-average probability of improving health and well-being. Yet, none guarantee prevention of disease, or aging, or death. It requires an act of faith that the pursuit of a healthy lifestyle will result in an actual extension of the human life span. Perhaps even more so, in this chapter, we discussed numerous chemical and technological ways in which people might attempt to extend their life spans (or at least their appearance of youth). Yet, there is even less evidence that antiaging drugs or the list of potential future technologies will result in any meaningful extension of the human life span. There are a great many people who are willing to invest their money in the promise. That is also a matter of faith—just of a different kind.

Perhaps, though, for most people, these deeper philosophical questions of material and immaterial realms are not all that important. Given the size and extent of the antiaging market, it seems more likely that most people are searching out the modern technological fountain of youth for far more mundane reasons. It may require faith to belief these treatments will actually extend life, but it does not require much evidence at all to see the immediate cosmetic effects of looking younger. Antiaging treatments that use cosmetic surgery, makeup, and hormone treatments to keep a tight and athletic body do not require much faith in the future; they only require immediate results. Most consumers are less concerned about adding extra years and more concerned about looking fit, youthful, and sexually attractive. In this case, the short-term benefits of HRT and hGH (and other cosmetic products) are visible and noticeable right away. Whether the singularity ever occurs in the future, there is little question that the cosmetic side of the antiaging movement will continue to grow and thrive.

SECTION THREE

Views from the Experts: An Anthology of Views on the Implications of a Successful Antiaging Movement from a Spectrum of Disciplines

As the 21st century unfolds, the antiaging movement no longer relies on myths, superstition, or magic to promise youth and vitality. Modern researchers and entrepreneurs, including many influential public figures, sincerely believe in the practical potential for radically extending human life span. Every year, billions of dollars are poured into antiaging research, and public agencies have begun to place greater priority on finding solutions to the potential social changes that may follow increasing numbers of older adults. In some sectors, the question is not *if* but *when* will aging become a treatable and perhaps curable ailment?

There is no successful antiaging solution now, but what if that changes? How might society change as a result? The impact of an ever-increasing elder population is a separate subject in and of itself, and quite often it is framed in terms of public health, the economy, and the costs of elder care. The essays in this section are less focused on governmental policy debate and are directed more toward the interpersonal implications of extremely long lives. How does a long life span and extended youth affect our daily routines, our life decisions, and our very philosophy?

This section includes essays from experts in a variety of disciplines: biology, sociology, psychology, philosophy, history, art, and theology. The writers rely on the presumptions of their field, so the essays are factually and logically consistent. Yet, they were also encouraged to bring their own opinions to their answers. There is no successful antiaging solution now, so these writers can only speculate. Their arguments cannot be based on proven evidence, as none yet exists. Nevertheless, they rely on the logic and perspectives of their given disciplines. Their interpretations of antiaging dilemmas reflect their diverse perspectives.

Instead of a chapter format, the essays are arranged as questions, and each essay is labeled according to its general answer. The first question considers the practical reality of radical life extension based on current science. It is answered by two experts (in biology and biodemography and sociology). The second and third questions consider the impact of prolonged youthfulness and life spans on social interaction and cultural values. They are answered with six essays from a psychologist, visual artist, a historian, and two philosophers. The final category, and perhaps the most telling, asks how a successful antiaging movement might impact religious faith. These last essays are drawn from leading voices among the three dominant faiths in the Western world: Judaism, Christianity (Catholicism and Protestantism), and Islam. The final two experts reflect the voices of those who may question, or completely deny, the reality of God and religious conviction.

In the antiaging movement (as well as in most academia), the line between factual certainty and philosophical speculation is often blurred. These essays are arranged in a way that reflects the transition from quantitative speculation to more philosophical argumentation. The first essays rely heavily on science and the social sciences, while the final essays reflect explicit positions of faith. Each expert is unavoidably colored by the presuppositions of his or her particular discipline. It could be argued that all the essays reflect opinions and views of some sort of personal faith—whether the faith is based on scientific beliefs or on immaterial beliefs is a matter for further discussion.

Question

Can Science Really Develop a Fountain of Youth?

Fundamental to any question about the implications of antiaging in a modern society is the larger question of whether it is possible to radically extend the human life span? Critics of the antiaging movement and its goals come from a variety of sources—from those who fear that ever-increasing ages will lead to overpopulation and environmental disruption, to those who fear that an excessive preoccupation with life on earth will lead to neglected concern for spiritual life after death. One source of criticism has remained constant throughout the last 500 years that the antiaging movement has grown and developed in Western society: there are those who simply do not believe it is possible. Either they believe that the human life span is fixed (for biological or religious reasons), or they believe that the physical conditions of the material world simply do not allow for eternal things. These critics may be religious or atheistic. It is not a matter of faith but a question of practical realities. Often the debate stems from scientists who share most of the same beliefs on other matters of scientific interest, but who disagree on the existing and theoretical potential of particular technologies.

There are two dimensions to this debate. First, do the laws of physics and biochemistry permit a (more or less) permanent extension of human life? It may be that the medical community has not discovered the solution to radical extension of human life, but an affirmative answer presumes that at some point, in some future, those laws will be better understood, and radical life extension will become both possible, and commonplace. A negative answer presumes that, though the average human life span may fluctuate and the duration of healthy living may expand, the basic span of human life is fixed, and no amount of time or scientific discovery will significantly change that.

The second dimension to this question relates to the intersection between scientific optimism and economic opportunism. Even if you believe there is a theoretical possibility (however small) of increasing the human life span, you might also be convinced that such biomedical breakthroughs are so far away that they are not at all practical in the short-term, and they may even be impractical for the foreseeable future. This sort of realism unavoidably colors the assessment of the antiaging marketplace, which depends on the promise of scientific breakthroughs sooner rather than later. Consumers who spend money on antiaging treatments or who invest in antiaging technologies must believe that the breakthroughs will come during their lifetimes. The realist would conclude that the marketplace is fundamentally deceptive and based on the exploitation of false hopes. By contrast, the scientific optimist might recognize deceptive marketing campaigns among certain individuals, but would nevertheless contend that the promise and the goals are real and practically achievable.

Two scholars weigh in on this question. Both are very well-known within the antiaging community, yet neither of them represent extreme views on either end of the spectrum. Dr. João Pedro de Magalhães is a biologist who heads a research lab at Liverpool University and is heavily involved in comparative genetics, which is a specialty in genetic markers that effect aging. He is an expert in the field who seeks to understand the genetic limitations of any life span for any life-form.

Dr. S. Jay Olshansky is a sociologist from the University of Chicago and chief scientist at Lapetus Solutions, which is a private firm that specializes in using modern technology to predict life-cycle events in real time (critical for insurance underwriting). He is an expert in the field of biodemography, which seeks to identify biological factors that might influence demographic patterns, including birthrates, death rates, longevity, and aging.

Given the multidimensional aspect of this question, these answers cannot be reduced to a simple "yes" or a "no." Nevertheless, the two authors disagree on fundamental presumptions and provide contrasting answers to the question.

YES—THE PROSPECT OF EVENTUALLY FINDING A SCIENTIFIC EQUIVALENT OF THE FOUNTAIN OF YOUTH IS POSSIBLE, EVENTUALLY.
João Pedro de Magalhães

Qin Shi Huang, the first emperor of the Qin Dynasty, tried to achieve immortality by taking mercury pills prepared by his court physicians. Unfortunately, and ironically, he reportedly died of mercury poisoning in 210 BCE. According to legend, Ponce de León discovered Florida in 1513 while searching for the fountain of youth. Russian Bolshevik revolutionary and physician Alexander Bogdanov self-experimented with blood transfusions with the hope that this would rejuvenate him. He died in 1928 when he received blood from a student suffering from malaria and tuberculosis. These are just a few examples of the many who throughout history have sought eternal life. "The meaningless absurdity of life is the only incontestable knowledge accessible to man," wrote Leo Tolstoy. Not surprisingly, the inevitability of aging and death can be terrifying, leading many to search for eternal life.

Early attempts to discover the fountain of youth, from alchemists to the Holy Grail, were more mystical than scientific enterprises. Bogdanov's experiments were arguably the first based on a scientific model. Interestingly, even though a lack of knowledge of the potential harms of blood transfusions eventually cost him his life, there is now evidence from mouse studies that young blood could have rejuvenating properties, and clinical trials are currently underway to determine whether this might be true for humans as well. Besides, in recent decades, research into the biological determinants of aging has made important strides, opening the door for real antiaging interventions.

We now know that aging is neither inevitable nor universal. Some species of animals appear not to age at all. These include simple species such as hydra as well as more complex vertebrates, such as some species of fish, turtles, and salamanders. Even among mammals, although all are thought to age, there are huge variations in life span, from a few years for mice and rats to over 200 years for the bowhead whale. This massive range of life spans, also reflected in the physiological rates of aging (a mouse ages 20–30 times faster than a human being), show that aging can be modulated by evolution.

One of the greatest discoveries in the biology of aging is that aging can be manipulated by diet and by genetic interventions in short-lived model organisms such as flies, worms, and mice. By changing a single gene in worms, it is possible to extend their life span by tenfold! The process of aging is surprisingly plastic. A growing number of labs in academia and biotech companies are now building on these discoveries to develop interventions, including drugs that retard human aging. We have come from trying to locate the fountain of youth to crafting it in high-tech research labs.

What are the prospects of curing aging? In the short-term, I think they are negligible. Although we can retard aging in short-lived animal models, reversing aging has not been demonstrated. Aging is a complex process involving multiple changes that affect virtually all organs. Intervening in specific age-related changes, such as skin aging, is possible and often labeled "anti-aging medicine." But some experts consider that misleading because such interventions only affect very specific aspects of aging, so real antiaging therapies capable of reversing the whole aging process have not yet been established. Furthermore, the retardation of aging in model organisms still needs to be demonstrated in more complex humans, which is likely not a simple step. And while I am optimistic that findings from model systems can be translated to improve human health and life by delaying aging, their benefits will still fall well short of curing aging. Life-extending interventions in mammals, typically rodents, extend life span up to 50 percent. Although this would be remarkable, even if only a fraction could be applicable to human beings, for example in the form of longevity drugs or gene therapy, it is still very far from curing aging.

Emerging technologies like genome editing and regenerative medicine hold great promise, but their potential in tackling aging is still unproven. When looking decades ahead there is room for great progress. Given that aging is malleable and some animals avoid it entirely, there is no reason to think it cannot be cured, even if it may be decades or centuries from now.

We have come a long way since Qin Shi Huang took his mercury pills. No longer are we taking shots in the dark regarding what may or may not work to prevent aging. The biology and genetics of aging have opened avenues for developing longevity drugs that I am convinced will have unprecedented medical benefits. There is also a growing cultural current for developing life-extending rejuvenation technologies, mostly driven by atheist and agnostic techies. For centuries, religion has offered the promise of eternal life, but now science is taking over that role. In the foreseeable future, modest extensions of human health and life from retarding aging are likely to become a reality. Centuries from now, aging and death may well be sad past tales.

NO—THE HUMAN LIFE SPAN IS NOT EASILY ADJUSTABLE, BUT LONGER LIVES OF HEALTHY LIVING ARE POSSIBLE.
S. Jay Olshansky

Boastful claims of miracle cures for every disease that has plagued humanity have been part of folklore dating back thousands of years. The promise of immortality, or at least radical life extension, has also been a common theme in books, movies, and most religions. By way of example, ancient Egyptians claimed miracle balms could restore youthful appearance. Chinese and Indian sages asserted that death could be forestalled by controlling how rapidly we breathe. Alchemists from the Middle Ages concocted "scientific" potions to combat diseases. Physicians in the early 20th century grafted the glands from animals onto older men with claims of rejuvenation, while modern equivalents with impressive academic or medical degrees (some obtained legitimately, others not so much) assert that immortality is within reach. It should therefore be no surprise that similar claims have been made in the modern era about aging itself—the underlying risk factor for most of what goes wrong with our bodies as we grow older.

If any of these declarations of disease eradication or radical life extension were actually true, there would be no disease, no aging, and no death. The fact that all three are still with us has not deterred the hucksters and their true believers throughout the centuries. In fact, the long line of what has come to be known as prolongevists that have surfaced through history, and which exist in abundance today, seem to share one common characteristic beyond their collective fantasy: they are all dead or heading in that direction. They are trying to make a living off our fear of death, and in many ways, they're succeeding.

In modern times, aging hucksterism is called "antiaging medicine," which is an unfortunate phrase, as scientists who study aging are actually not against growing older—we just dislike the infirmities that often accompany it. In fact, growing old is a privilege that has been denied to most throughout history. The fact that there are no proven aging interventions in existence today does not seem to deter its proponents. The more closely the nail of reality approaches the heart of aging hucksters, the louder they pronounce that a conspiracy is afoot that scientists won't release the cure for cancer or the "aging disease" as a way to keep the public in need of us all. After all, immortality would put the health care industry out of business. I personally can't think of anything more I'd like to see happen.

So, let's be clear. The modern version of history's longstanding notion of anti-aging medicine and all of the unfounded promises that go along with it is, quite simply, the second-oldest profession.

Having burst the bubble of the past and present antiaging medicine movement, there is nevertheless important good news. There is no need to exaggerate or over-state the case by promising that we are all about to live hundreds or thousands of years or achieve immortality. And although there are no magical potions that exist today that can even come close to fulfilling the claims of immortalists past and present, scientists are on the verge of breakthroughs that may enable many of us today to drink from a modest equivalent of a fountain of youth. The scientific study of aging is at an exciting precipice, with new evidence emerging daily about successful research efforts to extend life and slow aging in other species. There is every reason to believe the same can be accomplished in people. There is even a movement afoot, now supported by scientific evidence, to suggest that even a minor success in slowing aging would yield huge health and economic dividends to individuals and societies today and for decades into the future. This is known as the Longevity Dividend Initiative (LDI) or Geroscience, and this movement has taken on a life of its own.

Although immortality or radical life extension may not be in the cards, the time may come soon when the means to make us healthier for a longer period of time will become readily available. Along with colleagues George Martin, from the University of Washington, and Jim Kirkland, from the Mayo Clinic, we just published an edited volume by Cold Spring Harbor Laboratory Press titled *Aging: The Longevity Dividend* (2015) in which we outline the various scientific pathways researchers are now taking to modulate aging and extend the period of healthy life. This is no longer theoretical—it's going to happen.

Immortality and eternal youth will remain wishful pursuits lacking scientific credibility and biological plausibility, but there is every reason to believe that prog-ress in reducing avoidable mortality at middle and older ages will continue. Mod-ern science has made progress in understanding the biological determinants of longevity and aging with the intent of eventually using that knowledge to improve quality of life by extending the period of healthy life. Aging interventions are about to become the new public health paradigm of the 21st century.

Question

Does Youthfulness Breed Recklessness?

Finding the fountain of youth often inspires positive images of increased energy, strength, and youthful beauty. Older adults might remember the advantages of their youth that they miss rather than the difficult challenges of their youth that they no longer fear. With age and experience comes wisdom, caution, and the advantages of hindsight. One of the concerns about medical breakthroughs that promise to extend youthful vitality into later years is that they may encourage a sort of recklessness that is most associated with youth. Addressing this concern requires answers to other related questions. Is recklessness a by-product of youthful hope, which comes from knowing that there is a very long future ahead? Or is recklessness strictly a by-product of biological immaturity? Will experience and years automatically inspire wisdom? Or is it the decline of the human body or the fear of an impending death that inspires cautious living? Will the first two decades of life always be viewed in the same way, or does extending the average life span to 200, 400, or even 1,000 years necessarily change the definition of "youth"?

There are at least two approaches for answering these questions. The first is to consider the nature of human behavior and to decide whether "youth" is determined more by biological or psychological development. If youthful immaturity is a function of incomplete physiological development, then extended adulthood would have little impact on the behavioral expectations of later stages in the life cycle. Once the biological body reaches full maturity in adulthood, the psychological decision-making parts will begin to act predictably, and long periods of adulthood would have little effect on the probability of greater risk-taking. This view assumes behaviors are mostly determined by physiology. If, however, behaviors are a result of free will, then immaturity and reckless behaviors might arise at any age. Longer spans of healthy adulthood might lead to a greater variety of temptations and may lead to increasing trends of recklessness throughout society.

The second approach to these questions is to consider the nature of wisdom. If wisdom is defined by a sort of restraint that transcends youthful inexperience, then the definition of "recklessness" might conceivably change as the length of the average life span increases. Someone who is 350 years old might dismiss the actions of someone who is 120 years old as "reckless and immature." Even as an adult enters into older ages, the relative definitions of "cautious" and "restraint" would always be in flux. Alternatively, if wisdom is defined by more rigid standards of virtue and character, the age of an adult would have little to do with whether he or she were wise, or cautious, or reckless, or imprudent. A young person may be wise, if he or she adheres to the standards of restraint and prudence. Likewise, an older person may be reckless if he or she behaves unpredictably. Short lives or long lives would have little effect on these cultural standards.

These sorts of questions really reflect presumptions of human nature and cannot be answered decisively through science alone. The scholars for this question were drawn from fields of psychology, the visual arts, and history. Each discipline specializes in the study of human nature, though from a nonmechanical perspective. The psychologist Jill Rinzel tackles the question of youthful recklessness from the perspective of a social scientist and weighs the more predictable expectations of physiological development against the irregular patterns of adult decision making, which are often impulsive and capricious. The field of psychology provides a descriptive vocabulary based on quantitative research and then applies it to human behaviors, thereby bridging the divide between scientific determinism and human variability. Gregory Johnson is a visual artist who specializes in capturing the emotional aspects of human nature that are not quantifiable and often difficult to express or capture in words. He approaches the question by examining the examples of other artists and their works to reveal something about recklessness among those who express their emotions as a vocation. The last essay is written by Jeff Kleiman, who is an historian that studies human nature by tracing the trends and choices of those who have come before. He compares the motivations of figures in historic literature to the common clichés of modern society to highlight those universal characteristics of human recklessness that seem to continually perplex observers. By tracing the trends of human motivations in the past, he makes a prediction of potential expectations for similar decision-making processes in the future.

YES—IF SOCIETY REMAINS PREOCCUPIED BY YOUTHFUL LIFESTYLES AND NEGLECTS WISDOM, IT WILL BREED RECKLESSNESS.
Jill A. Rinzel

Youthfulness is certainly valued in American culture. Advertisements bombard us with thousands of products to help individuals look younger, feel younger, and act younger, but what does this mean to our culture as a whole? And why is this idea of youthfulness tied to ideas of recklessness? Is youthfulness the best goal? What are the repercussions of this type of focus?

There has been considerable research over the last few decades suggesting that brain development doesn't finish until the early twenties, and one of the last parts of the brain to fully develop is the prefrontal cortex, which helps weigh decisions, control impulses, and think about the consequences of possible actions. Additionally, teens seem to rely more on lower levels of the brain that rely on more gut-level responses and respond strongly to novelty and stimulation. Because of this, as well as other possible factors, teens are at a higher risk of behaving impulsively and recklessly. Does this mean that in order to be "youthful" one also needs to be reckless?

One major factor that has changed in the way we look at teens and adults, which plays into this, is society's definition of when "adulthood" begins. Adolescence was first popularized by Stanly G. Hall around 1900. This stage of life was used to refer to the time between childhood and adulthood, essentially extending the time period before truly becoming an adult. However, as society changed (delaying marriage and child-rearing, prolonging financial dependence and education, low-paying entry-level jobs, etc.), teens and individuals in their early twenties often remained dependent on their parents for longer and longer periods of time. In 1995, Jeffery Jensen Arnett used the term "emerging adulthood" to define the time after adolescence but before the individual is truly independent of his or her parents, approximately ages 18–25. During this time period, emerging adults are often dependent on their parents financially, emotionally, and socially. They are also more likely to engage in some risky behaviors. For example, they are more likely to engage in jobs that allow for large amounts of travel or involve risky behavior, known as *edgework*. While this time period connects well with the neuroscientific research on brain development, it also suggests an acceptance and encouragement of a prolonged youthful period of life and helps to explain why recklessness is associated with youthfulness.

This certainly suggests an acceptance of youthfulness and recklessness well into one's twenties, but does it continue due to society's idealization of youthfulness? Yes and no. Many types of reckless behavior drop off significantly after the teens and twenties, such as automobile accident rates and some risky driving habits. However, other types of behavior continue to be a problem and signal a more unconscious type of recklessness. For example, 68 percent of U.S. adults do not participate in employer-sponsored retirement plans, and those that do often do not save enough to sustain their standard of living in retirement. Additionally, only 26.3 percent of American adults surveyed had advanced directives in place. While these are not the same types of reckless behavior that teens engage in, it does suggest a lack of planning and forethought, which is similar to the type of thinking that is characteristic of youthfulness. American adults have been living longer, healthier lives than in the past, and this may be creating a focus on youth and immortality that, in combination with a society that values youthfulness, enables adults to put off thinking about major issues.

Feeling younger and healthier at older ages is wonderful, if adults still take responsibility and prepare appropriately for their futures. A society that encourages youthfulness by default downplays the importance in planning for the inevitable: aging and death. It is reckless for adults to fail to plan and save for the future, and it will end up causing problems for them and for society as a whole when aging adults end up relying more on public programs to support themselves in old age. Therefore, although recklessness in some overt ways decreases with age, it may take different forms as individuals age, with nonetheless serious outcomes.

This shift from more overt forms of recklessness to more unconscious forms (avoiding planning for the future) may be the point where brain development and societal values diverge. When the brain fully develops in one's early twenties, young adults are more capable of planning and forethought, and they are less likely to be highly influenced by the novelty of a risky situation. This explains the decline in reckless driving and accident rates, but the emphasis that society places on youthfulness, tempered by a fully developed brain, allows for a continuation of denial that aging and death will occur. Until our society embraces more of a drive and appreciation for the wisdom, experience, and responsibilities of adulthood, it is likely that large proportions of our society will continue to engage in the fallacy of eternal youthfulness and the risky behavior that goes along with it.

MAYBE—PERSISTENT YOUTHFUL IMMATURITY IS DETERMINED BY INDIVIDUALS' CHARACTER, NOT AGE.

Gregory Nathan Johnson

What will those of the future find in 2525? Laibach, the genre transgressive, politically influential musicians from Slovenia ask this question in their song titled "2525." The song lyrics foretell a future marred by war and imply that we will forget and not learn from the past. Those of a certain age may remember Laibach's lyrics as a parody of the earlier Zager and Evans 1969 Billboard smash hit "In the Year 2525." Ironically, it is an open question whether either song will be remembered in a half of a millennium. It doesn't take old age to forget—only the ignorance of youth. As Sigmund Freud said, "If youth knew, if age could."

As these songs suggest, humanity may well repeat the same selfish mistakes despite having access to technology that improves the conditions of daily life. New advances in science propose an extended youthfulness in our bodies or a delay of our deathly decay, yet will our minds and hearts also become purified? For many, this kind of advancement would seem like a Utopian dream, and the world would be better because of it. However, can our culture really survive extended youthfulness? It is my belief that we should be wary of confusing a longer, younger, or even immortal life with a better life. It may even be the case that if we were to live a long, healthy life as an eternal twenty-something, we may hurt our ability to be self-reflective and to grow in character.

The challenge in making this argument is that we have no direct evidence. We cannot pick up the phone and call a 200-year-old person or an immortal human being and question them on their quality of life and character. We can however look to the stories we tell each other and, in doing so, see the perceived concerns we have with extended youthfulness or an immortal life.

Superhero comics are a great place to set our sights. The Marvel Comics character Deadpool, in the 2016 self-titled film, starts as a wisecracking mortal human with a high degree of cynicism, neurosis, and moral ambiguity. Deadpool then acquires super-healing powers that grant him near immortality. Even with death conquered, he still remains a neurotic, cynical, and morally unclear individual. The Marvel Comics character Wolverine exhibits the same healing conditions and similar personality. Yet, virtual immortality provides no cure to either Deadpool's or Wolverine's troubled emotional states or character flaws. Deadpool and Wolverine are both "blessed" with nearly immortal bodies, but, unfortunately, their characters also have monstrous appearances: Deadpool is scarred by severe burns, and Wolverine has large metal claws.

The theoretical experience of a long life, where one never grows old yet is also beautiful, has been explored in the popular mythology of the eternal and always beautiful elves. The Western concept of the elves is molded by J.R.R Tolkien's *Lord of the Rings* trilogy. Tolkien's concept of the elves was then appropriated in many other authors' literary works, including Gary Gygax's *Dungeons & Dragons* role-playing game system. In Gygax's fantasy world, elves live long, youthful lives and may not reach adulthood until around 100 years old. It is assumed that, with immortality, the elves are slow learners, and their mental or physical maturity is curbed. As any college student knows, deadlines are the best motivators. If the antiaging movement does produce significantly longer periods of youthfulness (thereby pushing the mortal deadline further from our sight), humanity might become hedonistic. We may become too sluggish to grow up and become responsible women and men.

We do not all respond to the deadline of death the same. Some respond to the transition from youth to adulthood under the inevitability of death with positive action. Others respond with resolute hedonism and little self-reflection. In the 18th-century rococo period of art history, many artists valued youthful beauty and hedonism. Examples are found in Jean-Honoré Fragonard's paintings of drunken satyrs, porcelain-skinned maidens, and sexual fantasies in pastel lighting. The neoclassical period followed and purged rococo style through the use of somber color, reasoned restraint, and strong compositions of vertical and horizontal lines. It also returned to premodern moralizations found in Greek and Roman mythology. The rococo-influenced painter turned neoclassicist Jacques-Louis David, in his twenties, wrote, "I realized, that to proceed like the ancients, and be like Raphael [a Renaissance artist]—that was truly to be an artist. . . . I had confidence that I would save myself, and the ardor [coarse grains] of my will did not rest." Despite his youthful angst and coarse will, we see a young man recalling past cultures, fusing the old and new by emulating the ancient styles with his own voice. The hope was to build upon the shoulders of giants and make the world a better place. His effectiveness can be debated, but the intention was honorable.

David was by no means perfect or without criticism; one only needs to look at his misplaced support of Napoleon. He was, however, motived to build his character and move past his youthful desires. The 20th-century artist Pablo Picasso's long and relatively healthy life stands in contrast. On a self-portrait created in his youth, Picasso declared himself, *"Yo el Rey"* (I the King). Like a king, he indulged in sexual fantasies and violence, even in old age. His art from the beginning was inextricably bound to his youthful virility. Picasso's primary self-identity was often made manifest in the image of the Minotaur, the mythological half man, half bull that was appeased by the sacrifice of young maidens. Tragically, Picasso's firm hold on youth gave him little honest self-reflection and self-knowledge nor empathy for others.

Picasso's emotional maturity can be questioned. Like a child, he harbored uncontrolled self-indulgence. Old age provided him little in humility or genuine kindness. Like a vampire, he mixed carnal sexual love with violence. For Picasso, love was mostly physical. He devoured his lovers for inspiration in his artwork, and when his carnal love faded, he left his wife or mistress for a younger woman to mistreat. Each time, he left the woman on his terms. Perhaps each affair offered an opportunity for Picasso to forget his own passage of time and renewed feelings of youthfulness. Many women were hurt by Picasso, either through physical abuse or through rejection after years of dedication to him.

This pattern continued until his mistress Françoise Gilot and their two children left him in 1953. The result was like a castration, though the event wasn't enough for Picasso to end his delusion. Picasso was reflective throughout his career, but when he turned the mirror unto himself, I believe he was only looking for self-gratification and self-glory, like the wicked witch questioning the mirror, "Who is the fairest of them all?" This is illustrated in Pablo's *The Theater of Picasso*, an etching made in 1970 when he was close to 90 years old. Simon Schama's analysis of this artwork in his article "How Matisse and Picasso Turned Old Age into Art" (drawing from Janie Cohen's original research essay "Picasso's Dialogue with Rembrandt's Art") reveals the work is designed after Rembrandt's work titled *Ecco Homo*. In the center of Picasso's etching stands a representation of himself in the role of a guilt-less Jesus Christ surrounded by Picasso's numerous past mistresses, models, and wives. These women assume the role of the crowd surrounding Christ, demanding his death. The hubris and misplaced self-pity is overwhelming. For nearly 90 years of active life, Picasso remained Picasso.

It would be dangerous for us to believe that the promises made by the antiaging movement to extend life would make us any better as people. This belief may lead to a new kind of hubris. A long life valuing youthful culture doesn't mean we won't succumb to the folly of past mistakes. The stories we tell warn us that immortality will not cure us of our character flaws. If technology develops as the antiaging movement promises, we may live longer than any generation before and even hold onto our teenage appearance into adulthood. If any of us live to see the year 2525, let us not become elvish—beautiful but stunted in maturity. If science gives us near immortality, let us not become like Deadpool—neurotic and incapable of change in character. Rather, let's live knowing death is around the corner and become motivated to do the right thing now for ourselves, the ones we love, and humanity.

NO–AN OLDER POPULATION WILL LIKELY RESULT IN MORE CONSERVATIVE BEHAVIORS.
Jeffrey Kleiman

Few people will recall that Jonathan Swift wrote about extreme longevity. In *Gulliver's Travels*, we encounter a group of people born with a special mark signifying them as an elite of their society. These men and women live to an incredible age, yet they despise this opportunity. For them, this was no gift; rather, it is a curse. Old age means extended decrepitude, senility, and a desire to die that remains unfulfilled. An extended old age becomes ever more problematic. Swift's commentary here is obvious. Many people wish for extended life, but only under ideal conditions of physical and mental health. They would be forever vital, energetic, and capable.

However, let us assume for the moment that such a bounty of extended life with some guarantee of mental acuity and physical health is attainable. What then? How would life proceed? There are several approaches to ponder as we consider an unimaginably extended life span.

First, would life be extended in all its phases? We might ask if people were to live hundreds of years whether a more extended period of infancy, adolescence, maturity, middle age, and such become necessary preconditions. Instead of the terrible twos, do we dread the terrible 200s? Should we look forward to a century of teenaged rebellion and anxiety as a step toward several decades of high school and then college education? Intellectual and cognitive development cannot be rushed. Today, the evidence strongly suggests that brain maturity, especially the frontal lobes that guide rational decision making, do not ripen until the early-to-mid-twenties. Men generally take longer than women to achieve this state of higher executive functions. Would there be an eternity of spring break madness and never-ending requests of, "May I have the keys to the car tonight?" We might have a society where the ravages of puberty, accompanied by immature risk-taking, carries on beyond decades. How many of us would want to consider dozens of years as a midlife crisis or celebrate a centennial anniversary of achieving menarche?

Second, economic considerations loom large in our thoughts. How quickly would economic activity need to expand to accommodate an unprecedented long-lived population—how long would an average career span? Even with the possibility of good physical health, we, as a species, may not be equipped to cover a millennium of daily work routine. In difficult economic times, when people tend to hold on to secure jobs longer, there would likely be decades of "younger" folks circling, vulture-like, around the want ads, anxiously looking for impending retirements. Unless economic expansion occurred a regular pace, with provisions for fewer births, a stagnant economy would produce centuries of unemployment or minimum-wage jobs. Without sufficient economic growth, what would be the point of an extended life in poverty? Without sufficient opportunities, who would be content for a longer life struggling to survive?

A third consideration becomes retirement. In a greatly extended life span, when does retirement become a serious consideration? Will we be constrained by issues of health, the need to vacate a post to create job openings, our own whims based on a desire for a career change—of having changed careers too often? In a world of the super old, even with dynamic intervention to deal with replacement parts, corrective surgery, artificial this and that, we will face a longer period of retirement. During that time, people will be forced to reflect on how they have used their extra decades, if not centuries. Beyond the issues of introspection, there is the reality of being able to afford not working. After all, unless extended life spans are only for the very wealthy, ordinary folks will have to deal with a pension that must keep pace with 50 years or more of inflation.

Finally, we imagine a world of constant and bold innovation. Yet, most ordinary people embrace an increasingly conservative outlook as they age. Resistance to technological change becomes more pronounced. Recall the wave of jokes about older people many years ago when the programmable VCR first appeared. These wonderful new machines sat there flashing "12:00" for hours on end. Even today, it is not unusual for many older people turn to a younger generation for help with the perpetual updates that accompany the electronic features of our world. It is likely that as more people live longer and increase in greater numbers, this conservatism would find expression in the marketplace of goods and ideas. Politics of the super elderly would dominate the national agenda. And they would be heard, because older people are the most consistently organized voters.

There is much to consider in the drive to extend lifetimes. Impacts and unintended consequences abound. Even if we reject Swift's description of extended life span as an unalterable curse of perpetual infirmity and senility, we must reason through some likely consequences of living longer.

Question

Will the Benefits of Very Long Life Spans Outweigh the Social Costs?

At first glance, it would make sense to expect that a long life of health and well-being should automatically be welcomed as a social good. The alternative of a short life with sickness and disease is hardly a better option. The champions of antiaging technology uniformly agree. Life is good, sickness and death are evil, and society should do everything in its power to extend the first and eliminate the second. And yet, there remains considerable disagreement about whether significantly extending human life beyond current expectations is good for society. The question is not really about whether it is good to live a long and healthy life using the terms by which we know of life now. Rather, the deeper question is whether we would prefer to change the very conditions of life so that sickness and death are eliminated. That involves a much greater commitment to radical change.

The full implications of radical life extension must be considered before the technology exists to realize it. As Leon Kass wrote, "Conquering death is not something that we can try for a while and then decide whether the results are better or worse." If the medical technology necessary to eliminate sickness and to limit the power of death is discovered, it becomes a permanent innovation and cannot be unlearned. The unintended consequences become unavoidable once the technology is proven to be effective. What would such an innovation cost in terms of human resources, and do the potential benefits outweigh those costs? Is sickness and disease less desirable than the other consequences that may come from radically changing human life span? Are there enough resources to support more people? Would human society have to limit individual freedom to preserve the necessary resources? Would people be willing to make such sacrifices? Would this help or hinder the development of human moral reasoning? The answers to these questions should be considered before the technology is developed, because once the innovations are discovered, the unintended consequences become unavoidable.

At the same time, though, fear of unknown consequences should not overshadow the potential for known benefits. Historically speaking, humankind has always suffered sickness and death, and much suffering has come as a result of it. The actual experience of suffering and loss is a known quantity, so it is reasonable to assume that reducing sickness and diminishing the incidents of unexpected deaths would surely serve to alleviate some of that suffering. How can we justify not pursuing medical breakthroughs that would lead to greater health and longer lives?

These are philosophical questions that require insight into human nature. If we can assume that human nature is more or less positive, we should welcome longer lives to express it. We might also have greater faith in human ingenuity to solve the unintended problems that could arise from radically extended life spans. At the same time, if we are unsure about human nature or about humankind's ability to fix its own errors, then extending the life span may invite more problems than answers. The fear of unexpected and unintended consequences will outweigh the expected benefits of long life and healthy living.

These essays are weighted slightly in favor of the realists, rather than the optimists. The first two are written by philosophers who identify potential costs of radically long life spans, which are considered less often. Nicholas Agar is a philosopher from New Zealand who specializes in questions that ask how technological enhancements might change human nature and human virtue. Dale Murray is a philosopher from Wisconsin who specializes in environmental ethics and the intersection with human intervention into the natural order. The last expert is a historian, Jeff Kleiman, who specializes in the nightmares of human history, particularly the Jewish Holocaust during the World War II. Of the three writers, his essay is the most optimistic.

NO—THE PRICE OF RADICAL LIFE EXTENSION IS GREATER THAN MERE MONEY.
Nicholas Agar

Life extension seems to be an uncontroversial good. Almost all of us enjoy being alive, most of the time. As life extension promises more life, it must surely be good. In what follows, I suggest that we should think differently about what we might call moderate life extension, which produces life spans up to and somewhat beyond those currently experienced by humans, and radical life extension, which produces life spans well beyond those currently experienced by humans. The longest confirmed human life span was the 122 years and 164 days, enjoyed by Frenchwoman Jeanne Calment. This would make life extension up to and slightly beyond that age moderate. The maverick gerontologist Aubrey de Grey seeks rejuvenation therapies that could offer life expectancies of 1,000 years. His aspiration is clearly to radically extend human life spans. The categories of moderate and radical life extension lack precise boundaries. There's a degree of vagueness between moderate and radical life extension, just as there is some vagueness between those who belong to the class of bald people and those who are properly classed as hirsute. It's likely that life spans of 140 years fall within a region of vagueness between the moderate and the radical. This vagueness does not prevent us from using the distinction between moderate and radical life extension to capture differences between proposals to lengthen human lives, just as hairstylists respond differently to requests from the bald and the hirsute.

The most popular way to achieve moderate life extension is to live what we intuitively acknowledge as a healthy life. You should refrain from smoking, take regular exercise, eat a moderate and varied diet, and not holiday in known war zones. A slightly longer life span is one result among other benefits predictably conferred by a healthy lifestyle. Radical life extension promises life spans well beyond the longest lives enjoyed by humans up until now. It is unlikely to occur as the result of regular morning jogs and diets rich in leafy green vegetables. Rather, it is likely to require intervention in the fundamentals of human biology.

To see this, it's useful to consider a prominent recent proposal about how to achieve radical life extension. De Grey hopes to achieve radical life extension by ending aging. There is no possibility of a pill that will magically end aging. Aging is a by-product of being alive. Human bodies wear out in much the same way as driving wears out parts of cars. You can nevertheless keep a car on the road indefinitely by repairing the damage as it accumulates. De Grey wants to pursue the same approach to damage that accumulates in human bodies. There are numerous systems in the human body that accrue damage as we live. De Grey seeks to make his task manageable by focusing on the cellular level. He proposes that the multitude of life-shortening diseases reduce to seven types of damage that either occur to cells or affect the ways in which cells relate to each other. De Grey expects repairs of the seven causes of aging to yield indefinite life spans. Someone with an indefinite life span might expect to live up to a thousand years. These rejuvenation therapies will not come cheap. De Grey argues that the problem of aging requires the kind of coordination of effort and resources that put humans on the moon. It's likely to be the most expensive cooperative endeavor ever attempted by humans.

How should we think about this proposal? De Grey treats aging as a technological problem with a very costly technological solution. He rates aging as "humanity's worst problem" and is therefore confident the money is worth spending. Evaluation of this claim requires us to move beyond very general questions about whether life extension is good or bad. The decision to end aging does not occur in a vacuum. We must ask how worthy a pursuit of radical life extension is when compared with all of the other things we might do. Trade-offs occur on both the individual and societal level.

De Grey goes into some detail on one such trade-off. Suppose that we do achieve radical life extension. There is an expected problem of overpopulation. The burden of humanity on the earth's fragile ecosystems will increase significantly if the global birthrate continues as it is, but the rate at which people die greatly slows. If would be reckless to radically extend our life spans and simply hope for the best. De Grey suggests that the price for an indefinite life span should be childlessness. Those who want to confront the future with a clear conscience must choose between living indefinitely and having kids. To make this decision, you must do more than acknowledge the abstract attractiveness of a radically extended life span. You must consider the relative values of (1) living indefinitely and having possibly many children while overburdening the biosphere, (2) living an indefinite childless existence with a clear conscience, or (3) accepting only moderate life extension, having children, and having a clear conscience. Even if you really enjoy living and would like to live longer, it does not seem prudentially irrational to prefer option 3.

It's also important to consider trade-offs at the societal level. De Grey is asking for large sums of money to realize his vision of agelessness. More money on rejuvenation therapies means less money on other things, such as fighting poverty or ameliorating climate change. Again, one can acknowledge the abstract appeal of indefinite life spans for all who desire them while rejecting the suggestion that radical life extension ranks particularly high on our civilization's list of priorities.

In this short essay, I have suggested that good decisions about radical life extension must take account of the context in which they are taken. We must go beyond acknowledging the abstract appeal of agelessness to consider other values and goals that predictably conflict with radical life extension. What might be a priority for other societies at morally better times should not be viewed as particularly important for us here and now.

NO—THE OVEREMPHASIS ON VITALITY WILL LIKELY UNDERMINE THE SUBTLE NATURE OF MORAL CHARACTER.

Dale Murray

Through a range of dietary, pharmacological, and genetic interventions, the antiaging movement has perpetuated the promise of a fountain of youth. This seems to heavily involve an emphasis on vitality and has already, in some respects, changed the way that the young interact with the old, especially in the West. It may also involve how older people regard themselves and other elders. But what could possibly be culturally risky about extending vitality? After all, some of the interventions seeking to cure diseases and alleviate unnecessary suffering have admirable characteristics.

How *vitality* is understood is important. Part of it seems to involve energized capacities, but all too often, the expectation of popular culture translates "vitality" into "attractive outward appearance." With that, an emboldened antiaging movement could bring about unanticipated, ancillary hardships to the elderly. The zeal for reversing the aging process seems to contain within it an implicit message: Those who are not as quick, agile, virile, or who reveal the weather-worn creases and sags of age have not merely lost those abilities and physical attributes. It is as if they have somehow relinquished their value *as subjects* who previously harbored those traits. There already appears to be public obsession in the West with outward appearance. It's reasonable to speculate that its continuation may lead to greater disregard of those unable or unwilling to meet ideal societal expectations.

All of this could erode the importance of moral character. The worry of overemphasizing the appearance of things is that it might replace the intrinsic value that comes from excellence of internal character, which could be defined as action in accordance with the virtues. Constant expansion of the life span could undermine a mind-set of respectful acceptance of our limitations. It runs the risk of distracting us from what genuinely matters and what could enrich *both* youth culture and its more mature counterpart.

Are the premises behind the antiaging movement morally laudable? Which virtues are in peril? One is humility. Michael Sandel has recently decried the onslaught of genetic enhancements, noting that such interventions do not pay proper respect to the gifted nature of our talents. However, I want to take humility from a slightly different perspective. Sandel combats hubris—humans overreaching their bounds. I am thinking more of humility as acceptance of people "where they are." That one needn't be a supermodel or have had the latest Botox surgery to live a satisfying life. However, what may be considered staid, slow, inactivity of elders actually might reflect careful contemplation. Not rushing to judgment before speaking has value. This quiet reserve resists hasty generalizations. This is a good lesson to learn, one that we often try to teach our students. Counter to this is the quick and sometimes impulsive attitude toward embracing the next flashy, transitory thing embraced by the antiaging movement and its allies.

For Aristotle, magnanimity was a virtue of self-esteem. Its importance lies in brave acceptance, generosity, and action for noble purposes. Moreover, it is a resistance to vanity. Reversing the aging process with an eye on constantly remaking oneself could suggest that one is "winning at life" by being "pristine and unblemished," reflecting a vain temperament. However, one might take confidence in having faced adversity and showing some of the scars from it, recognizing that failure is an essential quality of learning. Fanatical efforts to look and feel young are attempts to escape the "failures" of aging. Assuming that learning is a key component to a well-lived life, and acknowledging that failure teaches myriad lessons, this would suggest that having a magnanimous character inherently (and justifiably) involves failures and flaws.

A third virtue at risk, prudence, crosses several generations, but it could be cast in terms of stewardship. Stewardship in this sense means maintaining the value of what we already possess. It is striking how, when comparing the features of the antiaging movement's celebration of youth culture, there is a paucity of essential and lasting characteristics. This seems to lack a certain authenticity. Radical extension of life could also have adverse environmental consequences as longer-lived generations place stresses on ecosystems worldwide.

Though it is unclear that vitality *inevitably* changes how we interact with old people, there is good reason to believe that it will. That is enough to warrant a closer examination of the question.

YES—EXTENDED LIFE SPANS WILL NOT SUBSTANTIALLY CHANGE HUMAN NATURE.

Jeffrey Kleiman

Life span origins have at least two major explanations. The first, found in evolutionary biology, suggests that we live long enough to reproduce, care for our offspring, and then shuffle off this mortal coil. The second, according to biblical accounts, states that our life span is 70 years (three score and ten), with a provisional blessing reserved for the most wonderful of people to live to 120. But that is neither here nor there. At this point, we speculate about longer life spans than even myths describe.

Author Alan Lightman, in his book *Einstein's Dreams*, speculates about human behavior if given the option of eternal life. For him, the world divides into two major groups: the "laters" and the "nows." As the names suggest, the first group of people postpone life's adventures and labors to spend time with friends and family. They sit about the cafes and read, talk, and generally enjoy life at a leisurely pace. There will always be tomorrow. The second group is animated. They are up and about to pursue many careers and a range of marriages and families, constantly learning, inventing, and tinkering.

Let us vary Lightman's premise a moment to ask about a greatly extended life span rather than immortality. Might we find the same two groups dominating the social landscape with similar outcomes? Given additional time for life, is it reasonable to assume that human behavior would vary any differently than it does today or has in the past? Or is the promise of an extended life span predicated on a series of false assumptions that perhaps our world today would be different if people had longer lives? We might ask whether longevity of an unimagined length would necessarily change the basic patterns of how we behave among family and friends.

Comedian Mel Brooks worked with Carl Reiner to develop the character of the 2,000-year-old man. It is very funny, very clever, and in many ways, very thoughtful. One of the routines Brooks and Reiner perform deals with the likelihood that a man this ancient had many, many children over the millennia. As the interviewer, Reiner asks about the thousands of children, and Brooks, as a typical parent, complains, "They never call, they never write, they don't visit, they don't keep in touch," and so on. How far might this be from the truth? Does the guarantee of an extended lifetime horizon lessen the bonds of human connection derived by birth or friendship?

Perhaps it is life's fragility and uncertainty that gives it value. Ajit Varki and Danny Brower, scientists from different fields, pondered whether the human proclivity to deny unpleasant truths had its origins in our species' awareness of death. Denial, they speculate, emergences from the reality of our short lives. Denial appears as a response to acknowledge mortality and all its consequences; once we deny the power of death, we can go on to deny thousands of things that happen in our world for which we are the authors. By the same token, the struggle to perpetuate memory through monumental works of art and architecture involves a degree of denial; we can live forever with these physical reminders. After all, what other purpose do cemeteries, crypts, vaults, and gravestones serve for most of us? Maybe the compulsion to create in order to be remembered would find more constructive uses of energy.

Human life span has grown across the millennia, ever since the agricultural revolution. Thirty-five years used to be considered a pretty decent life under the Mesopotamian kings or the Egyptian pharaohs. Not much changed through antiquity in the classical world, although, when Julius Caesar died at age 55, he was still considered a man in his prime. Life in post-Roman medieval Europe didn't do much to push the boundaries. Indeed, it was not until the world of secure nutrition, preventative medicine, and other interventions that ordinary people could expect to live into their late sixties and seventies with any assurance. Today, in the United States, the fastest-growing subset of elderly is the "super-old": folks aged 80 and beyond. Many advances help them to sustain physical and mental agility.

We may want to ask ourselves whether lives are better just because they are longer. It may be that a life lived in poverty for centuries really does not differ from living in want for 60 years. It may not be reasonable to expect that extended lifetimes would offer the occasion for people to seek a kinder or gentler approach to living with their fellows, especially if resources such as food and energy fell into short supply. On what basis can we expect people driven by the desire to control others, obsessed with greed, power hungry, and corrupt to abandon these obsessions if granted longer lives.

In the quest to extend life span, the issues of human nature can receive short shrift. Is it reasonable to expect that longer life spans will lead to different forms of human activity? Will our current inclination to denial and fear give way suddenly to perpetual hope and kindness? I don't know. Maybe when the kids start to call, write, and visit on regular basis.

Question

How Would a Successful Antiaging Technology Affect Faith?

One of the constant themes that emerges from the history of prolongevity and the modern antiaging movement is the tension between the goals of radically extending human life span and the goals of personal religious faith. There is nothing irreligious about a search for healthy living and long life, and yet there is often an unspoken competition between the priorities of life on earth versus the priorities of life hereafter. If we pursue human perfection on earth, are we abandoning the quest for immortal perfection in heaven? Other related issues of contention involve the ultimate source of life, the nature of human consciousness and free will, and the morality of experimenting with human biological potential. These are questions that reach beyond the quantitative standards of natural sciences and require systematic metaphysical reasoning.

The question of how a successful radical life-extension solution might affect religious faith cannot be answered with a simple "yes" or "no." We gathered leaders and experts from among the most common religious traditions in the West (Judaism, Islam, and Christianity—both Catholic and Protestant) and have asked them to comment on how their religious faith interprets the modern pursuit of a technological fountain of youth. These essays provide particular points of view from each major tradition. Nevertheless, there is also strong commonality between the traditions of faith. We also include an agnostic academic and a champion for atheism and transhumanism. The perspectives from the nonreligious voices are clearly distinct from the voices that presume divine revelation.

The essays are ordered in rough chronology, based on when the religious tradition (or nonreligious tradition) first emerged in human history. The voice of Judaism comes from a Chabad rabbi in the Chasidic tradition who is head of a yeshiva in Israel. A yeshiva is where men go to learn the Talmud and to become future leaders of their faith. Chasidic Judaism is relatively recent as a distinct branch from Judaism, but it is known for its strict observance to the most ancient Jewish traditions. Bishop Robert Morlino is the head of the Madison diocese in Wisconsin. In Catholicism, a bishop is the modern equivalent of one of Christ's apostles and is responsible for teaching and protecting doctrine, protecting the sacraments, conferring Holy Orders to priests, and administrating the Catholics within his district. Amer

Haleem is an Islamic scholar. Islam does not have an ordained clergy in the same way that Jewish or Christian faiths do. Instead, Islamic communities recognize certain political leaders and other scholars of the faith who serve roles as teachers and guides for the practice of the faith. Certain titles may be conferred (imam, which means "leader"), but all Muslims are expected to learn their faith on their own as well as in community. Amer Haleem is one of the few scholars who has translated the Koran into English. Reverend Louis Kinsley is a minister in the Church of Scotland. Protestant ministers are ordained, and the church is collectively governed by the elders (or ministers) of each church parish. They distinguish themselves from the Catholic faithful as part of the "reformed tradition," which means they do not recognize a single leader (patriarch, or pope) as the vicar of Christ and believe that God inspires the church through the entire community of believers, rather than through singular intermediaries. On most fundamental doctrines of Christian faith, Protestants and Catholics are united. They differ primarily on matters of practice, administrative leadership, and other particular points of theology. All four of these religious writers share a common belief that God is personally involved in the course of human life and that, ultimately, the unseen realm of the immaterial world is more significant than the created realm of the material world.

The final two writers do not claim any particular faith. Jeff Kleiman writes from an agnostic tradition, which neither affirms nor rejects the reality of God or the immaterial realm. Agnostics belief that there is no evidence to support or refute such beliefs, and therefore they do not include them in their considerations. The term *agnostic* was originally coined by Thomas Huxley (friend of Charles Darwin) and used to justify the theory of natural selection as an alternative explanation for human origins. Academics who trust only in empirical evidence for their theories often write from an agnostic perspective, regardless of their personal beliefs. Zoltan Istvan is the 2016 U.S. presidential nominee for the Transhumanist Party. He is a vocal advocate for antiaging research and the technologies that expand human capabilities. His presidential platform focused on prioritizing the majority of federal funding toward finding health care solutions and other antiaging research. Istvan is an atheist, and his faith in empirical science largely guides his activism for humanist achievements. The idea of atheism dates back to ancient times, but it has only been accepted as a serious alternative to religion in the most recent centuries.

JEWISH VIEW—IMMORTALITY IS PROMISED BY GOD, BUT ONLY FAITH CAN SECURE IT.

Rabbi Tuvia Bolton

Due to the recent advancements in science, medicine, and technology, the idea has arisen that possibly man can find a "cure," or rather a way to infinitely delay or perhaps totally eradicate, death. This is not a new idea; indeed, it was suggested by the snake to Eve (Chava) when he promised that she could eat from the tree and not die (Gen. 3:4).

In fact, G-d Himself also offered this possibility by creating the "tree of life" (2:9), but He so feared that man would partake therefrom after disobeying Him (Gen. 3:22) that He drove Adam from the garden and closed the way to the tree of life with a "revolving sword" (3:24). The reason was that death was caused by sin, false egotism, and selfishness, and if Adam ate from the tree of life *after* sinning, it would make these things so similar to holiness that it would make repentance impossible.

To explain, the world was created in six days, and the last creation was man, who, unlike everything else, was created in G-d's image (Gen. 1:26–27). One implication of this is that man would live forever. Just as G-d is eternal and not limited in any way, neither by time, place, or even spirit, so man would live eternally in a physical body without ever dying. Therefore, He warned Adam not to eat from the tree of knowledge lest he die (2:17), because death, at that time, did not exist for man. But when man disobeyed G-d's will and ate from the tree (just hours after he was created), he declared independence from the eternal Creator, became dependent on the temporal creation, broke his link to eternal life, and inherited death.

In other words, death has nothing to do with health or aging. Rather, it is only due to the decree of G-d and will only cease by the decree of G-d. To emphasize this, a midrash states that in the period from the 2,000 years after Adam until Jacob (the last forefather of Judaism), everyone would die suddenly and without any warning. But due to the prayers of Jacob, G-d had mercy on mankind and brought disease, etc., so man could prepare for and repent before death. Also, in the Talmud are mentioned several perfectly holy Jews that despite their total spiritual purity died *only* due to the sin of Adam. In other words, eliminating illness and lengthening life, or even eliminating sin, will not and cannot eliminate death.

Indeed, there is a story about a Chabad Chassid who was offered by his Rebbe a blessing for long life, to which he replied, "But not a life void of meaning, being blind and deaf to G-d etc." Simply put, every *moment* of life is infinite and eternal regardless of how *many* moments there are. Indeed, (as Prof. Victor Frankl teaches) the *last* moment of life can be more meaningful than the 80 or 90 years before it. Some say that this is hinted at by the sentence in Psalms (144:4), "Adam is like Hevel." Hevel means "wind," but it also is the name of Cain's brother whom he killed (or Abel). So, "Adam is like Hevel" means Adam, who lived 930 years at his last moment, was just like Hevel, who lived only a few hours. So, our quest should not be to end death but rather to enliven *life* so that every moment of life should be meaningful and treated as a miracle filled with mystery and responsibility to improve ourselves and the world around us.

But this is not to say that death itself will never cease. Indeed, 2 of the 13 basic principles of faith that Judaism is built upon is the arrival of Moshiach and the raising of the dead. So death *will* cease. But it will only happen when Moshiach changes the priorities of *all* mankind and brings them to realize their responsibility, compliance, partnership and unity with G-d's will (as it was in the beginning), which will eventually result in the "raising of the dead."

CATHOLIC VIEW—THE QUEST FOR LIFE ON EARTH DISTRACTS FROM THE ULTIMATE REALITY OF LIFE IN HEAVEN.

Bishop Robert Morlino

The interplay between an antiaging movement and the Catholic faith can be considered on two levels. On the first level, there is a practical consideration of the present science of these endeavors and their ethical impact on the community of human persons. On the second level, there is the deeper, existential consideration of the concepts of aging, suffering, and even death as seen through the eyes of faith.

On the first level, I'd like to speak briefly about the interaction between the antiaging movement and ethical concerns for the present day. These ethical issues speak not only to the Catholic person of faith, but they should really resonate with any person of goodwill. It's simply incumbent on the church to raise such ethical issues in every age.

In the first place, it would be reckless not to note that a number of the present technologies being touted for their antiaging qualities are being derived from fetal tissue procured by means of abortion. I must be very clear regarding the church's absolute opposition to the use of aborted fetal tissue for these purposes. Without getting into all the distinctions in this regard, it should be clear to anyone paying attention that the Catholic Church—not to mention the laws of human ecology—decries the sacrificing of one segment of humanity for the end benefit of another (whether that benefit be perceived or real, and regardless the degree of benefit).

Aside from those means, which are never justified, there is another level of consideration in the area of bioethics and antiaging research when it comes to means that an ethicist would call "morally neutral" in and of themselves. Here we are left to consider both the ends involved and the just use of resources to achieve those ends.

When speaking of antiaging, it would seem that ends can fall in a spectrum ranging from the prevention of cosmetic effects of aging, to diminishing human suffering, to extending life expectancy. Taking into account the relative weight of the ends to be achieved, one can then consider and discern the just use of resources to achieve those ends. For instance, if the end of particular antiaging research is an end to human suffering in one way or another, clearly it would have a much greater value for humanity than something more superficial.

Nevertheless, for those who claim the end is the prolonging of human life, an honest consideration of the just use of resources is also in order. Is it just, for example, to expend countless dollars and hours of human ingenuity to achieve five years of added life expectancy for some while others starve to death? Is this a good and just use of resources? Many of these questions come down to prudential judgments of individuals, but they are questions of ethics that should enter into the discussion. For Catholics (and others) interested in a consistent examination of ethical concerns applied to particular new technologies and areas of research, institutions such as the National Catholic Bioethics Center provide tremendous resources.

The above questions are challenging to many and worthy of consideration. On a completely other level, however, bodily aging, dying, and death itself do not matter to the Catholic Christian. Christians believe in a God who has assumed a human body, who has suffered, and who has died. In so doing, Jesus Christ has transformed suffering and death and the very meaning of human existence to the point that, for the Christian, the notion of an antiaging movement is ultimately of little consequence.

Most Christians have traditionally held to an anthropology in which bodily corruption and aging were not originally in the plan of God. However, with free will and the fall, the plan of God as regards humanity was frustrated, and humankind was met with corruption, disease, pain, aging, and death. There was disharmony in the natural order of things, and even the smallest instance of that initial disharmony has resonated and grown through all of human history in a way that no one, save God Himself, could set it aright again.

Of course, the end of the story is that God Himself did set it aright again, and He gave all humankind a way of once again experiencing the world as it was meant to be. In and through Jesus Christ, mankind can once again experience a perfected life, one absent of corruption, disease, pain, or aging. However, that life is in a world to come. In the present world, we continue to experience that which sin has wrought, passing through the Cross of Christ to experience perfection—a new life. Christianity expects suffering and death in this world but sees those things as a glorified means of attaining union with God.

In his letter to the church at Philippi, the Apostle Paul writes,

> My eager expectation and hope is that I shall not be put to shame in any way, but that with all boldness, now as always, Christ will be magnified in my body, whether by life or by death. For to me life is Christ, and death is gain. If I go on living in the flesh, that means fruitful labor for me. And I do not know which I shall choose. I am caught between the two. I long to depart this life and be with Christ, [for] that is far better. Yet that I remain [in] the flesh is more necessary for your benefit. (Philippians 1:20–24)

So long as Christians live, they are called to magnify Christ. In this sense, it does not matter whether the Christians age or not, nor whether they die or not—so long as they strive to magnify Christ in all that they do.

As a final point, I would add that for many a faithful Christian—Pope St. John Paul II and St. Mother Teresa of Calcutta are recent, excellent examples—aging can provide a tremendous opportunity to magnify Christ and to witness to the hope that a Christian has in the life to come. This witness was given in 2008 by renowned professor and priest Cardinal Avery Dulles. In his final address at Fordham University (which was read in his presence, due to his inability to speak), Dulles declared,

> Suffering and diminishment are not the greatest of evils, but are normal ingredients in life, especially in old age. They are to be accepted as elements of a full human

346 FINDING THE FOUNTAIN OF YOUTH

existence. Well into my 90th year I have been able to work productively. As I become increasingly paralyzed and unable to speak, I can identify with the many paralytics and mute persons in the Gospels, grateful for the loving and skillful care I receive and for the hope of everlasting life in Christ. If the Lord now calls me to a period of weakness, I know well that his power can be made perfect in infirmity. "Blessed be the name of the Lord!"

ISLAMIC VIEW—MORTAL DEATH IS INEVITABLE, AND THE PROMISE OF A FOUNTAIN OF YOUTH IS DECEPTIVE TO BOTH FAITH AND MAN.
Amer Haleem

And give glad tidings to those who believe and do righteous deeds that for them are Gardens beneath which rivers flow. Whenever they are provided of the fruit of them as provision, they shall say: This is the very like we were provided in the world before. And so shall it be given them, in full resemblance, yet perfected in delectation. Even thus, for them therein are wives of perfect purity—and therein shall they abide together forever. (Surat Al-Baqarah 2:25)

Islam, like the religions of Heavenly Revelation that it consummates, has no issue whatever with the perpetuity of human life. Indeed, from it stems two major faith tenets. First, God hallows human life as sacred. As such, He burdens each soul with the moral obligation to preserve its own life—"and do not cast yourselves, by your own hands, into destruction" (Sûrat Al-Baqarah 2:195)—and also to strive in sustaining the lives of all others—"and whoever saves a life, it shall be as he has saved the life of all humankind" (Sûrat Al-Mâ'idah 5:32). In Islam specifically (and this is significant), the command to conserve human life includes medicinal intervention, which it unprecedentedly incorporates as part of its Divine Moral Law, the *Sharî'ah*. Second, from the first man to the last, the ineluctable destiny of every human being is life everlasting in one of only two outcomes: Admission by the grace of God to His Paradise, or internment in Hellfire for rejecting God as One without partner, associate, or relation, for this eviscerates any good one may have done in life and bars all possibility of divine forgiveness and salvation.

Yet, Islam takes issue categorically with the belief that *any* living creature or lifeform can escape death, whatever the substance of its creation or the essence of its spirit, and no matter if it is part of the perceptible world or hidden in the unseen from the senses of other beings. "Every single soul shall taste death" (Sûrat Al-Anbiyyâ' 21:35), not only humans, but the animals, plants, angels, *jinn* (the race from which Satan comes), even the mountains, earth, and sky—every fashioned thing; for God tells us that the creations our narrow empiricism dismisses as inanimate, He has enchanted with life in a manner beyond the apprehension of our senses.

This brings us to the central problem of the burgeoning prolongevity and antiaging movements, which have coalesced at the confluence of three conjectures, all of them pillars of the modern project and principally rooted in the radically reactionary intellectualism of Europe's post-Reformation 18th century: the doctrines of phenomenalism and humanism and the idea of progress. In a word, the leaders of the quest for indefinite life without infirmity believe that all knowledge (indeed, existence itself) arises from human sensory experience, making man the prime being and focal point of the world. Luckily (for in this view it is purely fortuitous), man is possessed of the supreme faculty, the human intellect, enabling him to solve any question of his concern, uppermost of these, of course, being his (until now?) assured mortality.

The antiaging believer has abiding faith in another transformative power intervening on his behalf, and by which man is, after all, a special species: the inevitability of continuous improvement, expansion, and capacitation of the human condition because of cumulative scientific innovation—the exponential advancement in technology constituting for him proof that this is an axiomatic truth. Never mind that this argument is itself an infinite loop, beginning and ending with human sensory-limited rationality. The fact is the strict literalist interpretations of these secular dogmas render these death-defying movements dangerously extremist expressions of humanist fundamentalism. Simply put, they see the human being—as one of their torchbearers, Aubrey de Grey likens it—as a mere body that is nothing more than a "very complicated machine [that] can be subjected to maintenance and repair in the same way as a simple machine, like a car body." In this view, technology is transcendence, as inventor Ray Kurzweil explains it. Immortality is only a matter of creating nanotechnologies to perform "more pervasive systemic interventions that maintain the integrity . . . [of] our bodies and brains," similar to what we already do with "complex information systems." Is it any wonder that these movements' founders and leading advocates are technologists, futurists, and data specialists?

I call these enterprises dangerous (and make no mistake, they are lucrative enterprises, indeed) because they sell the false promise of life happily ever after on earth to a people desperate with the fear of death but rendered scripturally illiterate by an age that has absolutely erased from our hearts the objective correlatives of Divine Revelation as a legitimate source of knowledge, let alone a higher source, thus turning the reports of the Heavenly Books and the witness of the prophets of the coming Judgment and the life Hereafter into "nothing but tales of the ancients" (see Sûrat Al-Mutaffifîn 83:10–13).

What those who yet study the revealed verses of God know is that the human body, though originally shaped to perfect soundness by the two Right Hands of God "from a clay of aged, black mud" (Sûrat Al-Hijr 15:28), lay lifeless until He "breathed of His spirit into him" (Sûrat Al-Sajdah 32:9). It is this that gives man life, not the mere body but the spirit with which God ensouls it, the nature of which, and how He sews it into our forms and unknits it, being of His exclusive province. "The spirit is of the affair of my Lord alone. Nor have you been given of knowledge more than very little" (Sûrat Al-Isrâ' 17:85). Hence, it is the very soul of man that these would-be technicians of unfailing earthly life deny, with no hint of being conscious of the irony.

It is precisely as an antidote to such astounding arrogance and ingratitude that the Prophet Muhammad, on him be peace, advised us: "Remember often the ender of pleasures." For death is the great "remembrancer" of human beings, whose collective name in Arabic, *al-insân*, is an emphatic of the root "to forget," making us literally "forgetting-kind." And how well named we are. We forget that we were originally dead. "Has it occurred to man that there were eons in time when he was not even a thing to be mentioned?" (Sûrat Al-Insân 76:1). We forget our humble origins. "We created you from dust" (Sûrat Al-Hajj 22:5). We forget our testimony. "And He made them bear witness to their own souls: Am I not your Lord? They said: O yes, indeed! We do so bear witness!" (Sûrat Al-A'râf 7:172). We forget why God made us ("I have not created . . . human beings but to worship Me alone" (Sûrat Al-Dhâriyât, 51:56)); the purpose of our fleeting earthly lives ("We but test you in life with evil and good as a trial"); and the eternal consequence of this sojourn ("Then it is to Us you shall all be returned for recompense (Sûrat Al-Anbiyyâ' 21:35)).

In this light, death is a literal godsend, for it makes faith's most persistent and eloquent argument. Behold this inert-limbed flesh, this insentient, stilled body that only just before lived, loved, looked, laughed—springing endlessly creative language and even new life. What escaped it? Who took it? From where did it come? To where did it go? To this end, the Koran interrogates us. If we as human beings deny God's promise to resurrect us for Judgment, "then why do you not hold back the soul of the dying when it reaches the throat? Yet all the while you are helplessly looking on" (Sûrat Al-Wâqi'ah 56:83–84).

No, death we cannot outrun. "Indeed, the death from which you flee shall most surely catch you up" (Sûrat Al-Jumu'ah 62:8). But neither do we deserve the life God breathed into us. "How can you disbelieve in God when you were lifeless and He gave you life" (Sûrat Al-Baqarah 2:28)? Here, then, are twin blessings, each in its turn removing the veil from our eyes to behold the One All-Living who never dies.

Then which of your Lord's blessings will either of you belie? All who are upon the earth shall pass away, but everlasting is the Face of your Lord—the Possessor of All Majesty and Honor. (Sûrat Al-Rahmân 55:25–27)

PROTESTANT VIEW—THE FOUNTAIN OF YOUTH ATTEMPTS TO SUBSTITUTE DIVINE SALVATION WITH HUMAN SALVATION.

Rev. Louis Kinsey

Reformed theology will not be found cheerleading the antiaging movement. At best, it will be indifferent to the notion that scientific medicine be deployed in an effort to capture eternal youth. At worst, it will be antagonistic toward any argument or movement, the implication of which is to suggest that the poor continue to live in a daily struggle for survival while a wealthy elite is able to purchase the prolongation of life or even physical immortality.

The root of such antagonism is in the Gospel, in which Christ has commanded us to love our neighbors: "You shall love the Lord your God with all your heart with all your soul, with all your strength, and with all your mind, and your neighbor as yourself" (Luke 10:27). Consolidating the means of longevity and physical immortality in the hands of the rich cannot be what he meant. Yet, the principal antipathy of reformed spirituality toward the aspirations of antiaging protagonists is theological. It concerns the purpose and meaning of life itself. Here it is worth remembering that it is not so long ago that even the youngest child brought up in a Scottish household knew the purpose of life, for in answer to that most elemental of all questions, "What is the chief end of man?," those raised in Presbyterian Scotland could answer with confidence, along with the 17th-century Westminster divines, "The chief end of man is to glorify God and to enjoy him forever" (from the *Westminster Shorter Catechism*).

The orientation of human life is Godward. The purpose of the creature is to live for the creator's glory, not to perpetuate one's own earthly existence. And if Scottish Calvinism is no longer able to successfully persuade of the theocentric purpose of human life, it could once. This is the reformed view of the world. The point of human existence is to manifest the goodness and grace of God in words and actions and to enjoy the friendship of God by means of repentance and faith alone.

If the first concern that reformed theology has with the antiaging movement is with the purpose of life itself, the second is that the effort to resist the aging process and to secure physical immortality represents a stubborn human refusal to accept the divinely ordained consequences of sin by attempting the impossible: to return in some sense to Eden itself and to make permanent our sinful estrangement from God (The Scots Confession of 1560). In the Genesis account of human origins, the first man and woman ate forbidden fruit and experienced alienation from God. They encountered God's justice and grace as a result. The justice of God was eviction from Eden. Paradise was over. By contrast, the grace of God was the placing of cherubim on Eden's boundary, that man would be prevented from returning to the garden, where he might eat from the tree of life and live forever at a sinful distance from a holy God.

> Then the Lord God said: "Behold, the man has become like one of us, to know good and evil. And now, lest he put out his hand and take also of the tree of life, and eat, and live forever"—therefore the Lord God sent him out of the garden of Eden to till the ground from which he was taken. So he drove out the man; and he placed cherubim at the east of the garden of Eden, and a flaming sword which turned every way, to guard the way to the tree of life. (Gen. 3:22–24)

Close on its heels is this Christian concern that the search for physical immortality is nothing less than the replacement of the divinely ordained means of salvation and immortality—dying with Christ and rising with him at the resurrection—with the human fruits of scientific medicine. In answer to the question, "How does Christ's resurrection benefit us?," the Heidelberg Confession answers, "First, by his resurrection he has overcome death, so that he might make us share in the righteousness he obtained for us by his death. Second, by his power we too are already raised to a new life." And here we come to one of the principal accusations offered by reformed theology: mankind seeks, in the search for physical immortality, to replace salvation as a gift of God with a form of salvation that outworks itself through human effort and scientific striving.

We are removed back to the pre-Reformation. Salvation is now by works, once more, not by faith in the promises of God. We are taken back to that default human position wherein we continually seek to save ourselves by our own efforts and achievements. Mankind can see no wisdom in dying in Christ, in being consigned to the ground or to the elements, in faith that when the last trumpet sounds, the dead will rise bodily, and when "the last enemy that will be destroyed is death" (1 Cor. 15:26). Yet this is precisely the orthodox Christian vision of immortality, the divinely appointed means by which this sinful flesh and blood, which we presently occupy, will one day inherit that eternal life that cannot be inherited in any other way (1 Cor. 25:50). It may sound wonderfully beneficent; yet, the scientific and medical model of physical immortality cannot realize the chief end of man, for it neither glorifies God whose salvific plan it rejects, nor does it offer everlasting enjoyment of God, for it seeks to return us to the tree of life, where we are invited to eat the fruit of life while still sinfully estranged from the divine life giver.

But let us not simply focus on the life to come. What is the human vision of the good life? What is the moral life, and how can we live it? The search for the fountain of youth is self-evidently a search for the continuation of the self. There may be many reasons and motives. Fear of death and dying may propel me on a quest to slow up the aging process. I may be moved by a compulsion to cultivate a certain aesthetic; the cult of the body and the pursuit of physical attractiveness press upon me, aware as I am of the influence of the media in a culture obsessed with celebrity and appearance. But will length of days, even immortality, bring me enjoyment of life?

To these questions, reformed Christian thought returns as always to the Holy Scriptures, where Jesus Christ holds out to us the key to happiness and human self-fulfillment: "Most assuredly, I say to you, unless a grain of wheat falls into the ground and dies, it remains alone; but if it dies, it produces much grain" (John 12:24). In this saying, Jesus explains that the pathway to salvation here and in the next life necessarily involves dying to one's selfish aspirations in an act of sacrificial abandonment; yet, the very act of such a death, for the sake of Christ and his truth claims, will bring about consequences that are morally good and worthy. A harvest of good will come forth. The life that is good cannot be found in the self-centered pursuit of immortality. Rather, it is in expending oneself in the service of the one who expended himself in crucifixion that true life blooms.

So, here it is, disclosed and revealed for the anthropocentric idolatry and moral distraction that it is. The antiaging movement is the misguided child of human wisdom and scientific accomplishment, looking for eternity in the wrong place, setting to one side the divine plan of repentance, faith, and resurrection through which, alone, true immortality might be found. Mankind is found to be striving against God himself, seeking to overpower the cherubim at last in a vain attempt to break back into the Garden of Eden to steal from the tree of life.

It is a curiously and largely Western form of human narcissism that can offer nothing of lasting universal benefit, except for an apocalyptic vision of overcrowding and the inevitably violent race to gather scarce resources. It is selfishness run rampant. We shall buy eternity, says a wealthy elite, simply because we can afford to. Meanwhile, heaven sighs, and the blood of Abel cries out from the ground (Gen. 4:10).

AGNOSTIC VIEW—EXTENDED LIFE PROVIDES NEW OPPORTUNITIES FOR LEARNING, RENDERING FAITH LESS NECESSARY.

Jeffrey Kleiman

What is a Faustian bargain? For Christopher Marlowe in the 17th century, the bargain entailed a straightforward trade between the devil and Faust. The former offered power and wealth and forbidden knowledge of "magic" about the world's mysteries in exchange for the latter's soul. At the end of the agreed upon period, the devil claimed Faust in a violent and frightening storm during darkest night. The moral of the tale in this version remained clear and simplistic: do not question the ways of God and faith. Keep away from the temptations of the devil.

Death, Christians learned, emerged as the punishment for rebellion against divine will in the Garden of Eden. Death became the price exacted by humanity for original sin, something that no human could ever hope to escape. During one's lifetime, prayer, charity, obedience to the church, and submission to sufferings offered by God would all find mitigation for life's perils after death. Attempting to alter, challenge, or avoid this fate could only bring terrible consequences. Faust became an object lesson in impiety through his acquisition of forbidden knowledge.

Yet, Johann von Goethe gave the tale a very different twist, one that may carry greater weight for us today. Faust, for Goethe, embodied human curiosity, knowledge for its own sake; experience should not be shunned, and questions should be asked. The world demanded exploration. Humans would fail. Unforeseen consequences will bring suffering to the innocent. Yet, should we surrender the desire for new knowledge and the lessons of experience for the safe haven of traditional ways and conventional morals?

It is Goethe's Faust that drives us today. For Goethe, in this world, God understands human weaknesses and, in the next, will offer forgiveness. Knowledge remains precious in its own right. In both accounts, Marlowe and Goethe supernaturally return youth to Faust so that his lifetime may be extended, a variant on the drive for longer life, antiaging if you will, taking the first steps toward immortality.

However, Goethe's Faust set only one condition to this devil's agreement: unlike Marlowe's Faust, where a term of years established the bargain, Mephistopheles could claim Faust's soul only when Faust had ceased to be curious. Faust noted that "should the hour should ever come when I say halt, I have had enough, I am satisfied, let this hour never end," then the devil could claim his due. Living forever in this instance did not serve as the chief goal in and of itself. Goethe certainly did not imagine a boundless pursuit of physical pleasures. For Goethe, insatiable curiosity drives humanity forward. Life should be as long as possible in pursuit of all strands of knowledge. With extended youth and staving off old age's infirmities, who would not want to engage in many wide-ranging experiences? Who would not want to understand the mysteries of how the world operates?

With modern science, we find ourselves broaching a Faustian bargain. As we move to increased mastery of genetic understanding of disease, artificial organs, growing new skin, or increasing resistance to disease, we have not debated fully the question of death. Annually, more and more of humanity move beyond survival. The older evolutionary imperative of living to reproduce while assuring the survival of offspring to maintain life fades a bit each year.

What will be the price we pay as we negotiate with death for a new Faustian bargain? Let us consider the two schools of thought expressed by Marlowe and Faust. Do we necessarily have to accept the role of a divinity in any of this? The belief in a God directly present in human life, who shapes our own lives as well as history, as was Marlowe's case, suggests it is wrong to challenge the world. Everything is as the divine shaped it. One may not properly doubt or question the life span of three-score-and-ten years. To push the bounds of a life span is a rebellion against the divine order.

Goethe's God is a distant god, one not necessarily wrapped up in human affairs on a daily basis, perhaps not even shaping human history. This deity is wise and forgiving, offering redemption, knowing that people are frail and prone to weaknesses of every sort. If we accept Goethe's vision, we are morally bound to embrace the adventure of discovery, unwrap the secrets of nature, and press against bounds that constrain a love of life. Living forever would not be a problem as long as we continue to be curious, active, probing. The price we would pay is small.

And what if we were uncertain about any divinity at all? Neither proof nor disproof of God bothers the mind; what if one remains neutral in these matters? *Agnostic* is the term commonly used to describe this outlook. How does this influence our interpretation of a Faustian Bargain? As an agnostic, one would likely endorse Goethe but necessarily embrace his optimism that knowledge of every sort is worth the price exacted. Skepticism is a traveling companion of the agnostic. Doubt and uncertainty shape the view.

For an agnostic is likely a pragmatic person unworried about heaven or hell, the fate of an eternal soul, or the direction of human history. Neither accepting nor dismissing the possibility of God means that different criteria color the appreciation of extending life. Rather, the costs would be weighed against benefits, risks against gains. Life span is merely a physical issue without spiritual consequence, a matter of mechanics. Is this attainable, to what degree, and what sort of impact?

For the agnostic, life is of more importance than any afterlife. Life is here and now and real; the afterlife is a vague promise without evidence. Postponing death might have little to do with spiritual or divine consequences.

ATHEIST VIEW – RELIGIOUS FAITH SUPPRESSES THE NATURAL EVOLUTION THAT HUMAN TECHNOLOGY PROMISES.

Zoltan Istvan

All around the world, religious terror is striking and threatening us. Whether in France, Istanbul, London, or the United States, the threat is now constant. We can fight it all we want. We can send out our troops; we can chip refugees; and we can try to monitor terrorists' every move. We can even improve trauma medicine to deal with the extreme violence they bring us. But none of this solves the underlying issue: Abrahamic religions such as Christianity and Islam are fundamentally violent philosophies with violent Gods. Sam Harris, Richard Dawkins, Christopher Hitchens, and others have all reiterated essentially the same thing.

Consider these verses from the Koran:

Koran (3:56): "As to those who reject faith, I will punish them with terrible agony in this world and in the Hereafter, nor will they have anyone to help."
Koran (8:12): "I will cast terror into the hearts of those who disbelieve. Therefore strike off their heads and strike off every fingertip of them."

And then consider these verses from the Bible:

Deuteronomy 17:12: "Anyone arrogant enough to reject the verdict of the holy man who represents God must be put to death. Such evil must be purged."
Numbers: 31:17: "Now therefore kill every male among the little ones, and kill every woman that hath known man by lying with him."

Of course, both the Koran and Bible have passages that highlight kindness too—but you don't get a get-out-of-jail-free card in the 21st century by being both violent and peaceful. If you beat your spouse, you're an abuser and can face jail time (even if you're a loving spouse other times). It's one or the other in the 21st century: If you're a warmonger, murderer, or a terrorist, you're a bona fide warmonger, murderer, or terrorist. And nothing is going to change that.

The fundamental problem with religion is that believers—about 5 billion people right now on Planet Earth—are so sure they're "correct" on anything and everything they believe. This is, of course, a sure sign of insanity, especially since most of what people believe was taught to them when they were children (and they had no way to filter it out or reason about it).

The only real truth out there, at least while our brains are just three-pound bags of meat (and our senses—like our eyes—see just 1 percent of the visible universe), is to know "absolute truth" is something way too complex to understand. The only real thing to understand right now is the scientific method—the holy grail of wisdom that reason advocates follow. It states that if you test a hypothesis enough times and the outcome seems to always be similar, you can utilize that as a semitruth and apply it functionally in one's life (but beware: it could change anytime, and it might). That's the language of reason—the language of science. It's the same method of thinking that explains why jet airplanes don't fall out of the sky. Or why skyscrapers keep standing through hurricanes. Or why we could put a man on the moon and bring him back.

However, it's not the thinking method that President Obama used to swear on a Bible to get his job on inauguration day. Or George W. Bush when he stopped life-saving stem-cell funding for seven years during his presidency. Or the Pope when he insists condom usage is a sin, despite it having the possibility of saving millions of lives from AIDS in Africa.

The scientific method is also not the thinking method of the pilots who flew into the World Trade Center. Or of the murderer who gunned down people in Orlando. And it's certainly not the method of thinking that the truck driver used to run down innocent people in Nice, France.

Like the hundreds of millions of other nonreligious people out there, it's hard for me to fathom how religious people got brainwashed into being this way—this ignorant. But bear in mind, it's not just religious terrorism that is literally killing us—it's much more.

Consider how many nonreligious secular people there are leading our nation right now. The answer is astonishing: it's zero (at least publicly). All 535 members of Congress, all 8 Supreme Court justices, and our president believe in God and an afterlife.

No wonder life extension and antiaging science is basically unfunded by the U.S. government. Why should the United States care about whether you live longer or can overcome disease when you're all going to wake up in Jesus's arms after you die? Or in some heavenly Islamic paradise with a bunch of virgins?

I'm a presidential candidate that wants you to live—not in some unknown paradise once you die that no one has ever seen before or can prove exists. I want you to live now, regardless of what craziness, disease, or tragedy the world can throw at you. I want your loved ones to live too—and not die because of aging, sickness, or terrorism. I want you all to survive as long as you want and to try to find a perfect world here on earth.

Transhumanist science can give that to us, and it will soon. Antiaging research is quickly improving and will soon be able to stop the aging process altogether. Science and radical medicine can eliminate all disease in the near future—but only if society and government give it the cultural support it needs and spend adequate resources to make this happen.

If you want to live—and not be killed or die—make a point to criticize and disavow religion and religious people for being deathist: the idea that death is either welcome or acceptable (whether it comes via terrorism, disease, or aging).

In the 21st century, fundamental religion is a form of mental disease. And, sadly, that disease continues to take lives everywhere, in the worst of ways.

References for Further Reading

In addition to nearly 600 articles taken from more than 200 scientific and popular journals, the following bibliography lists a selection of critical sources used for each of the history chapters in section one.

CHAPTER 1: MYTH, MAGIC, AND FOLKLORE: IMMORTALITY IN THE ERAS BEFORE SCIENCE

Barton, George A. *Archaeology and the Bible.* Philadelphia: American Sunday School Union, 1916.

Burgess, Glyn S., ed. *The Voyage of Saint Brendan: Representative Versions of the Legend in English Translation with Indexes of Themes and Motifs from the Stories.* Translated by W. R. S. Barron. Liverpool, UK: Liverpool University Press, 2005.

Carey, John. *Ireland and the Grail.* Aberystwyth, West Wales: Celtic Studies Publication, 2007.

de Boron, Robert. *Merlin and the Grail: Joseph of Arimathea, Merlin, Perceval.* Translated by Nigel Bryant. Rochester, NY: Brewer, 2001.

Ford, Patrick. *The Mabinogi, and Other Medieval Welsh Tales.* Berkeley: University of California Press, 1977.

Foster, Benjamin R. trans. *The Epic of Gilgamesh.* New York: Norton & Company, 2001.

Fuson, Robert H. *Juan Ponce de León and the Spanish Discovery of Puerto Rico and Florida.* Blacksburg, VA: McDonald & Woodward Publishing Company, 2000.

Geoffrey of Monmouth. *The History of the Kings of Britain.* Translated by Lewis Thorpe. New York: Penguin, 1966.

Heidel, Alexander. *The Gilgamesh Epic and Old Testament Parallels.* Chicago: University of Chicago Press, 1949.

Japan Society. *Wasobyoye: The Japanese Gulliver.* New York: Japan Society, 1933.

Livy. *History of Rome.* Edited by Ernest Rhys. Translated by Canon Roberts. New York: E. P. Dutton and Co., 1912.

Mackenzie, Donald A. *Egyptian Myth and Legend.* London: Gresham Publishing Company, 1913.

Mackenzie, Donald A. *Myths of China and Japan.* Boston: Longwood Press, 1923.

Mercer, Samuel A. B., trans. *The Pyramid Texts in Translation and Commentary.* New York: Longmans, Green & Co., 1952.

Newstead, Helaine. *Bran the Blessed in Arthurian Romance.* New York: Columbia University Press, 1939.

Post, Stephen G., and Robert H. Binstock, eds. *The Fountain of Youth: Cultural, Scientific, and Ethical Perspectives on a Biomedical Goal.* New York: Oxford University Press, 2004.

Pritchard, James B. *The Ancient Near East: An Anthology of Text and Pictures.* Princeton, NJ: Princeton University Press, 1975.

Slavicek, Louise Chipley. *Juan Ponce de León.* Philadelphia: Chelsea House, 2003.

Spence, Lewis. *The Myths of the North American Indians.* New York: T. Y. Crowell Company, 1914.

Swift, Jonathan. *Gulliver's Travels.* New York: Dover Publications, 1996.

Westervelt, W. D. *Legends of Ma-ui—A Demi God of Polynesia, and of His Mother Hina.* Honolulu: Hawaiian Gazette Co., 1910.

CHAPTER 2: CHANGES IN RELIGIOUS FAITH AND THE RISE OF ANTIAGING SCIENCE

Abu-Asab, Mones, trans. *Avicenna's Medicine: A New Translation of the 11th-century Canon with Practical Applications for Integrative Healthcare.* Rochester, VT: Healing Arts Press, 2013.

Ackerman, Jane. *Elijah, Prophet of Carmel.* Washington, D.C.: Washington Province of Discalced Carmelites, Inc., 2002.

Ashford, Ann. "Arab Civilization Found in Translation." *Socialist Review,* no. 282 (February 2004).

Balazs, Etienne. *Chinese Civilization and Bureaucracy.* New Haven, CT: Yale University Press, 1964.

Barnes, Jonathan, trans. *Complete Works of Aristotle.* New York: Oxford University, 1954.

Bettenson, Henry, trans. *Augustine of Hippo's City of God.* New York: Penguin Classics, 2004.

Birnbaum, Philip. *A Treasury of Judaism.* New York: Hebrew Publishing Co., 1957.

Borel, Henri, and Dwight Goddard, trans. *Laotzu's Tao and Wu Wei: Tao-Te Ching.* New York: Brentano's Publishers, 1919 [2008].

Bridges, Henry. *The "Opus Majus" of Roger Bacon.* Toronto: University of Toronto Libraries, 2011.

Budge, Ernest A. Wallis, ed. *The History of Alexander the Great, Being the Syriac Version of the Pseudo-Callisthenes.* Translated by E. H. Haight, A. M. Wolohojian, and E. A. W. Budge. New York: Cambridge University Press, 1889 [2003].

Budge, Ernest A. Wallis, ed. *The Life and Exploits of Alexander the Great: Being a Series of Translations of the Ethiopic Histories of Alexander by the Pseudo-Callisthenes and other Writers, with Introduction, Etc.* Palala Press, 1896 [2015].

Campany, Robert Ford. *To Live as Long as Heaven and Earth: A Translation and Study of Ge Hong's Traditions of Divine Transcendents.* Berkeley: University of California Press, 2002.

Constantine of Pisa. *The Book of the Secrets of Alchemy.* Translated by Barbara Obrist. New York: E. J. Brill, 1990.

Coomaraswamy, Ananda K. *"What Is Civilisation?" and Other Essays.* Cambridge, MA: Golgosova Press, 1989.

Eamon, William. *The Professor of Secrets: Mystery, Medicine, and Alchemy in Renaissance Italy.* Washington, D.C.: National Geographic Society, 2010.

Eliot, Charles, ed. *Letters of Marcus Tullius Cicero and Letters of Gaius Plinius Gaecilius Secundus.* New York: P. F. Collier & Son Corporation, 1937 [1965].

Graham, A. C., trans. *The Book of Lieh-tzŭ: A Classic of Tao.* New York: Columbia University Press, 1960 [1990].

Gruman, Gerald J. *A History of Ideas about the Prolongation of Life: The Evolution of Prolongevity Hypothesis to 1800.* New York: Arno Press, 1966 [1977]. (This reference was used for chapters 2, 3, 4, and 5.)

Grunar, O. Cameron, trans. *A Treatise on the Canon of Medicine of Avicenna.* London: Luzac & Co., 1930 [1984].

Guillaume, A., ed. *The Life of Muhammad: A Translation of Ishāq's* Sīrat Rasūl Allāh. Pakistan: Oxford University Press, 1955 [2004].

Haq, Syed Nomanul. *Names, Natures and Things: The Alchemist Jābir ibn Hayyān and His Kitāb al-Ahjār (Book of Stones).* Boston: Kluwer Academic Publishers, 1994.

Henry, John. *The Secret Life of an Alchemist: Francis Bacon's Real Philosophy of Nature.* Edinburgh, Scotland: Francis Bacon Society, 2006.

Holmyard, E. J., and Richard Russell, trans. *The Works of Geber.* Whitefish, MT: Kessinger Publishing, 1928 [1942].

Maspero, Henri. *Taoism and Chinese Religion.* Rev. ed. Translated by Frank A. Kierman, Jr. Melbourne, AUS: Quirin Press, 1950 [2014].

O'Shaughnessy, Thomas. *Muhammad's Thoughts on Death: A Thematic Study of the Qur'anic Data.* Leiden, Netherlands: E. J. Brill, 1969.

Palmer, Martin, trans. *The Book of Chuang Tzu.* New York: Penguin Books, 1996.

Pankhurst, Estelle Sylvia. *Ethiopia: A Cultural History.* Essex, UK: Lalibela House, 1959.

Polano, H. *The Talmud: Selections.* Charleston, SC: BiblioLife, 2009 [1876].

Principe, Lawrence M. *The Secrets of Alchemy.* Chicago: University of Chicago Press, 2013.

Robinet, Isabelle. *Daoism: Growth of a Religion.* Translated by Phyllis Brooks. Palo Alto, CA: Stanford University Press, 1997.

Sailey, Jay. *The Master Who Embraces Simplicity: A Study of the Philosopher Ko Hung, A.D. 283–343.* San Francisco: Chinese Materials Center, Inc., 1978.

Shah, Mazhar H. *The General Principles of Avicenna's Canon of Medicine.* Karachi, Pakistan: Naveed Clinic, 1966.

Silberer, Herbert. *Hidden Symbolism of Alchemy and the Occult Arts.* Translated by Smith Ely Jelliffe. New York: Dover Publications, Inc., 1917 [1971].

Sivin, Nathan. "On the *Pao P'u Tzu Nei P'ien* and the Life of Ko Hong (283–343)." *Isis* 60 (1976): 388–391.

Smith, Martin Ferguson, trans. *Lucretius on the Nature of Things.* Indianapolis: Hackett Publishing Company, 2001.

Stavenhagen, Lee, trans. *A Testament of Alchemy Being the Revelations of Morienus, Ancient Adept and Hermit of Jerusalem.* Hanover, NH: Brandeis University Press, 1974.

Stoneman, Richard. *Alexander the Great: A Life in Legend.* New Haven, CT: Yale University Press, 2008.

Stoneman, Richard, Kyle Erickson, and Ian Richard Netton, eds. *Alexander Romance in Persia and the East.* Eelde, Netherlands: Barkhuis, 2012.

Ware, James R. *Alchemy, Medicine & Religion in the China of A.D. 320: The Nei P'ien of Ko Hung.* New York: Dover Publications, Inc., 1981.

Wolohojian, Albert Mugrdich, trans. *The Romance of Alexander the Great by Pseudo-Calisthenes.* New York: Columbia University Press, 1969.

Yamanaka, Yuriko, and Nishio, Tetsuo. *The Arabian Nights and Orientalism: Perspectives from East and West.* New York: I. B. Tauris & Co. Ltd., 2006.

Yardley, J. C. *Curtius Rufus: Histories of Alexander the Great, Book 10.* New York: Oxford University Press, 2009.

Yu, David C. *History of Chinese Daoism.* Vol. 1. Lanham, MD: University Press of America, 2000.

CHAPTER 3: ENLIGHTENED AGING

Bacon, Francis. *The Historie of Life and Death.* New York: Da Capo Press, 1968.

Bacon, Roger. *The Cure of Old Age and the Preservation of Youth.* Regressed Publishing, 1683 [2013].

Barrett, Paul H., and R. B. Freeman, eds. *The Works of Charles Darwin.* Vol. 10, *The Foundations of the Origin of Species.* New York: New York University Press, 1987.

Becker, Carl. *The Heavenly City of the Eighteenth-century Philosophers.* New Haven, CT: Yale University Press, 1932 [2003].

Bichat, Xavier. *Physiological Researches on Life and Death.* Ulan Press, 2012.

Buffon, Georges Louis Leclerc. *The System of Natural History.* Los Angeles: University of California Libraries, 1814.

Cress, Donald A., trans. *René Descartes Discourse on Method.* 3rd ed. Indianapolis: Hackett Publishing Company, Inc., 1998.

Danto, Arthur, and Sidney Morgenbesser, eds. *Philosophy of Science.* New York: Meridian Books, 1960.

Darwin, Charles. *The Descent of Man and Selection in Relation to Sex.* Rev. ed. New York: D. Appleton and Company, 1897.

Darwin, Charles. *The Expression of the Emotions in Man and Animals.* 3rd ed. New York: Oxford University Press, 1889 [1998].

de Beer, Gavin, ed. *Charles Darwin and Thomas Henry Huxley: Autobiographies.* New York: Oxford University Press, 1983.

Ensor, George. *Inquiry Concerning the Population of Nations.* New York: Augustus M. Kelley, Publishers, 1818 [1967].

Godwin, William. *Of Population: An Enquiry Concerning the Power of Increase in the Numbers of Mankind.* New York: Augustus M. Kelley, 1820 [1964].

Greene, John C. *The Death of Adam: Evolution and Its Impact on Western Thought.* Ames: The Iowa State University Press, 1959 [1974].

Haller, Albertus. *First Lines of Physiology.* New York: Johnson Reprint Corporation, 1786 [1966].

Hawking, Stephen, ed. *On the Revolutions of Heavenly Spheres by Nicolaus Copernicus.* Philadelphia: Running Press, 2002.

Horstmanshoff, Manfred, Helen King, and Claus Zittel, eds. *Blood, Sweat, and Tears: The Changing Concepts of Physiology from Antiquity to Early Modern Europe.* Boston: Brill Publishers, 2012.

Hufeland, Christopher Wilhelm. *Art of Prolonging Life.* Translated by Erasmus Wilson. London: Forgotten Books, 2012.

Huxley, Thomas H. *Science and Education Essays.* New York: D. Appleton and Company, 1894.

Jacque, D. H. *The Philosophy of Human Beauty; Or Hints Two Physical Perfection.* Wood & Holbrook Publishers, 1871.

Levi, Honor, trans. *Blaise Pascal Pensées and Other Writings.* New York: Oxford University Press, 1995 [2008].

Malthus, Thomas Robert. *An Essay on the Principle of Population.* Edited by Philip Appleman. W. W. Norton & Company, 1976.

Meek, Ronald L., ed. *Marx and Engels on Malthus.* Translated by Dorothea L. Meek and Ronald L. Meek. London: Lawrence and Wishart, 1953.

Metchnikoff, Élie. *The Nature of Man: Studies in Optimistic Philosophy.* Translated by P. Chalmers Mitchell. New York: Arno Press, 1910 [1977].

Metchnikoff, Élie. *The Prolongation of Life: Optimistic Studies.* Translated by P. Chalmers Mitchell. New York: Arno Press, 1908 [1977].

Price, Richard. *The Evidence for a Future Period of Improvement in the State of Mankind, with the Means and Duty of Promoting It.* HardPress Publishing, 2012.

Priestly, Joseph. *An Essay on the First Principles of Government; and on the Nature of Political, Civil, and Religious Liberty.* Gail ECCO, 2010.

Robinson, Daniel, ed. *Significant Contributions to the History of Psychology, 1750–1920.* Washington, D.C.: University Publications of America, 1978.

Schäfer, Daniel. *Old Age and Disease in Early Modern Medicine.* New York: Pickering & Chatto, 2011.

Sweetsers, William. *Mental Hygiene; Or an Examination of the Intellect and Passions, Designed to Illustrate Their Influence on Health and Duration of Life.* Ulan Press, 2012.

Thoms, William J. *Human Longevity, Its Facts and Its Fictions; Including an Inquiry into Some of the More Remarkable Instances.* Whitefish, MT: Kessinger Publishers, 1873 [2007].

Thomson, J. Arthur. *Herbert Spencer.* New York: E. P. Dutton & Co., 1906.

Walsh, James J. *The Popes and Science: The History of the Papal Relations to Science during the Middle Ages and Down to Our Own Time.* New York: Fordham University Press, 1908.

Weismann, August. *Essays upon Heredity and Kindred Biological Problems.* London: Oxford Clarendon Press, 1891.

CHAPTER 4: ANTIAGING IN THE INDUSTRIAL AGE

Anderson, Barbara Gallatin. *The Aging Game: Success, Sanity, and Sex after 60.* New York: McGraw-Hill Book Company, 1979.

Appleman, Philip. *The Silent Explosion.* Boston: Beacon Press, 1965.

Arking, Robert. *Biology of Aging.* 2nd ed. Sunderland, MA: Sinauer Associates, Inc., 1998.

Ayala, Francisco, chair, Committee on the Conduct of Scientists. *On Being a Scientist.* Washington, D.C.: National Academy Press, 1989.

Ayala, Francisco J., and John A. Kiger, Jr. *Modern Genetics.* Menlo Park, CA: The Benjamin/Cummings Publishing Company, Inc., 1980.

Ayala, Francisco Jose, and Theodosius Dobzhansky. *Studies in the Philosophy of Biology: Reduction and Related Problems.* Los Angeles: University of California Press, 1974.

Baillie, John. *The Belief in Progress.* New York: Charles Scribner's Sons, 1951.

Barlow, Connie, ed. *Evolution Extended: Biological Debates on the Meaning of Life.* Cambridge, MA: MIT Press, 1994.

Barlow, Connie, ed. *From Gaia to Selfish Genes: Selected Writings in the Life Sciences.* Cambridge, MA: MIT Press, 1991.

Bengtson, Vern L., and W. Andrew Achenbaum, eds. *The Changing Contract across Generations.* New York: Aldine de Gruyter, 1993.

Bergson, Henri. *Creative Evolution.* Translated by Arthur Mitchell. New York: Henry Holt and Company, 1911.

Bergson, Henri. *An Introduction to Metaphysics.* Translated by T. E. Hulme. New York: G. P Putnam's Sons, 1912.

Bergson, Henri. *Mind-energy: Lectures and Essays. H.* Translated by Wildon Carr. London: MacMillan and Co. Lmtd., 1921.

Bergson, Henri. *Time and Free Will: An Essay on the Immediate Data of Consciousness.* Translated by F. L. Pogson. New York: Humanities Press Inc., 1910 [1971].

Braithwaite, Richard Bevan. *Scientific Explanation: A Study of the Function of Theory, Probability and Law in Science.* New York: Cambridge University Press, 1953 [1968].

Bury, John B. *The Idea of Progress: An Inquiry into Its Origin and Growth.* New York: Dover Publications, Inc., 1932 [1955].

Child, Charles Manning. *Senescence and Rejuvenescence.* New York: Arno Press, 1979.

Choron, Jacques. *Death and Western Thought.* New York: Collier Books, 1963.

Choron, Jacques. *Modern Man and Mortality.* New York: Macmillan Company, 1964.

Clark, Robert L., and Joseph J. Spengler. *The Economies of Individual and Population Aging.* New York: Cambridge University Press, 1980.

Comfort, Alex. *The Biology of Senescence.* 3rd ed. New York: Elsevier, 1956 [1979].

Condorcet, Antoine-Nicholas. *Outlines of an Historical View of the Progress of the Human Mind.* G. Langer, 2009.

Davis, Richard H., and Margaret Neiswender, eds. *Aging: Prospects and Issues.* Los Angeles: Ethel Percy Andrus Gerontology Center, University of Southern California, 1973.

Dawkins, Richard. *The Selfish Gene.* New York: Oxford University Press, 1976 [2006].

de Ropp, Robert S. *Man against Aging.* New York: Grove Press, 1959 (1962).

Eisele, Frederick R., ed. *Political Consequences of Aging.* Philadelphia: American Academy of Political and Social Science, 1974.

Finch, Caleb E. *Longevity, Senescence, and the Genome.* Chicago: University of Chicago Press, 1990.

Fries, James F., and Lawrence M. Crapo. *Vitality and Aging: Implications of the Rectangular Curve.* San Francisco: W. H. Freeman and Company, 1981.

Fromm, Erich H. *Escape from Freedom.* New York: Henry Holt and Company, LLC, 1965.

Fuller, Steve. *Kuhn vs. Popper: The Struggle for the Soul of Science.* New York: Columbia University Press, 2004.

Gallagher, Idella J. *Morality in Evolution: The Moral Philosophy of Henri Bergson.* The Hague, Netherlands: Martinus Nijhoff, 1970.

Gardner, Martin, ed. *Great Essays in Science.* New York: Washington Square Press, Inc., 1957 [1963].

Ginsburg, Morris. *The Idea of Progress: A Revaluation.* Westport, CT: Greenwood Press, Publishers, 1953 [1972].

Goldman, Robert N. *Einstein's God: Albert Einstein's Quest as a Scientist and as a Jew to Replace a Forsaken God.* Northvale, NJ: Jason Aronson, Inc., 1997.

Goodway, David, ed. *Against Power and Death: The Anarchist Articles and Pamphlets of Alex Comfort.* London: Freedom Press, 1994.

Greene, John. *The Death of Adam: Evolution and Its Impact on Western Thought.* Ames: Iowa State University Press, 1959 [c.1976].

Gruman, Gerald J. *Charles Asbury Stephens: Natural Salvation—The Message of Science.* New York: Arno Press, 1956 [1977].

Gruman, Gerald J. *The "Fixed Period" Controversy: Prelude to Ageism.* New York: Arno Press, 1979.

Haavio-Mannila, Elina, Osmo Kontula, and Anna Rotkirch. *Sexual Lifestyles in the Twentieth Century.* New York: Palgrave, 2002.

Hall, G. Stanley. *Senescence: The Last Half of Life.* New York: Arno Press, 1922 [1972].

Harris, Diana K. *Sociology of Aging.* 2nd ed. New York: Harper & Row, Publishers, 1990.

Hawking, Stephen. *A Brief History of Time: Updated and Expanded Edition.* New York: Bantam Books, 1988 [1996].

Hawking, Stephen. *Hawking on the Big Bang and Black Holes.* New Jersey: World Scientific, 1993.

Hawking, Stephen, and Roger Penrose. *The Nature of Space and Time.* Princeton, NJ: Princeton University Press, 1996.

Hayflick, Leonard. *How and Why We Age.* New York: Ballantine Books, 1994.

Hess, Beth B., and Elizabeth W. Markson. *Growing Old in America.* 4th ed. New Brunswick, NJ: Transaction Publishers, 1991 [1993].

Horwich, Paul, ed. *World Changes: Thomas Kuhn and the Nature of Science.* Cambridge, MA: MIT Press, 1993.

Huxley, Aldous. *After Many a Summer Dies the Swan.* New York: Perennial Classic, 1965.

Huxley, Julian. *Essays of a Biologist.* Freeport, NY: Books for Libraries Press, 1923 [1970].

Huxley, Julian. *Evolution in Action.* New York: Harper & Row, Publishers, 1953.

Huxley, Julian. *Evolution: The Modern Synthesis.* New York: John Wiley & Sons, Inc., 1964.

Huxley, Julian. *New Bottles for the New Wine.* New York: Harper & Brothers Publishers, 1957.

Huxley, Julian. *Religion without Revelation.* London: C. A. Watts & Co. Ltd., 1967.

Huxley, Thomas H., and Julian Huxley. *Evolution and Ethics, 1893–1943.* London: Pilot Press, Ltd., 1947.

Huyck, Margaret Hellie. *Growing Older: Things You Need to Know about Aging.* Englewood Cliffs, NJ: Prentice-Hall, Inc., 1974.

Kallen, Horace Meyer. *William James and Henri Bergson: A Study in Contrasting Theories of Life.* Chicago: University of Chicago Press, 1914 [1980].

Kanungo, M. S. *Genes and Aging.* New York: Cambridge University Press, 1994.

Klatz, Ronald, and Robert Goldman. *Stopping the Clock: Why Many of Us Will Live Past 100—And Enjoy Every Minute!* New Canaan, CT: Keats Publishing, Inc., 1996.

Kohn, Robert R. *Principles of Mammalian Aging.* Englewood Cliffs, NJ: Prentice-Hall, Inc., 1971.

Kuhn, Thomas S. *The Structure of Scientific Revolutions.* Chicago: University of Chicago Press, 1962 [2012].

Le Roy, Edouard. *A New Philosophy: Henri Bergson.* Translated by Vincent Benson. New York: Henry Holt & Company, 1913.

Masoro, Edward J., ed. *Handbook of Physiology.* Sect. 11, *Aging.* New York: Oxford University Press, 1995.

Medawar, Peter. *The Limits of Science.* New York: Oxford University Press, 1984 [1987].

Medawar, Peter B. *The Future of Man: The BBC Reith Lectures 1959.* New York: Basic Books, Inc., Publishers, 1959 [1961].

Medawar, Peter B., and Jean S. Medawar. *The Life Science: Current Ideas of Biology.* London: Wildwood House Ltd., 1977.

Minkler, Meredith, and Carroll L. Estes, eds. *Critical Perspectives on Aging: The Political and Moral Economy of Growing Old.* Amityville, NY: Baywood Publishing Company, Inc., 1991.

Neugarten, Bernice L., and Robert J. Havighurst, eds. *Extending the Human Life Span: Social Policy and Social Ethics.* Chicago: Committee on Human Development, University of Chicago, 1977.

Niebuhr, Reinhold. *Faith and History: A Comparison of Christian and Modern Views of History.* New York: Charles Scribner's Sons, 1949.

Pearson, Durk, and Sandy Shaw. *Life Extension: A Practical Scientific Approach.* New York: Warner Books, 1981.

Picart, Caroline Joan "Kay" S. *The Darwinian Shift: Kuhn vs. Laudan.* Acton, MA: Copley Custom Publishing Group, 1997.

Quetelet, Lambert Adolphe Jacques. *A Treatise on Man and the Development of his Faculties.* New York: Cambridge University Press, 1871 [2013].

Rose, Michael R. *Darwin's Spectre: Evolutionary Biology in the Modern World.* Princeton, NJ: Princeton University Press, 1998.

Rose, Michael R. *Evolutionary Biology of Aging.* New York: Oxford University Press, 1991.

Rosenfeld, Albert. *Prolongevity.* New York: Alfred A. Knopf, 1976.

Ruse, Michael. *Mystery of Mysteries: Is Evolution a Social Construction?* Cambridge, MA: Harvard University Press, 1999.

Salmon, Arthur E. *Alex Comfort.* Boston: Twayne Publishers, 1978.

Sartre, Jean-Paul. *Nausea.* New York: Penguin, 2000.

Schneider, Edward L., and John W. Rowe, eds. *Handbook of the Biology of Aging.* 3rd ed. New York: Academic Press, Inc., 1990.

Sears, Robert R., and S. Shirley Feldman, eds. *The Seven Ages of Man.* Los Altos, CA: William Kaufmann, Inc., 1964 [1973].

Shock, Nathan W., ed. *Perspectives in Experimental Gerontology: A Festschrift for Doctor F. Verzár.* New York: Arno Press, 1966 [1980].

Simmons, Leo W. *The Role of the Aged in Primitive Society.* New York: Archon Books, 1945 [1970].

Simpson, George Gaylord. *The View of Life: The World of an Evolutionist.* New York: Harcourt, Brace & World, Inc., 1947 [1964].

Smith, Homer. *From Fish to Philosopher: The Story of Our Internal Environment.* Andesite Press, 1953 [2015].

Smith, Homer. *Man and His Gods.* Boston: Little & Brown, 1952.

Solnick, Robert L. *Sexuality and Aging.* Rev. ed. Los Angeles: Ethel Percy Andrus Gerontology Center, University of Southern California Press, 1978.

Strehler, Bernard L. *The Biology of Aging: A Symposium.* Washington, D.C.: American Institute of Biological Sciences, 1957.

Strehler, Bernard L. *Time, Cells, and Aging.* New York: Academic Press, 1962 [1977].

Thomson, J. Arthur. *Concerning Evolution.* New Haven, CT: Yale University Press, 1925.

Thomson, J. Arthur. *Darwinism and Human Life.* 3rd ed. London: Andrew Melrose, Ltd., 1910 [1916].

Thomson, J. Arthur. *Heredity.* 5th ed. New York: R. V. Coleman, 1908 [1926].

Thomson, J. Arthur. *The Outline of Science: A Plain Story Simply Told.* 4 vols. New York: G. P. Putnam's Sons, 1922.

Thomson, J. Arthur. *Riddles of Science.* Rev. ed. Greenwich, CT: Fawcett Publications, 1958 [1962].

Thomson, J. Arthur. *What Is Man?* New York: G. P. Putnam's Sons, 1924 [1925].

Tuveson, Ernest Lee. *Millennium and Utopia: A Study in the Background of the Idea of Progress.* New York: Harper & Row, Publishers, 1949 [1964]

Weindruch, Richard, and Roy L. Walford. *The Retardation of Aging and Disease by Dietary Restriction.* Springfield, IL: Charles C. Thomas, Publishers, 1988.

Wilde, Oscar. *The Picture of Dorian Gray.* New York: W. W. Norton, 2006.

Wise, David A., ed. *Issues in the Economics of Aging.* Chicago: University of Chicago Press, 1990.

Woodruff, Diana S., and James E. Birren. *Aging: Scientific Perspectives and Social Issues.* Monterey, CA: Brooks/Cole Publishing Company, 1983.

Wray, K. Brad. *Kuhn's Evolutionary Social Epistemology.* New York: Cambridge University Press, 2011.

CHAPTER 5: ANTIAGING IN THE 21ST CENTURY: FROM THEORY TO PRACTICE

The following list also includes the references for selected chapters in section two.

Agar, Nicholas. *Humanity's End: Why We Should Reject Radical Enhancement.* Cambridge, MA: MIT Press, 2010.

Agar, Nicholas. *The Sceptical Optimist: Why Technology Isn't the Answer to Everything.* New York: Oxford University Press, 2015.

Agar, Nicholas. *Truly Human Enhancement: A Philosophical Defense of Limits.* Boston: MIT Press, 2013.

Anton, Ted. *The Longevity Seekers: Science, Business, and the Fountain of Youth.* Chicago: University of Chicago Press, 2013.

Applewhite, Ashton. *This Chair Rocks: A Manifesto against Ageism.* Networked Books, 2016.

Auerbach, Alan J., and Ronald D. Lee. *Demographic Change and Fiscal Policy.* New York: Cambridge University Press, 2001.

Austad, Steven N. *Why We Age: What Science Is Discovering about the Body's Journey through Life.* New York: John Wiley & Sons, Inc., 1997.

Avise, John C., and Francisco J. Ayala, eds. *In the Light of Evolution.* Vol. 1, *Adaptation and Complex Design.* Washington, D.C.: National Academies Press, 2006.

Ayala, Francisco J. *Am I a Monkey?: Six Big Questions about Evolution.* Baltimore: Johns Hopkins University Press, 2010.

Ayala, Francisco J. *Darwin's Gift to Science and Religion.* Washington. D.C.: Joseph Henry Press, 2007.

Bell, Trudy E., and Dave Dooling. *Engineering Tomorrow: Today's Technology Experts Envision the Next Century.* New York: IEEE Press, 2000.

Bergeman, Cindy S. *Aging: Genetic and Environmental Influences.* Thousand Oaks, CA: SAGE Publications, 1997.

Birren, James, and K. Warner Schaie. *Handbook of the Psychology of Aging.* 5th ed. New York: Academic Press, 1977 [2001].

Bludau, Juergen. *Aging, but Never Old: The Realities, Myths, and Misrepresentations of the Antiaging Movement.* Denver: Praeger, 2010.

Bostrum, Nick. "A History of Transhumanist Thought." *Journal of Evolution and Technology* 14, no. 1 (April 2005).

Brockman, John, ed. *What We Believe but Cannot Prove: Today's Leading Thinkers on Science in the Age of Certainty.* New York: Harper Perennial, 2006.

Broderick, Damien. *The Spike: How Our Lives Are Being Transformed by Rapidly Advancing Technologies.* New York: Tom Doherty Associates Book, 2001.

Broderick, Damien. *Year Million: Science at the Far Edge of Knowledge.* New York: Atlas & Co., Publishers, 2008.

Butler, Robert. *Why Survive?: Growing Old in America.* New York: Johns Hopkins University Press, 1975 [2002].

Carr, Deborah S. *Encyclopedia of Life Course and Human Development.* New York: Macmillan, 2008.

Cave, Stephen. *Immortality.* New York: Crown Publishers, 2012.

Clark, William R. *A Means to an End: The Biological Basis of Aging and Death.* New York: Oxford University Press, 1999.

Common Sense Media. *Children, Teens, Media, and Body Image: A Common Sense Media Research Brief.* San Francisco: Common Sense Media, 2015.

Dawkins, Richard, ed. *The Oxford Book of Modern Science Writing.* New York: Oxford University Press, 2008.

De Grey, Aubrey D. N. *Strategies for Engineered Negligible Senescence: Why Genuine Control of Aging May Be Foreseeable.* New York: New York Academy of Sciences, 2004.

De Grey, Aubrey, and Michael Rae. *Ending Aging: The Rejuvenation Breakthroughs That Could Reverse Human Aging in Our Lifetime.* New York: St. Martin's Press, 2007.

Enyeart, Stacy. *The Ageless Obsession: Finding the Fountain of Youth.* Denver: Outskirts Press, 2014.

Finch, Caleb. *The Biology of Human Longevity: Inflammation, Nutrition, and Aging in the Evolution of Life Spans.* New York: Elsevier, 2007.

Fry, Prem S., and Corey L. M. Keyes, eds. *New Frontiers in Resilient Aging: Life Strengths and Well-being in Late Life.* New York: Cambridge University Press, 2010.

Gillick, Muriel R. *The Denial of Aging: Perpetual Youth, Eternal Life, and Other Dangerous Fantasies.* Cambridge, MA: Harvard University Press, 2006.

Gosden, Roger. *Cheating Time: Science, Sex, and Aging.* New York: W. H. Freeman and Company, 1996.

Gosden, Roger. *Designing Babies: The Brave New World of Reproductive Technology.* New York: W. H. Freeman and Company, 1999.

Gould, Stephen Jay. *The Structure of Evolutionary Theory.* Cambridge, MA: Harvard University Press, 2002.

Gupta, Sanjay. *Chasing Life: New Discoveries in the Search for Immortality to Help You Age Less Today.* New York: Warner Wellness, 2007.

Haag, James W., Gregory R. Peterson, and Michael L. Spezio, eds. *The Routledge Companion to Religion and Science.* New York: Routledge, 2012.

Hall, Stephen S. *Merchants of Immortality: Chasing the Dream of Human Life Extension.* New York: Houghton Mifflin Company, 2003.

Hawking, Stephen, ed. *A Stubbornly Persistent Illusion: The Essential Scientific Works of Albert Einstein.* Philadelphia: Running Press, 2007.

Hung, Edwin H.-C. *Beyond Kuhn: Scientific Explanation, Theory Structure, Incommensurability and Physical Necessity.* Burlington, VT: Ashgate Publishing Company, 2006.

Institute of Medicine. *Extending Life, Enhancing Life.* Washington D.C.: Institute of Medicine, 1991.

Jenkins, Jo Ann. *Disrupt Aging: A Bold New Path to Living Your Best Life at Every Age.* New York: Public Affairs, 2016.

Kelder, Peter. *Ancient Secret of the Fountain of Youth.* New York: Doubleday, 1998.

Klatz, Ronald, and Carol Kahn. *Grow Young with HGH.* New York: Harper Collins Books, 1997.

Kohlbacher, Florian, and Cornelius Herstatt, eds. *The Silver Market Phenomenon: Business Opportunities in an Era of Demographic Change.* Berlin: Springer-Verlag, 2008.

Kurzweil, Ray. *The 10% Solution for a Healthy Life: How to Eliminate Virtually All Risk of Heart Disease and Cancer.* New York: Crown Publisher, Inc., 1993.

Kurzweil, Ray. *The Age of Spiritual Machines: When Computers Exceed Human Intelligence.* New York: Viking, 1999.

Kurzweil, Ray. *How to Create a Mind: The Secret of Human Thought Revealed.* New York: Penguin Books, 2012.

Kurzweil, Ray. *The Singularity Is Near: When Humans Transcend Biology.* New York: Viking, 2005.

Kurzweil, Ray, and Terry Grossman. *Fantastic Voyage: Live Long Enough to Live Forever.* London: Rodale International Ltd., 2005.

March, J., J. L. McGaugh, and S. B. Kiesler, eds. *Aging: Biology and Behavior.* New York: Academic Press, 1982.

Medina, John J. *The Clock of Ages: Why We Age—How We Age—Winding Back the Clock.* New York: Cambridge University Press, 1996.

Minker, Meredith, and Carroll L. Estes, eds. *Critical Perspectives on Aging: The Political and Moral Economy of Growing Old.* Amityville, NY: Baywood Publishing, 1991.

Moody, Harry. *Aging Concepts and Controversies.* Thousand Oaks, CA: Pine Forge Press, 2009.

More, Max, and Natasha Vita-More, eds. *The Transhumanist Reader.* Malden, MA: John Wiley & Sons, Ltd., 2013.

Mueller, Laurence D., Casandra L. Rauser, and Michael R. Rose. *Does Aging Stop?* New York: Oxford University Press, 2011.

National Institute on Aging. *Our Future Selves.* Washington, D.C.: National Institute on Aging, 1978.

National Institute on Aging. *Toward and Independent Old Age: A National Plan for Research on Aging.* Washington, D.C.: National Institute on Aging, 1982.

Overall, Christine. *Aging, Death, and Human Longevity: A Philosophical Inquiry.* Los Angeles: University of California Press, 2003.

Oz, Mehmet C., and Michael F. Roizen. *You Staying Young: The Owner's Manual for Extending Your Warranty.* New York: Free Press, 2007.

Post, Stephen G., and Robert H. Binstock, eds. *The Fountain of Youth: Cultural, Scientific, and Ethical Perspectives on a Biomedical Goal.* New York: Oxford University Press, 2004.

Powell, Lane H., and Dawn Cassidy. *Family Life Education: Working with Families across the Life Span.* 2nd ed. Longrove, IL: Waveland Press, 2006.

Raymer, Steve, and Peter Healey, eds. *Unnatural Selection: The Challenges of Engineering Tomorrow's People.* Sterling, VA: Earthscan, 2009.

Razin, Assaf, and Efraim Sadka, with Chang Woon Nam. *The Decline of the Welfare State: Demography and Globalization.* Cambridge, MA: MIT Press, 2005.

Rhode, Deborah L. *The Beauty Bias: The Injustice of Appearance in Life and Law.* New York: Oxford University Press, 2010.

Richards, Jay W. *Are We Spiritual Machines?: Ray Kurzweil vs. the Critics of Strong A.I.* Seattle: Discovery Institute, 2002.

Ricklefs, Robert E., and Caleb E. Finch. *Aging: A Natural History.* W. H. Freeman & Co., 1995.

Rockstein, M., and M. L. Sussman, eds. *Nutrition, Longevity and Aging.* New York: Academic Press, 1976.

Rose, Michael R. *Evolutionary Biology of Aging.* New York: Oxford University Press, 1991.

Rose, Michael R. *The Long Tomorrow: How Advances in Evolutionary Biology Can Help Us Postpone Aging.* New York: Oxford University Press, 2005.

Rose, Michael, Hardip B. Passananti, and Margarida Matos. *Methuselah Flies: A Case Study in the Evolution of Aging.* River Edge, NJ: World Scientific Publishing Co., Pte. Ltd., 2004.

Rothblatt, Martine. *Virtually Human: The Promise and the Peril of Digital Immortality.* New York: St. Martin's Press, 2014.

Sandler, Ronald L., ed., *Ethics and Emerging Technologies.* New York: Palgrave MacMillan, 2014.

Scommegna, P. M. *Death and Taxes: The Public Policy Impact of Living Longer*. Washington, D.C.: Population Reference Bureau, Inc., 1984.

Shostak, Stanley. *Becoming Immortal: Combining Cloning and Stem-cell Therapy*. Albany, NY: State University of New York Press, 2002.

Shostak, Stanley. *The Evolution of Death: Why We Are Living Longer*. Albany, NY: State University Press, 2006.

Shostak, Stanley. *Evolution of Sameness and Difference: Perspectives on the Human Genome Project*. Amsterdam: Harwood Academic Publishers, 1999.

Silvertown, Jonathan. *The Long and the Short of It: The Science of Life Span and Aging*. Chicago: University of Chicago Press, 2013.

Singham, Mano. *Quest for Truth: Scientific Progress and Religious Beliefs*. Bloomington, IN: Phi Delta Kappa Educational Foundation, 2000.

Stipp, David. *The Youth Pill: Scientists at the Brink of an Anti-aging Revolution*. New York: Current, 2010.

Stock, Gregory. *Redesigning Humans: Our Inevitable Genetic Future*. Boston: Houghton Mifflin Company, 2002.

Stove, David. *Scientific Irrationalism: Origins of a Postmodern Cult*. New Brunswick, NJ: Transaction Publishers, 2001.

Susskind, Leonard. *The Black Hole War: My Battle with Stephen Hawking to Make the World Safe for Quantum Mechanics*. New York: Little, Brown and Company, 2008.

Swarts, Katherine, ed. *The Aging Population*. New York: Greenhaven Press, 2009.

Walford, R. L. *Maximum Life Span*. New York: Norton, 1983.

Wilkinson, David. *God, Time and Stephen Hawking*. Grand Rapids, MI: Monarch Books, 2001.

Wilson, David Sloan. *Darwin's Cathedral: Evolution, Religion, and the Nature of Society*. Chicago: University of Chicago Press, 2002.

Young, Simon. *Designer Evolution: A Transhumanist Manifesto*. Amherst, NY: Prometheus Books, 2006.

Zorea, Aharon. *Birth Control (Health and Medical Issues Today)*. Westport, CT Greenwood Press, 2012.

Zorea, Aharon. *Steroids (Health and Medical Issues Today)*. Westport, CT: Greenwood Press, 2014.

About the Author and Contributors

Author

Aharon W. Zorea, PhD, is professor of history at the University of Wisconsin–Richland. His published works include *In the Image of God: A Christian Response to Capital Punishment*; Greenwood's *Birth Control* and *Steroids*; and more than 60 articles on politics and legal and social policy. Zorea holds a master's degree from Purdue University and a doctorate in policy history from Saint Louis University. He maintains his website at ZoreaNotes.com.

Contributors

Nicholas Agar, PhD, of the Australian National University, earned his bachelor's and master's degrees at Victoria University of Wellington, New Zealand, and currently serves there as a professor in the School of History, Philosophy, Political Science & International Relations. He is the author of half a dozen books, including *The Sceptical Optimist* (Oxford University Press, 2015); *Truly Human Enhancement* (MIT Press, 2013); and *Humanity's End* (MIT Press, 2010). His current project presents an ethical evaluation of technological revolutions, from the Neolithic to the digital.

Rabbi Tuvia Bolton received his bachelor of arts in philosophy from the University of Michigan. He is a pupil of Rabbi Yisroel Jacobson and a graduate of Hadar HaTorah Yeshiva, New York. Rabbi Bolton holds three rabbinical ordinations from leading Israeli halachic authorities. He has over 35 years of teaching experience at the Chabad Torah Academy "Yeshiva Ohr Tmimim" in Kfar Chabad, Israel, and currently serves as its director (Rosh Yeshiva). More information about the yeshiva can be found at www.ohrtmimim.org/Yeshiva. Rabbi Bolton can be contacted at ravbolton@gmail.com.

Amer Haleem, MSJ, writes and speaks on Islam and Muslims and their American experience. He has been the editor of the two foremost English-language magazines for Muslims. He was senior editor of *The Gracious Quran: A Modern-phrased Interpretation in English*, a translation of the scripture of Islam with a major introduction and extensive notes; Abu Hamid Al-Ghazali's (Algazel's) seminal work on the theoretical foundations of Islamic Law, *The Quintessence of the Science of the Principles* (*Al-Mustasfa min 'Ilm Al-Usul*); and *Lasting Prayers of the Quran and the Prophet Muhammad*. He is currently editing the classic Islamic juristic primer of Ibn Rushd (Averroes), *The Beginning of the Independent Jurist* (*Bidayat Al-Mujtahid*).

Zoltan Istvan received his bachelor of arts in philosophy and religious studies from Columbia University. Istvan served as the 2016 Transhumanist Party presidential candidate, has worked as a journalist for National Geographic Channel, and has served as a director for the international conservation group WildAid. He has appeared in dozens of television stories, articles, and Web casts as a futurist and the best-selling author of *The Transhumanist Wager*, which is a fictional thriller about philosopher Jethro Knights and his unwavering quest for immortality via science and technology. Istvan has been featured by CNN, Fox News, RT, the *New Times*, the *San Francisco Chronicle*, *Outside*, *Slate*, the *Huffington Post*, *Wired UK*, BBC Radio, the Travel Channel, and other media.

Gregory Nathan Johnson, MFA, is a visual artist and lecturer at the University of Wisconsin Colleges–Richland Center. Mr. Johnson's artwork primarily focuses on figurative painting and an exploration of the ethics of contemporary art, while being aware of his own implicit connection within his own critiques. Beyond conceptual figure painting, Johnson is also an illustrator and graphic artist. His work and more information can be found at his Web site: gregorynathanjohnson.com.

Louis Kinsey received his bachelor of arts from the Universities of Edinburgh and Aberdeen and is a Church of Scotland minister in Aberdeen, Scotland, where he serves as a parish minister to a congregation on the northern side of the city. He is a British Army Reserve chaplain who has served in Iraq and Afghanistan. In addition, he serves as a chaplain in a correctional facility within the context of a multifaith chaplaincy team and is also a school chaplain. His particular interests include Jewish religion and culture during the late Second Temple period, synagogue studies, early church history, reformed worship and liturgy, the development of hymnody, and chaplaincy and institutions. He has a special interest in the Wycliffe Bible Translators, working to offer the Bible to the 1,800 language groups that still have no copy of the Holy Scriptures in their own tongue (https://www.wycliffe.org.uk).

Jeffrey Kleiman, PhD, earned his degree from Michigan State and has taught for the University of Wisconsin colleges for more than 25 years. In that time, he has won recognition for his teaching from students, along with two Fulbright Awards to Eastern Europe. Originally trained as an American urban historian, Professor Kleiman has turned to Holocaust research and is currently completing the translation of a survivor's diary from Yiddish.

João Pedro de Magalhães, PhD, graduated with a degree in microbiology in 1999 from the Escola Superior de Biotecnologia, in his hometown of Porto, Portugal, and then obtained his PhD in 2004 from the University of Namur, Belgium. Following a postdoc with genomics pioneer Professor George Church at Harvard Medical School, in 2008, Dr. de Magalhães was recruited to the University of Liverpool. He is now a senior lecturer and leads the Integrative Genomics of Ageing Group (pcwww.liv.ac.uk/~aging). The group's research broadly focuses on understanding the genetic, cellular, and molecular mechanisms of aging.

Robert Morlino, PhD, was installed as the fourth bishop of the Dioceses of Madison, Wisconsin, in 2003. He earned his bachelor's degree in philosophy from Fordham University; a master's degree in philosophy from the University of Notre Dame; the master of divinity degree from the Weston School of Theology in Cambridge, Massachusetts; and a doctorate in moral theology from the Gregorian University in Rome, with specialization in fundamental moral theology and bioethics. Bishop Morlino was ordained a Jesuit priest in 1974 and has taught philosophy at Loyola College in Baltimore; St. Joseph University in Philadelphia; Boston College; and the University of Notre Dame and St. Mary's College in Indiana. He also served as the ninth bishop of the Dioceses of Helena, Montana, from 1999 to 2003.

Dale Murray, PhD, is an associate professor of philosophy with a joint appointment with the University of Wisconsin–Richland and the University of Wisconsin–Baraboo/Sauk County. His published works include a book, *Nozick, Autonomy, and Compensation*, as well as several research articles and book reviews in such journals as *Teaching Philosophy*, *Journal of Value Inquiry*, *Journal of Medicine and Philosophy*, *American Journal of Bioethics—Neuroscience*, and the *Internet Encyclopedia of Philosophy*. He has teaching and research interests in social and political philosophy and applied ethics. He is currently working on a book-length manuscript titled *The Global and the Local: An Environmental Ethics Casebook*.

S. Jay Olshansky, PhD, is a professor of public health at the University of Illinois at Chicago; chief scientist at Lapetus Solutions, Inc.; and a research associate at the Center on Aging at the University of Chicago and at the London School of Hygiene and Tropical Medicine. The focus of his research to date has been on estimates of the upper limits to human longevity, exploring the health and public policy implications associated with individual and population aging; forecasts of the size, survival, and age structure of the population; the pursuit of the scientific means to slow aging in people (The Longevity Dividend); and the global implications of the reemergence of infectious and parasitic diseases. Dr. Olshansky is a fellow of the Gerontological Society of America and is on the Board of Directors of the American Federation of Aging Research. He is the first author of *The Quest for Immortality: Science at the Frontiers of Aging* (Norton, 2001) and *A Measured Breath of Life* (2013) and coeditor of *Aging: The Longevity Dividend* (Cold Spring Harbor Laboratory Press).

Jill A. Rinzel, PhD, is an associate professor of psychology and education at the University of Wisconsin–Waukesha in Waukesha, Wisconsin. Her research is focused on the impact of various childhood sports experiences on their social and academic skills and on how memories of childhood sports experiences influence adult levels and types of physical activities. Her research interests also include the influence of service learning on critical thinking and academic engagement.

Index

Chesterton, G.K., 59, 307
Children: cognitive development of, 209–210;
    with growth disorders, 287, 289; obese, 198;
    sleep requirements of, 201–202
China: animism in, 41; Confucianism in,
    41–42; historical pursuit of life extension in,
    9, 10, 16; and the idea of reincarnation, 40;
    immortality legends in, 23–24; Taoism in,
    39, 41–47, 49, 51, 55–56, 90; timeline, 42
Chinese legends: "Islands of the Blest," 36–37;
    story of Xu Fu, 24–25, 44
Chinese medicine (TCM), 268, 269
Chocolate, 245, 275
Cholesterol: high, 116, 201, 268; high-density
    lipoprotein (HDL), 246, 260; low, 225;
    low-density lipoprotein (LDL), 225, 246,
    249, 250, 261; lowering, 250, 253, 254,
    258, 261, 275; normal, 201; regulation of,
    225, 250, 272; as a steroid, 121; synthesizing
    vitamin D from, 262
Choline, 267
Chondroitin sulfate, 272–273, 275
Christian realism, 101
Christianity, 25, 39, 40, 49, 64, 101, 156, 318,
    341, 342, 353; and humanism, 59–60; under
    Muslim rule, 49; Orthodox, 254; sacred
    texts, 49; in Spain, 53. See also Catholicism;
    Protestantism
Chromium, 263, 265
Chromosomes, 108, 131–132
Chronic diseases, 214–215. See also Age-related
    conditions; Age-related diseases
Chronic inflammation, 240
Chronic obstructive pulmonary disease
    (COPD), 230, 231
Church of Scotland, 342
Ciba Pharmaceuticals, 122, 123
Cicirelli, Victor C., 113
Cinnabar, 46, 51
City of God (Augustine), 63
Clark, William, 133, 146
Clarke, Arthur C., 160
Clement IV (pope), 62
Cloning, 258, 300–302, 303; human, 164
Cobalamin, 261–262, 266, 274
Cobalt, 263
Coenzyme Q10 (CoQ10), 272
Coffee, 246–247, 251
Cohen, Janie, 330
Collagen, 190–191
Collins, Francis, 312
Columbus, Christopher, 12, 28, 37, 55

Columbus, Diego, 12
Common Sense (Paine), 76
Comparative biology, 7
Condorcet, Marquis de, 75–77
Confucianism, 41–42
Congestive heart failure, 226
Conservation movement, 105
Constantine V (Byzantine emperor), 49–50
Cook, Howard, 132
Copper, 263, 264, 267, 274
CoQ10 (coenzyme Q10), 272
Cordain, Loren, 257–258
Coronary artery disease, 225–226. See also
    Cardiovascular disease
Cortisone, 121
Cosmeceuticals, 183, 189–192
Cosmetic enhancements, 128, 202–204, 289.
    See also Plastic surgery
Cosmetic procedures: cosmeceuticals, 183,
    189–192; increase in rate of, 188; over-the
    counter, 189–192; prescription treatments,
    192–193; surgical procedures, 193–194.
    See also Plastic surgery
Cosmetic surgery. See Plastic surgery
Cosmetics industry, 3, 149, 183, 188–189, 315
Counterculture, 6
Cranberries, 245
Creutzfeldt-Jakob disease, 287
Crick, Francis, 131
Criminology, 93
CRISPR, 298
Cross-linkage theory, 175
Crusades, 53, 56
Cryo-Care (Arizona), 306
Cryogenics, 295, 305
Cryonics, 295, 304–306
Cryonics Institute, 305
Cryonics Society of California, 306
Cryonics Society of New York, 295, 306
Cuba, 13
Cultural stereotypes, 210
Curcumin, 297
Cuvier, Georges, 80, 81
Cybernetic implants, 213
Cytex, 219

D'Anghiera, Peter Martyr, 14, 15
Daniel Fast, 254
Dark chocolate (epicatechin), 245, 275
Darwin, Charles, 79, 82, 83–84, 85, 86, 87, 90,
    93, 100, 158; and the mind-body problem,
    88–89; theory of evolution, 83–85, 102, 103

Lifestyle changes, 239–243
Lightman, Alan, 338
Lindeberg, Staffan, 258
Lipofuscin, 292
Liposomes, 190, 191
Liposuction, 188, 193, 289
Lister, Joseph, 95
Liver disease, 287
Longevity. *See* Life expectancy
Longevity Dividend Initiative (LDI), 323
Longevity genes, 203, 257
Lord of the Rings trilogy (Tolkien), 329
Louis XIV (king of France), 65
Louis XV (king of France), 79
Louis XVI (king of France), 76
L-theanini, 271–272
Lucidril, 292
Lupus, 291
Lyell, Charles, 83

MacBride, Ernest, 85
Magalhães, João Pedro de, 143–144, 239, 320–322
Magnesium, 263
Mahoney, Suzanne Marie. *See* Somers, Suzanne
Major League Baseball, 123, 193
Male Hormone, The (de Kruif), 122
Malebranche, Nicolas, 65
Malthus, Thomas, 77–79, 83
Man against Aging (de Ropp), 107
Manganese, 263, 267
Manichaeism, 154
Manilius, Marcus, 167
Al-Mansūr (caliph), 49–50
Marcus Aurelius (Roman emperor), 50
Marlowe, Christopher, 351, 352
Martin, George, 323
Massachusetts Institute of Technology (MIT), 143
Massage therapy, 241
Master Miracle Supplement (MMS), 239
Materialism, 112, 303
Mathematics, 62
Matrix, The (film), 307, 309
McArthur Research Network on Successful Aging, 211
McGinn, Colin, 311
McGuire, Mark, 193
MD Longevity Clinics (San Francisco and New York), 283
Meaning of Evolution (Darwin), 103
Means to an End, A (Clark), 133, 146

Mechanics, 74
Mechanism, 72, 88, 109, 160, 164, 165
Meclofenoxate, 292
Medicine: ancient Greek and Roman writings, 66–67, 70; Ayurvedic, 268, 269; traditional Chinese, 268, 269. *See also* Antiaging medicine
Meditation, 241
Meditations on First Philosophy (Descartes), 73
Mediterranean diet, 250, 254–255, 258
Melanin, 222
Melatonin, 270–271, 294
Memoirs (Fontaneda), 13
Memorial Sloan-Kettering Cancer Center, 276
Men: and the antiaging market, 185, 188; bioidentical hormone therapies for, 283; breast reduction, 194; erectile dysfunction, 185, 271, 291; male enhancement, 185
Mendel, Johann Gregor, 131, 136
Menopause, 193, 233, 285
Mental aging: acting older and wiser, 209–210; daily routines, 206; and education, 208; gaining wisdom, 205; mental acuity in older ages, 205; myths of, 204–205; new learning, 206–209; and relationships, 207–208; and sexual activity, 208; and travel, 207; and work and vocation, 209
Merck Pharmaceutical Company, 121
Mercury: cosmeceuticals containing, 191; as elixir of immortality, 24, 44, 46, 47, 51; fatal ingestion of, 24, 44, 268, 320, 321; in fish, 272
Mesopotamia, 10, 16–18, 19–20
Mesopotamian legends: fountain of youth, 10; Gilgamesh, 16–20, 36–37; story of Gilgamesh and Enkidu, 16–18; Utnapishtim and the flood, 17
Metabolic theory of aging, 174
Metabolism, 120, 141, 171
Metaphysics, 74, 154
Metchnikoff, Élie, 98, 99, 259, 270
Meteorology, 80
Metformin, 145, 296
Methandrostenalone, 122
Methuselah Foundation, 142–143, 237
Microbiology, 228
Microdermabrasion, 188, 192
Microorganisms, 95, 96, 98, 99, 100, 157
Middle Ages, 39, 54–55
Middle East: fountain of youth myth in, 10; Islamic, 56; scholarship in, 39
Midlife Development in the United States (MIDUS) study, 197